Respiratory System

First and second edition authors:

Angus Jeffries

Andrew Turley

Pippa McGowan

Third edition authors:

Harish Patel

Catherine Gwilt

4th Edition

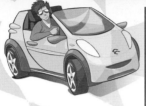

CRASH COURSE

SERIES EDITOR:
Dan Horton-Szar
BSc(Hons) MBBS(Hons) MRCGP
Northgate Medical Practice,
Canterbury,
Kent, UK

FACULTY ADVISOR:
Omar S Usmani
MBBS PhD FHEA FRCP
NIHR Career Development Fellow,
Clinical Senior Lecturer & Consultant Physician in Respiratory & Internal Medicine,
National Heart and Lung Institute,
Imperial College London and Royal Brompton Hospital,
London, UK

Respiratory System

Sarah Hickin
BSc(Hons) MBBS
Core Trainee, Royal Brompton and Harefield NHS Trust,
London, UK

James Renshaw
BSc(Hons) MBBS
Core Trainee,
South Thames, Deanery, London, UK

Rachel Williams
BSc(Hons) MBBS
F2, West Middlesex University Hospital,
London, UK

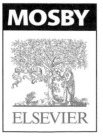

MOSBY
ELSEVIER

Edinburgh London New York Oxford Philadelphia St Louis Sydney Toronto 2015

ELSEVIER
MOSBY

Commissioning Editor: Jeremy Bowes
Development Editor: Helen Leng
Project Manager: Andrew Riley
Designer/Design Direction: Christian Bilbow
Icon Illustrations: Geo Parkin
Illustration Manager: Jennifer Rose

First edition 1999

Second edition 2003

Third edition 2008

Fourth edition 2013

Updated Fourth edition 2015

ISBN: 978-0-7234-3861-8

British Library Cataloguing in Publication Data
A catalogue record for this book is available from the British Library

Library of Congress Cataloging in Publication Data
A catalog record for this book is available from the Library of Congress

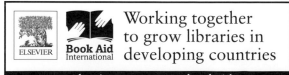

Series editor foreword

The *Crash Course* series was first published in 1997 and now, 16 years on, we are still going strong. Medicine never stands still, and the work of keeping this series relevant for today's students is an ongoing process. These fourth editions build on the success of the previous titles and incorporate new and revised material to keep the series up to date with current guidelines for best practice and recent developments in medical research and pharmacology.

We always listen to feedback from our readers, through focus groups and student reviews of the *Crash Course* titles. For the fourth editions, we have completely rewritten our self-assessment material to keep up with today's 'single-best answer' and 'extended matching question' formats. The artwork and layout of the titles have also been largely reworked to make the text easier on the eye during long sessions of revision.

Despite fully revising the books with each edition, we hold fast to the principles on which we first developed the series. *Crash Course* will always bring you all the information you need to revise in compact, manageable volumes that integrate basic medical science and clinical practice. The books still maintain the balance between clarity and conciseness, and provide sufficient depth for those aiming at distinction. The authors are medical students and junior doctors who have recent experience of the exams you are now facing, and the accuracy of the material is checked by a team of faculty advisors from across the UK.

I wish you all the best for your future careers!

Dr Dan Horton-Szar

Authors

Firstly, thank you for taking the time to open this latest version; we are very proud of this publication and we really hope you will find it as beneficial and user friendly as we set out to make it. Our aim was to add to the strengths of the previous edition but also to update the text to reflect changing medical school syllabuses and assessment styles.

We have once again revamped the layout, splitting the text into three sections following a 'bench to bedside' approach to respiratory medicine. Whilst each topic is accessible as a standalone resource, taken together we have tried to provide a coherent journey from basic science to clinical assessment of a patient and finally respiratory pathology. Cross referencing suggestions between sections and also up to date guidelines will enable you quickly to link relevant aspects of science and clinical medicine in an evidence-based manner. Lastly, you will find a range of multiple choice questions of the SBA and EMQ format in place of previous short answer and essay based assessments.

We strongly feel this book has a wide scope of application, whether you are revising for basic science exams, or are on the wards looking for clinical information with a pathophysiological focus, there is something for you. We hope you find this edition valuable in both study and working life and wish you all the best for your assessments!

Sarah Hickin, James Renshaw and Rachel Williams

Faculty Advisor

Crash Course is a unique series. The authors themselves have just completed their final year exams and are preparing for their first postgraduate exams and so, have a heightened knowledge and are experienced with the current requirements of the ever changing medical curriculum.

Sarah, Rachel and James have brought their own vision to this edition, focusing firmly on integrating basic science with clinical practice to make *Respiratory Medicine* an essential and enjoyable read. This edition has updated clinical guidelines and is extensively cross referenced, reinforcing the complementary information in the different chapters.

It has been a pleasure to work with the authors, whose momentum in keeping focused on this book was admirable, particularly in their first foundation year and especially after undertaking stretches of night's on-call, in order to keep to our deadlines!

I do hope you enjoy this edition.

Omar S Usmani

Acknowledgements

FIGURE ACKNOWLEDGEMENTS

Fig. 1.3 adapted with permission from Hlastala MP, Berger AJ (2001) Physiology of Respiration, 2nd edn. Oxford: Oxford University Press.

Fig. 1.5 adapted with permission from West JB (2001) Pulmonary Physiology and Pathophysiology: An Integrated, Case-Based Approach. Philadelphia: Lippincott Williams & Wilkins.

Figs 2.13 and 4.19 reproduced from Widdicombe JG, Davies A (1991) Respiratory Physiology (Physiological Principles in Medicine), 2nd edn. London: Hodder Arnold.

Fig. 2.14 reproduced from http://academic.kellogg.edu/herbrandsonc/bio201_mckinley/f25-9a_bronchioles_and__c.jpg © Copyright 1999, Kellogg Community College. Learning the Respiratory System Chapter 25

Fig. 2.15B adapted from StudyBlue, Australia, University of Queensland, Health & Disease, Respiratory System (II) Flashcards, How are the lungs innervated by the SNS? ©2012 STUDYBLUE Inc.

Figs 4.3, 16.2, 16.3 and 19.1 reproduced from Criner GJ, D'Alonzo GE (eds) (1999) Pulmonary Pathophysiology. Madison, WI: Fence Creek Publishing.

Figs 4.14, 4.16, 5.7, 5.8, 5.9 and 6.6 reproduced from Berne RM, Levy MN (1993) Physiology, Human Physiology – The Mechanisms of Body Function, 3rd edn. St Louis: Mosby.

Fig. 9.20 after Burton, Hodgkin & Ward (1977) Lippincott-Raven.

Fig. 9.21 reproduced from Munro & Campbell 2000, with permission of Churchill Livingstone.

Fig. 10.8 Reproduced from NICE guidelines http://www.nice.org.uk/usingguidance/commissioningguides/pulmonaryrehabilitationserviceforpatientswithcopd/mrc_dyspnoea_scale.jsp. Adapted from Fletcher CM, Elmes PC, Fairbairn MB et al. (1959) The significance of respiratory symptoms and the diagnosis of chronic bronchitis in a working population. British Medical Journal 2: 257–266.

Fig. 12.3 reproduced from: http://www.aafp.org/afp/2003/0115/p315.html.

Fig. 12.6 reproduced from: http://www.sciencephoto.com/media/260880/view.

Fig. 12.8 reproduced from: http://www.mdcalc.com/wells-criteria-for-pulmonary-embolism-pe/.

Fig. 14.8 reproduced from: the American Joint Committee on Cancer (AJCC).

Fig. 16.7 reproduced from http://www.patient.co.uk/health/Asthma-Peak-Flow-Meter.htm.

Fig. 16.8 reproduced from BTS guidelines as to how to treat a patient initially presenting with possible asthma. Available online at: http://www.brit-thoracic.org.uk/Portals/0/Guidelines/AsthmaGuidelines/sign101%20Jan%202012.pdf.

Fig. 18.2 reproduced from Kumar PJ, Clark ML (eds) (1994) Clinical Medicine: A Textbook for Medical Students and Doctors, 3rd edn. London: Baillière Tindall.

Fig. 20.8C reproduced with permission from Corne J, Pointon K (2010) Chest X-Ray Made Easy, 3rd edn. Edinburgh: Churchill Livingstone.

Contents

Contents

PART 1
BASIC SCIENCE AND PHYSIOLOGY

Overview of the respiratory system (1)

● **Objectives**

By the end of this chapter you should be able to:
- Describe how respiration is controlled.
- List the main functions of the respiratory system.
- Describe how breathing is brought about.
- Understand how defects in ventilation, perfusion and diffusion cause hypoxaemia.
- Know which structures are involved in gas exchange.
- Show the differences between restrictive and obstructive disorders.
- Show what happens if lung disease increases the work of breathing to excessive levels.

OVERALL STRUCTURE AND FUNCTION

Respiration

Respiration refers to the processes involved in oxygen transport from the atmosphere to the body tissues and the release and transportation of carbon dioxide produced in the tissues to the atmosphere.

Microorganisms rely on diffusion to and from their environment for the supply of oxygen and removal of carbon dioxide. Humans, however, are unable to rely on diffusion because:

- Their surface area:volume ratio is too small.
- The diffusion distance from the surface of the body to the cells is too large and the process would be far too slow to be compatible with life.

Remember that diffusion time increases with the square of the distance, and, as a result, the human body has had to develop a specialized respiratory system to overcome these problems. This system has two components:

1. A gas-exchange system that provides a large surface area for the uptake of oxygen from, and the release of carbon dioxide to, the environment. This function is performed by the lungs.
2. A transport system that delivers oxygen to the tissues from the lungs and carbon dioxide to the lungs from the tissues. This function is carried out by the cardiovascular system.

Structure

The respiratory system can be neatly divided into upper respiratory tract (nasal and oral cavities, pharynx, larynx and trachea) and lower respiratory tract (main bronchi and lungs) (Fig. 1.1).

Upper respiratory tract

The upper respiratory tract has a large surface area and a rich blood supply, and its epithelium (respiratory epithelium) is covered by a mucus secretion. Within the nose, hairs are present, which act as a filter. The function of the upper respiratory tract is to warm, moisten and filter the air so that it is in a suitable condition for gaseous exchange in the distal part of the lower respiratory tract.

Lower respiratory tract

The lower respiratory tract consists of the lower part of the trachea, the two primary bronchi and the lungs. These structures are contained within the thoracic cavity.

Lungs

The lungs are the organs of gas exchange and act as both a conduit for air flow (the airway) and a surface for movement of oxygen into the blood and carbon dioxide out of the blood (the alveolar capillary membrane).

The lungs consist of airways, blood vessels, nerves and lymphatics, supported by parenchymal tissue. Inside the lungs, the two main bronchi divide into smaller and smaller airways until the end respiratory unit (acinus) is reached (Fig. 1.2).

Acinus

The acinus is that part of the airway that is involved in gaseous exchange (i.e. the passage of oxygen from the lungs to the blood and carbon dioxide from the blood to the lungs). It begins with the respiratory bronchioles and includes subsequent divisions of the airway and alveoli.

3

Fig. 1.1 Schematic diagram of the respiratory tract.

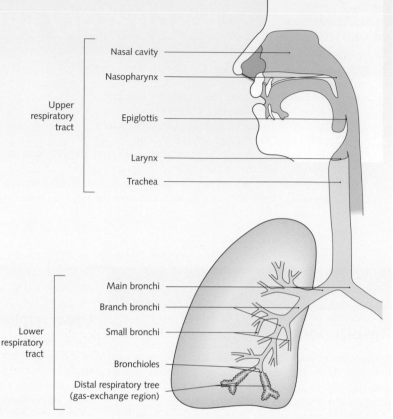

Upper respiratory tract
- Nasal cavity
- Nasopharynx
- Epiglottis
- Larynx
- Trachea

Lower respiratory tract
- Main bronchi
- Branch bronchi
- Small bronchi
- Bronchioles
- Distal respiratory tree (gas-exchange region)

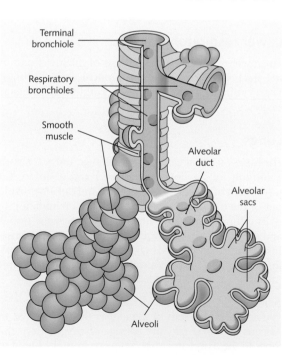

Terminal bronchiole

Respiratory bronchioles

Smooth muscle

Alveolar duct

Alveolar sacs

Alveoli

Fig. 1.2 The acinus, or respiratory unit. This part of the airway is involved in gas exchange.

Conducting airways

Conducting airways allow the transport of gases to and from the acinus but are themselves unable to partake in gas exchange. They include all divisions of the bronchi proximal to, but excluding, respiratory bronchioles.

Pleurae

The lung, chest wall and mediastinum are covered by two continuous layers of epithelium known as the pleurae. The inner pleura covering the lung is the visceral pleura and the outer pleura covering the chest wall and mediastinum is the parietal pleura. These two pleurae are closely opposed and are separated by only a thin layer of liquid. The liquid acts as a lubricant and allows the two surfaces to slip over each other during breathing.

BASIC CONCEPTS IN RESPIRATION

The supply of oxygen to body tissues is essential for life; after only a brief period without oxygen, cells undergo irreversible change and eventually die.

The respiratory system plays an essential role in preventing tissue hypoxia by optimizing the oxygen content of arterial blood through efficient gas exchange. The three key steps involved in gas exchange are:

1. Ventilation.
2. Perfusion.
3. Diffusion.

Together these processes ensure that oxygen is available for transport to the body tissues and that carbon dioxide is eliminated (Fig. 1.3). If any of the three steps are compromised, for example through lung disease, then the oxygen content of the blood will fall below normal (hypoxaemia) and levels of carbon dioxide may rise (hypercapnia) (Fig. 1.4). In clinical practice, we do not directly test for tissue hypoxia but look for:

- Symptoms and signs of impaired gas exchange (e.g. breathlessness or central cyanosis).
- Abnormal results from arterial blood gas tests.

Ventilation

Ventilation is the movement of air in and out of the respiratory system. It is determined by both:

- The respiratory rate (i.e. number of breaths per minute, normally 12–20).
- The volume of each breath, also known as the tidal volume.

(1) Ventilation
Air moves in and out of lungs

(3) Gas exchange
CO_2 and O_2 diffuse across the alveolar membrane

(2) Perfusion
Mixed-venous blood is delivered to the lungs from the right heart

(4) Gas exchange
CO_2 and O_2 diffuse between the tissue capillaries and cells

Fig. 1.3   Key steps involved in respiration. RA = right atrium; LA = left atrium; RV = right ventricle; LV = left ventricle.

Fig. 1.4 Common respiratory terms	
Hypocapnia	Decreased carbon dioxide tension in arterial blood (P_aCO_2 <4.8 kPa or 35 mmHg)
Hypercapnia	Increased carbon dioxide tension in arterial blood (P_aCO_2 >6 kPa or 45 mmHg)
Hypoxaemia	Deficient oxygenation of the arterial blood
Hypoxia	Deficient oxygenation of the tissues
Hyperventilation	Ventilation that is in excess of metabolic requirements (results in hypocapnia)
Hypoventilation	Ventilation that is too low for metabolic requirements (results in hypercapnia)

A change in ventilation, in response to the metabolic needs of the body, can therefore be brought about by either:

- Altering the number of breaths per minute.
- Adjusting the amount of air that enters the lungs with each breath.

In practice, the most common response to hypoxaemia is rapid, shallow breathing, which increases the elimination of carbon dioxide and often leads to hypocapnia. However, it should be noted that a raised respiratory rate, or tachypnoea, is not the same as hyperventilation. The term hyperventilation refers to a situation where ventilation is too great for the body's metabolic needs.

The mechanisms of ventilation

The movement of air into and out of the lungs takes place because of pressure differences caused by changes in lung volumes. Air flows from a high-pressure area to a low-pressure area. We cannot change the local atmospheric pressure around us to a level higher than that inside our lungs; the only obvious alternative is to lower the pressure within the lungs. We achieve this pressure reduction by expanding the size of the chest.

The main muscle of inspiration is the diaphragm, upon which the two lungs sit. The diaphragm is dome-shaped; contraction flattens the dome, increasing intrathoracic volume. This is aided by the external intercostal muscles, which raise the ribcage; this results in a lowered pressure within the thoracic cavity and hence the lungs, supplying the driving force for air flow into the lungs. Inspiration is responsible for most of the work of breathing; diseases of the lungs or chest wall may increase the workload so that accessory muscles are also required to maintain adequate ventilation.

Expiration is largely passive, being a result of elastic recoil of the lung tissue. However, in forced expiration (e.g. during coughing), the abdominal muscles increase intra-abdominal pressure, forcing the contents of the abdomen against the diaphragm. In addition, the internal intercostal muscles lower the ribcage. These actions greatly increase intrathoracic pressure and enhance expiration.

Impaired ventilation

There are two main types of disorder which impair ventilation. These are:

1. Obstructive disorders:
   - Airways are narrowed and resistance to air flow is increased.
   - Mechanisms of airway narrowing include inflamed and thickened bronchial walls (e.g. asthma), airways filled with mucus (e.g. chronic bronchitis, asthma) and airway collapse (e.g. emphysema).

2. Restrictive disorders:
   - Lungs are less able to expand and so the volume of gas exchanged is reduced.
   - Mechanisms include stiffening of lung tissue (e.g. pulmonary fibrosis) or inadequacy of respiratory muscles (e.g. Duchenne muscular dystrophy).

Obstructive and restrictive disorders have characteristic patterns of lung function, measured by pulmonary function tests.

Ventilatory failure occurs if the work of breathing becomes excessive and muscles fail. In this situation, or to prevent it from occurring, mechanical ventilation is required.

Perfusion

The walls of the alveoli contain a dense network of capillaries bringing mixed-venous blood from the right heart. The barrier separating blood in the capillaries and air in the alveoli is extremely thin. Perfusion of blood through these pulmonary capillaries allows diffusion, and therefore gas exchange, to take place.

Ventilation:perfusion inequality

To achieve efficient gaseous exchange, it is essential that the flow of gas (ventilation: V) and the flow of blood (perfusion: Q) are closely matched. The V/Q ratio in a normal, healthy lung is approximately 1. Two extreme scenarios illustrate mismatching of ventilation and perfusion (Fig. 1.5). These are:

- Normal alveolar ventilation but no perfusion (e.g. due to a blood clot obstructing flow).
- Normal perfusion but no air reaching the lung unit (e.g. due to a mucus plug occluding an airway).

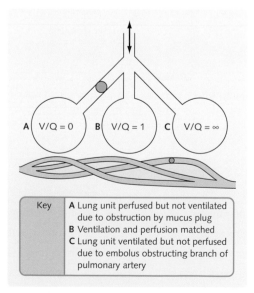

Key	A Lung unit perfused but not ventilated due to obstruction by mucus plug
	B Ventilation and perfusion matched
	C Lung unit ventilated but not perfused due to embolus obstructing branch of pulmonary artery

Fig. 1.5 Ventilation:perfusion mismatching.

Ventilation:perfusion inequality is the most common cause of hypoxaemia and underlies many respiratory diseases.

Diffusion

At the gas-exchange surface, diffusion occurs across the alveolar capillary membrane. Molecules of CO_2 and O_2 diffuse along their partial pressure gradients.

Partial pressures

Air in the atmosphere, before it is inhaled and moistened, contains 21% oxygen. This means that:

- 21% of the total molecules in air are oxygen molecules.
- Oxygen is responsible for 21% of the total air pressure; this is its partial pressure, measured in mmHg or kPa and abbreviated as PO_2 (Fig. 1.6).

Partial pressure also determines the gas content of liquids, but it is not the only factor. Gas enters the liquid as a solution, and the amount that enters depends on its solubility. The more soluble a gas, the more molecules that will enter solution for a given partial pressure. The partial pressure of a gas in a liquid is sometimes referred to as its tension (i.e. arterial oxygen tension is the same as P_aO_2).

As blood perfusing the pulmonary capillaries is mixed-venous blood:

- Oxygen will diffuse from the higher PO_2 environment of the alveoli into the capillaries.
- Carbon dioxide will diffuse from the blood towards the alveoli, where PCO_2 is lower.

Blood and gas equilibrate as the partial pressures become the same in each and gas exchange then stops.

Oxygen transport

Once oxygen has diffused into the capillaries it must be transported to the body tissues. The solubility of oxygen in the blood is low and only a small percentage of the body's requirement can be carried in dissolved form. Therefore most of the oxygen is combined with haemoglobin in red blood cells. Haemoglobin has four binding sites and the amount of oxygen carried by haemoglobin in the blood depends on how many of these sites are occupied. If they are all occupied by oxygen the molecule is said to be saturated. The oxygen saturation (S_aO_2) tells us the relative percentage of the maximum possible sites that can be bound. Note that anaemia will not reduce S_aO_2; lower haemoglobin means there are fewer available sites but the relative percentage of possible sites that are saturated stays the same.

The relationship between the partial pressure of oxygen and percentage saturation of haemoglobin is represented by the oxygen dissociation curve.

Diffusion defects

If the blood–gas barrier becomes thickened through disease, then the diffusion of O_2 and CO_2 will be impaired. Any impairment is particularly noticeable during exercise, when pulmonary flow increases and blood spends an even shorter time in the capillaries, exposed to alveolar oxygen. Impaired diffusion is, however, a much less common cause of hypoxaemia than ventilation:perfusion mismatching.

CONTROL OF RESPIRATION

Respiration must respond to the metabolic demands of the body. This is achieved by a control system within the brainstem which receives information from various sources in the body where sensors monitor:

- Partial pressures of oxygen and carbon dioxide in the blood.
- pH of the extracellular fluid within the brain.
- Mechanical changes in the chest wall.

HINTS AND TIPS

It is easy to get confused about P_aO_2, S_aO_2 and oxygen content. P_aO_2 tells us the pressure of the oxygen molecules dissolved in plasma, not those bound to haemoglobin. It is not a measure of how much oxygen is in the arterial blood. S_aO_2 tells us how many of the possible haemoglobin binding sites are occupied by oxygen. To calculate the amount of oxygen you would also need to know haemoglobin levels and how much oxygen is dissolved. Oxygen content (C_aO_2) is the only value that actually tells us how much oxygen is in the blood and, unlike P_aO_2 or S_aO_2, it is given in units which denote quantity (mL O_2/dL).

Fig. 1.6	Abbreviations used in denoting partial pressures.
PO_2	Oxygen tension in blood (either arterial or venous)
P_aO_2	Arterial oxygen tension
P_vO_2	Oxygen tension in mixed-venous blood
P_AO_2	Alveolar oxygen tension
Carbon dioxide tensions follow the same format (PCO_2, etc.)	

On the basis of information they receive, the respiratory centres modify ventilation to ensure that oxygen supply and carbon dioxide removal from the tissues match their metabolic requirements. The actual mechanical change to ventilation is carried out by the respiratory muscles: these are known as the effectors of the control system.

Respiration can also be modified by higher centres (e.g. during speech, anxiety, emotion).

OTHER FUNCTIONS OF THE RESPIRATORY SYSTEM

Respiration is also concerned with a number of other functions, including metabolism, excretion, hormonal activity and, most importantly:

- The pH of body fluids.
- Regulation of body temperature.

Acid–base regulation

Carbon dioxide forms carbonic acid in the blood, which dissociates to form hydrogen ions, lowering pH. By controlling the partial pressure of carbon dioxide, the respiratory system plays an important role in regulating the body's acid–base status; lung disease can therefore lead to acid–base disturbance. In acute disease it is important to test for blood pH and bicarbonate levels, and these are included in the standard arterial blood gas results.

Body temperature regulation

Body temperature is achieved mainly by insensible heat loss. Thus, by altering ventilation, body temperature may be regulated.

Metabolism

The lungs have a huge vascular supply and thus a large number of endothelial cells. Hormones such as noradrenaline (norepinephrine), prostaglandins and 5-hydroxytryptamine are taken up by these cells and destroyed. Some exogenous compounds are also taken up by the lungs and destroyed (e.g. amfetamine and imipramine).

Excretion

Carbon dioxide and some drugs (notably those administered through the lungs, e.g. general anaesthetics) are excreted by the lungs.

Hormonal activity

Hormones (e.g. steroids) act on the lungs. Insulin enhances glucose utilization and protein synthesis. Angiotensin II is formed in the lungs from angiotensin I (by angiotensin-converting enzyme). Damage to the lung tissue causes the release of prostacyclin PGI_2, which prevents platelet aggregation.

Organization of the respiratory tract ②

● **Objectives**

By the end of this chapter you should be able to:
- Appreciate the differences between the upper and lower respiratory tract, in terms of both macroscopic structure and cellular make-up.
- Be familiar with the bronchial tree and the acinar unit and how these relate to gas exchange at the blood–air interface.
- Briefly describe physical, humoral and cellular pulmonary defence mechanisms.

THE RESPIRATORY TRACT

The respiratory tract is the collective term for the anatomy relating to the process of respiration, from the nose down to the alveoli. It can be considered in two parts: that lying outside the thorax (upper tract) and that within the thorax (lower tract) (see Fig. 1.1). These will be considered in turn, detailing both macroscopic and microscopic structure.

Macroscopic structure

Upper respiratory tract

Nose and nasopharynx
The nose is the part of the respiratory tract superior to the hard palate. It consists of the external nose and the nasal cavities, which are separated into right and left by the nasal septum. The main functions of these structures are olfaction (not detailed) and breathing.

The lateral wall of the nasal cavity consists of bony ridges called conchae or turbinates (Figs 2.1 and 2.2), which provide a large surface area covered in highly vascularized mucous membrane to warm and humidify inspired air. Under each turbinate there is a groove or meatus. The paranasal air sinuses (frontal, sphenoid, ethmoid and maxillary) drain into these meatuses via small ostia, or openings.

Nasal neurovascular supply and lymphatic drainage
The terminal branches of the internal and external carotid arteries provide the rich blood supply for the internal nose. The sphenopalatine artery (from the maxillary artery) and the anterior ethmoidal artery (from the ophthalmic) are the two most important branches.

Sensation to the area is provided mainly by the maxillary branch of the trigeminal nerve. Lymphatic vessels drain into the submandibular node, then into deep cervical nodes.

Pharynx
The pharynx extends from the base of the skull to the inferior border of the cricoid cartilage, where it is continuous anteriorly with the trachea and posteriorly with the oesophagus. It is described as being divided into three parts: the nasopharynx, oropharynx and the laryngopharynx, which open anteriorly into the nose, the mouth and the larynx, respectively (Fig. 2.3). The pharynx is part of both the respiratory and gastrointestinal systems.

The nasopharynx is situated above the soft palate and opens anteriorly into the nasal cavities at the choanae (posterior nares). During swallowing, the nasopharynx is cut off from the oropharynx by the soft palate. The nasopharynx contains the opening of the eustachian canal (pharyngotympanic or auditory tube) and the adenoids, which lie beneath the epithelium of its posterior wall.

Musculature, neurovascular supply and lymphatic drainage
The tube of the pharynx is enveloped by the superior, middle and inferior constrictor muscles, respectively. These receive arterial blood supply from the external carotid through the superior thyroid, ascending pharyngeal, facial and lingual arteries. Venous drainage is by a plexus of veins on the outer surface of the pharynx to the internal jugular vein. Both sensory and motor nerve supplies are from the pharyngeal plexus (cranial nerves IX and X); the maxillary nerve (cranial nerve V) supplies the nasopharynx with sensory fibres. Lymphatic vessels drain directly into the deep cervical lymph nodes.

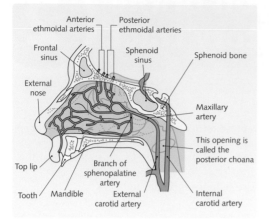

Fig. 2.1 Lateral view of the nasal cavity showing the rich blood supply.

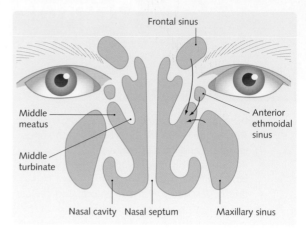

Fig. 2.2 Frontal view of the nasal cavity drainage sites of the paranasal sinuses.

Fig. 2.3 Schematic diagram showing midline structures of the head and neck.

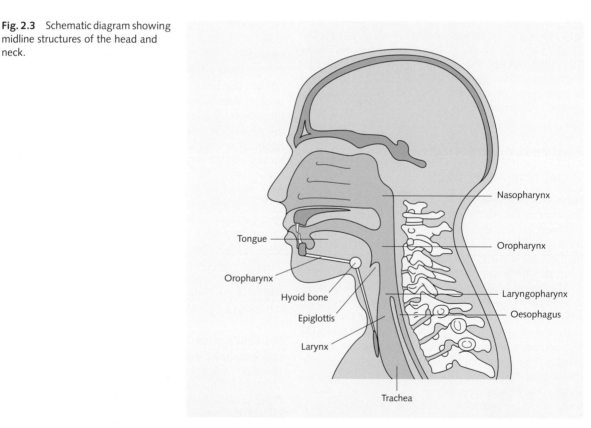

Larynx

The larynx is continuous with the trachea at its inferior end. At its superior end, it is attached to the U-shaped hyoid bone and lies below the epiglottis of the tongue. The larynx consists of a cartilaginous skeleton linked by a number of membranes. This cartilaginous skeleton comprises the epiglottis, thyroid, arytenoid and cricoid cartilages (Fig. 2.4). The larynx has three main functions:

1. As an open valve, to allow air to pass when breathing.
2. Protection of the trachea and bronchi during swallowing. The vocal folds close, the epiglottis is pushed

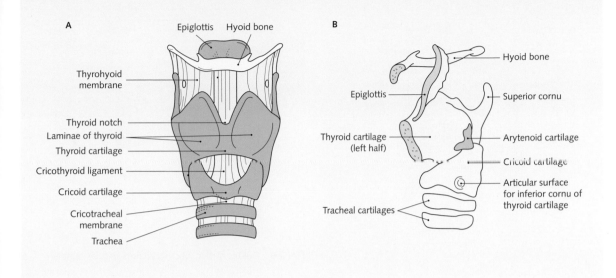

Fig. 2.4   The larynx. (A) External view – anterior aspect. (B) Median section through the larynx, hyoid bone and trachea.

back covering the opening to the larynx, and the larynx is pulled upwards and forwards beneath the tongue.

3. Speech production (phonation).

Musculature

There are external and internal muscles of the larynx. One external muscle, the cricothyroid, and numerous internal muscles attach to the thyroid membrane and cartilage. The internal muscles may change the shape of the larynx: they protect the lungs by a sphincter action and adjust the vocal folds in phonation.

Blood and nerve supply and lymphatic drainage

The blood supply of the larynx is from the superior and inferior laryngeal arteries, which are accompanied by the superior and recurrent laryngeal branches of the vagus nerve (cranial nerve X). The internal branch of the superior laryngeal nerve supplies the mucosa of the larynx above the vocal cords, and the external branch supplies the cricothyroid muscle. The recurrent laryngeal nerve supplies the mucosa below the vocal cords and all the intrinsic muscles apart from the cricothyroid. Lymph vessels above the vocal cords drain into the upper deep cervical lymph nodes; below the vocal cords, lymphatic vessels drain into the lower cervical lymph nodes.

Trachea

The trachea is a cartilaginous and membranous tube of about 10 cm in length. It extends from the larynx to its bifurcation at the carina (at the level of the fourth or fifth thoracic vertebra). The trachea is approximately 2.5 cm in diameter and is supported by C-shaped rings of hyaline cartilage. The rings are completed posteriorly by the trachealis muscle. Important relations of the trachea within the neck are:

1 The thyroid gland, which straddles the trachea, with its two lobes positioned laterally, and its isthmus anterior to the trachea with the inferior thyroid veins.
2 The common carotid arteries, which lie lateral to the trachea.
3 The oesophagus, which lies directly behind the trachea, and the recurrent laryngeal nerve, which lies between these two structures.

Lower respiratory tract

The lower respiratory tract is that contained within the thorax, a cone-shaped cavity defined superiorly by the first rib and inferiorly by the diaphragm. The thorax has a narrow top (thoracic inlet) and a wide base (thoracic outlet). The thoracic wall is supported and protected by the bony thoracic cage consisting of:

* Thoracic vertebrae.
* Manubrium.
* Sternum.
* Twelve pairs of ribs with associated costal cartilages (Fig. 2.5).

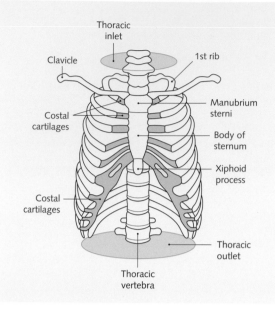

Fig. 2.5   The thoracic cage.

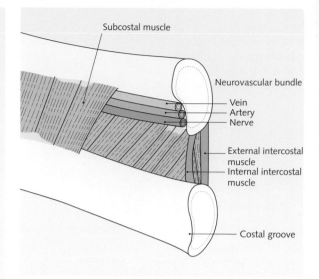

Fig. 2.6   Details of the subcostal neurovascular bundle.

Each rib makes an acute angle with the spine and articulates with the body and transverse process of its equivalent thoracic vertebra, and with the body of the vertebra above. The upper seven ribs (true ribs) also articulate anteriorly through their costal cartilages with the sternum. The eighth, ninth and 10th ribs (false ribs) articulate with the costal cartilages of the next rib above. The 11th and 12th ribs (floating ribs) are smaller and their tips are covered with a cap of cartilage.

The space between the ribs is known as the intercostal space. Lying obliquely between adjacent ribs are the internal and external intercostal muscles. The intercostal muscles support the thoracic cage; their other functions include:

- External intercostal muscles – raise the ribcage and increase intrathoracic volume.
- Internal intercostal muscles – lower the ribcage and reduce intrathoracic volume.

Deep to the intercostal muscles and under cover of the costal groove lies a neurovascular bundle of vein, artery and nerve (Fig. 2.6). This anatomy is important during some procedures (e.g. when inserting a chest drain, this is done above the rib to minimize damage to the neurovascular bundle).

Mediastinum
The mediastinum is situated in the midline and lies between the two lungs. It contains the:

- Heart and great vessels.
- Trachea and oesophagus.
- Phrenic and vagus nerves.
- Lymph nodes.

Pleurae and pleural cavities
The pleurae consist of a continuous serous membrane, which covers the external surface of the lung (parietal pleura) and is then reflected to cover the inner surface of the thoracic cavity (visceral pleura) (Fig. 2.7), creating a potential space known as the pleural cavity. The visceral and parietal pleurae are so closely apposed that only a thin film of fluid is contained within the pleural cavity. This allows the pleurae to slip over each other during breathing, thus reducing friction. Normally, no cavity is actually present, although in pathological states this potential space may expand, e.g. pneumothorax.

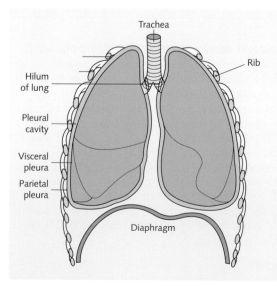

Fig. 2.7   The two pleurae form a potential space called the pleural cavity.

Where the pleura is reflected off the diaphragm on to the thoracic wall, a small space is created which is not filled by the lung tissue; this space is known as the costodiaphragmatic recess. At the root of the lung (the hilum) in the mediastinum, the pleurae become continuous and form a double layer known as the pulmonary ligament.

The parietal pleura has a blood supply from intercostal arteries and branches of the internal thoracic artery. Venous and lymph drainage follow a return course similar to that of the arterial supply. Nerve supply is from the phrenic nerve; thus, if the pleura becomes inflamed this may cause ipsilateral shoulder-tip pain. Conversely, the visceral pleura receives its blood supply from the bronchial arteries. Venous drainage is through the bronchial veins to the azygous and hemiazygous veins. Lymph vessels drain through the superficial plexus over the surface of the lung to bronchopulmonary nodes at the hilum. The visceral pleura has an autonomic nerve supply and therefore has no pain sensation.

Lungs

The two lungs are situated within the thoracic cavity either side of the mediastinum and contain:

- Airways: bronchi, bronchioles, respiratory bronchioles, alveolar ducts, alveolar sacs and alveoli.
- Vessels: pulmonary artery and vein and bronchial artery and vein.
- Lymphatics and lymph nodes.
- Nerves.
- Supportive connective tissue (lung parenchyma), which has elastic qualities.

Hilum of the lung

The hilum or root of the lung (Fig. 2.8) consists of:

- Bronchi.
- Vessels: pulmonary artery and vein.

- Nerves.
- Lymph nodes and lymphatic vessels.
- Pulmonary ligament.

Bronchopulmonary segments

The trachea divides to form the left and right primary bronchi, which in turn divide to form lobar bronchi, supplying air to the lobes of each lung. The lobar bronchi divide again to give segmental bronchi, which supply air to regions of lung known as bronchopulmonary segments. The bronchopulmonary segment is both anatomically and functionally distinct. This is important because it means that a segment of diseased lung can be removed surgically (e.g. in tuberculosis).

Surface anatomy

The surface anatomy of the lungs is shown in Figures 2.9–2.11.

Microscopic structure

Here differing tissue and cell types are discussed, moving from the nose down to the alveoli. An overview in the differences in structure throughout the bronchial tree is shown in Figure 2.15.

Upper respiratory tract

Nose and nasopharynx

The upper one-third of the nasal cavity is the olfactory area and is covered in yellowish olfactory epithelium.

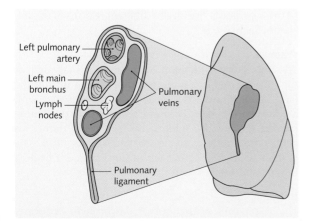

Fig. 2.8 Contents of the hilum.

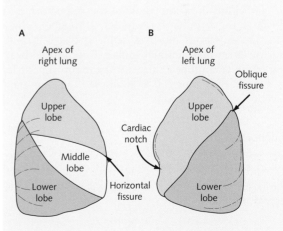

Fig. 2.9 Lateral aspect of the lungs. The outer surfaces show impression of the ribs. (A) Right lung; (B) left lung.

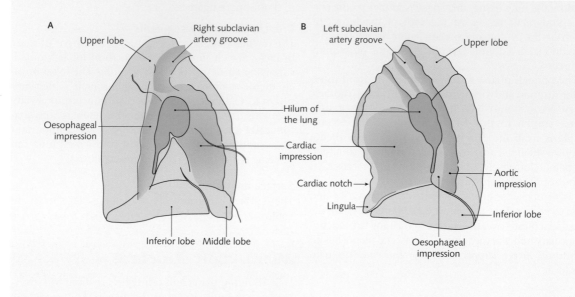

Fig. 2.10 Relations of the lung. (A) Right lung; (B) left lung.

The nasal sinuses and the nasopharynx (lower two-thirds of the nasal cavity) comprise the respiratory area, which is adapted to its main functions of filtering, warming and humidifying inspired air. These areas are lined with pseudostratified ciliated columnar epithelium (Fig. 2.12), also known as respiratory epithelium. With the exception of a few areas, this pattern of epithelium lines the whole of the respiratory tract down to the terminal bronchioles. Throughout these cells are numerous mucus-secreting goblet cells with microvilli on their luminal surface. Coordinated beating of the cilia propels mucus and entrapped particles to the pharynx, where it is swallowed, an important defence against infection.

Adenoids
The nasopharyngeal tonsil is a collection of mucosa-associated lymphoid tissue (MALT) that lies behind the epithelium of the roof and the posterior surface of the nasopharynx.

Oropharynx and laryngopharynx
The oropharynx and laryngopharynx have dual function as parts of both the respiratory and alimentary tracts. They are lined with non-keratinized stratified squamous (NKSS) epithelium several layers thick and are kept moist by numerous salivary glands.

Larynx and trachea
The epithelium of the larynx is made up of two types: NKSS epithelium and respiratory epithelium. NKSS epithelium covers the vocal folds, vestibular fold and larynx above this level. Below the level of the vestibular fold (with the exception of the vocal folds, which are lined with keratinized stratified squamous epithelium), the larynx and trachea are covered with respiratory epithelium.

Lower respiratory tract
The basic structural components of the walls of the airways are shown in Figure 2.13, though the proportions of these components vary in different regions of the tracheobronchial tree.

Trachea
The respiratory epithelium of the trachea is tall and sits on a thick basement membrane separating it from the lamina propria, which is loose and highly vascular, with a fibromuscular band of elastic tissue. Under the lamina propria lies a loose submucosa containing numerous glands that secrete mucinous and serous fluid. The C-shaped cartilage found within the trachea is hyaline in type and merges with the submucosa.

Bronchi
The respiratory epithelium of the bronchi is shorter than the epithelium of the trachea and contains fewer

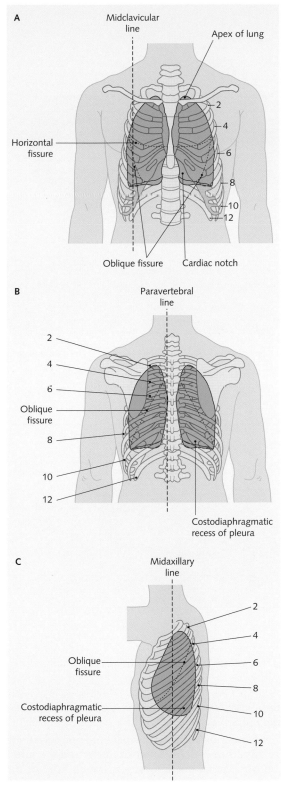

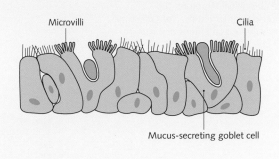

Fig. 2.12 Respiratory epithelium.

goblet cells. The lamina propria is denser, with more elastic fibres and it is separated from the submucosa by a discontinuous layer of smooth muscle. It also contains mast cells. The cartilage of the bronchi forms discontinuous flat plates and there are no C-shaped rings.

Tertiary bronchi
The epithelium in the tertiary bronchi is similar to that in the bronchi. The lamina propria of the tertiary bronchi is thin and elastic, being completely encompassed by smooth muscle. Submucosal glands are sparse and the submucosa merges with surrounding adventitia. MALT is present.

Bronchioles
The epithelium here is ciliated cuboidal but contains some Clara cells, which are non-ciliated and secrete proteinaceous fluid. Bronchioles contain no cartilage, meaning these airways must be kept open by radial traction and there are no glands in the submucosa. The smooth-muscle layer is prominent. Adjusting the tone of the smooth-muscle layer alters airway diameter, enabling resistance to air flow to be effectively controlled.

Respiratory bronchioles
The respiratory bronchioles are lined by ciliated cuboidal epithelium, which is surrounded by smooth muscle. Clara cells are present within the walls of the respiratory bronchioles. Goblet cells are absent but there are a few alveoli in the walls; thus, the respiratory bronchiole is a site for gaseous exchange.

Alveolar ducts
Alveolar ducts consist of rings of smooth muscle, collagen and elastic fibres. They open into two or three alveolar sacs, which in turn open into several alveoli.

Alveoli
An alveolus is a blind-ending terminal sac of respiratory tract (Fig. 2.14). Most gaseous exchange occurs in the alveoli. Because alveoli are so numerous, they provide the majority of lung volume and surface area. The

Fig. 2.11 Surface anatomy of the lungs and pleura (shaded area). (A) Anterior aspect; (B) posterior aspect; (C) lateral aspect. Numbering relates to relative rib position.

Fig. 2.13 Structure of the airways: (A) bronchial structure; (B) bronchiolar structure. *Note there are no submucosal glands or cartilage in the bronchiole.*

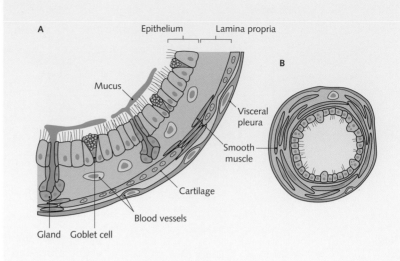

Fig. 2.14 The relationship of the alveoli to the respiratory acinus.

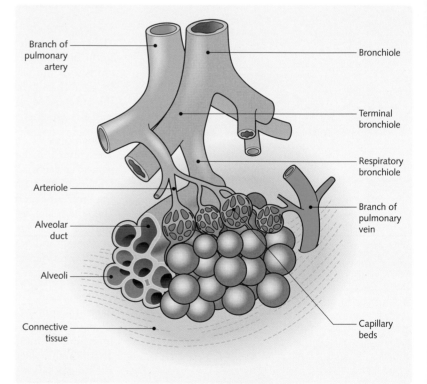

majority of alveoli open into the alveolar sacs. Communication between adjacent alveoli is possible through perforations in the alveolar wall, called pores of Kohn. The alveoli are lined with type I and type II pneumocytes, which sit on a basement membrane. Type I pneumocytes are structural, whereas type II pneumocytes produce surfactant.

Type I pneumocytes

To aid gaseous diffusion, type I pneumocytes are very thin; they contain flattened nuclei and few mitochondria. Type I pneumocytes make up 40% of the alveolar cell population and 90% of the surface lining of the alveolar wall. Cells are joined by tight junctions.

Fig. 2.15A An overview of the respiratory tree. Differences in structure of the airways

Airway	Generation No.	Lining	Wall structure	Diameter	Function	Contractile
Trachea	0	Respiratory epithelium	Membranous tube supported by C-shaped rings of cartilage, loose submucosa and glands	25 mm	Con	No
Bronchus	1–11	Respiratory epithelium	Fibromuscular tubes containing smooth muscle are reinforced by incomplete rings of cartilage and express β-receptors	1–10 mm	Con	Yes
Bronchiole	12–16	Simple ciliated cuboidal epithelium and Clara cells	Membranous and smooth muscle in the wall; no submucosal glands and no cartilage	1.0 mm	Con	Yes
Respiratory bronchiole	18+	Simple ciliated cuboidal epithelium and Clara cells	Merging of cuboidal epithelium with flattened epithelial lining of alveolar ducts; membranous wall	0.5 mm	Con/Gas	Yes
Alveolar duct	20–23	Flat non-ciliated epithelium; no glands	Outer lining of spiral smooth muscle; walls of ducts contain many openings laterally into alveolar sacs	0.5 mm	Gas	Yes
Alveolus	24	Pneumocytes types I and II	Types I and II pneumocytes lie on an alveolar basement membrane; capillaries lie on the outer surface of the wall and form the blood–air interface	75–300 mm	Gas	No

Con = conduction; Gas = gas exchange.

Type II pneumocytes

Type II pneumocytes are surfactant-producing cells containing rounded nuclei; their cytoplasm is rich in mitochondria and endoplasmic reticulum, and microvilli exist on their exposed surface. These cells make up 60% of the alveolar cell population, and 5–10% of the surface lining of the alveolar wall.

Alveolar macrophages

Alveolar macrophages are derived from circulating blood monocytes. They lie on an alveolar surface lining or on alveolar septal tissue. The alveolar macrophages phagocytose foreign material and bacteria; they are transported up the respiratory tract by mucociliary clearance. They are discussed later in this chapter.

Mucosa-associated lymphoid tissue

Mucosa-associated lymphoid tissue (MALT) is non-capsulated lymphoid tissue located in the walls of the respiratory tract. It is also found in the gastrointestinal and urogenital tract. MALT is a specialized local system of concentrated lymphoid cells in the mucosa, and has a major role in the defence of the respiratory tract against pathogens (see below).

The respiratory tree and blood–air interface

Respiratory tree

Inside the thorax, the trachea divides into the left and right primary bronchi at the carina. The right main bronchus is shorter and more vertical than the left (for this reason, inhaled foreign bodies are more likely to pass into the right lung). The primary bronchi within each lung divide into secondary or lobar bronchi. The lobar bronchi divide again into tertiary or segmental bronchi. The airways continue to divide, always splitting into two daughter airways of progressively smaller calibre until eventually forming bronchioles.

Figure 2.15A outlines the structure of the respiratory tree. Each branch of the tracheobronchial tree can be classified by its number of divisions (called the

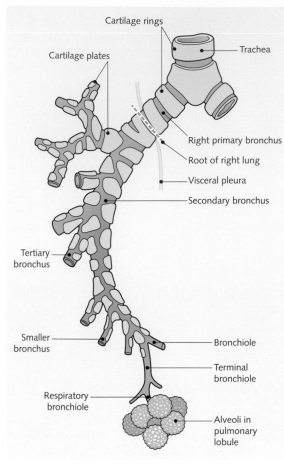

Fig. 2.15B Visual representation of the bronchial tree

generation number); the trachea is generation number 0. The trachea and bronchi contain cartilage in their walls for support and to prevent collapse of the airway. At about generation 10 or 11, the airways contain no cartilage in their walls and are known as bronchioles. Airways distal to the bronchi that contain no cartilage rely on lung parenchymal tissue for their support and are kept open by subatmospheric intrapleural pressure (radial traction).

Bronchioles continue dividing for up to 20 or more generations before reaching the terminal bronchiole. Terminal bronchioles are those bronchioles which supply the end respiratory unit (the acinus).

The tracheobronchial tree can be classified into two zones:

1. The conducting zone (airways proximal to the respiratory bronchioles), involved in air movement by bulk flow to the end respiratory units.
2. The respiratory zone (airways distal to the terminal bronchiole), involved in gaseous exchange.

As the conducting zone does not take part in gaseous exchange, it can be seen as an area of 'wasted' ventilation and is described as anatomical dead space.

Acinus

The acinus is that part of the airway that is involved in gaseous exchange (i.e. the passage of oxygen from the lungs to the blood and carbon dioxide from the blood to the lungs). The acinus consists of:

- Respiratory bronchioles, leading to the alveolar ducts.
- Alveolar ducts, opening into two or three alveolar sacs, which in turn open into several alveoli. Note: alveoli can also open directly into alveolar ducts and a few open directly into the respiratory bronchiole.

Multiple acini are grouped together and surrounded by parenchymal tissue, forming a lung lobule (Fig. 2.15B). Lobules are separated by interlobular septa.

The blood–air interface

The blood–air interface is a term that describes the site at which gaseous exchange takes place within the lung.

The alveoli are microscopic blind-ending air pouches forming the distal termination of the respiratory tract; there are 150–400 million in each normal lung. The alveoli open into alveolar sacs and then into alveolar ducts. The walls of the alveoli are extremely thin and are lined by a single layer of pneumocytes (types I and II) lying on a basement membrane. The alveolar surface is covered with alveolar lining fluid. The walls of the alveoli also contain capillaries (Fig. 2.16). It should be noted that:

- Average surface area of the alveolar–capillary membrane = 50–100 m^2.
- Average thickness of alveolar–capillary membrane = 0.4 mm.

This allows an enormous area for gaseous exchange and a very short diffusion distance.

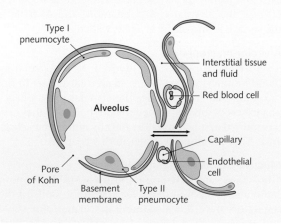

Fig. 2.16 The alveolus.

Pulmonary defence mechanisms

Overview

The lungs possess the largest surface area of the body in contact with the environment and, therefore, are extremely susceptible to damage by foreign material and provide an excellent gateway for infection. The lungs are exposed to many foreign materials, e.g. bacteria and viruses, as well as dust, pollen and pollutants. Defence mechanisms to prevent infection and reduce the risk of damage by inhalation of foreign material are thus paramount (Fig. 2.17). There are three main mechanisms of defence:

1. Physical.
2. Humoral.
3. Cellular.

Physical defences are particularly important in the upper respiratory tract, whilst at the level of the alveoli other defences, such as alveolar macrophages, predominate.

Physical defences

Entry of particulates to the lower respiratory tract is restricted by the following three mechanisms:

1. Filtering at the nasopharynx – hairs within the nose act as a coarse filter for inhaled particles; sticky mucus lying on the surface of the respiratory epithelium traps particles, which are then transported by the wafting of cilia to the nasopharynx; the particles are then swallowed into the gastrointestinal tract.
2. Swallowing – during swallowing, the epiglottis folds back, the laryngeal muscles constrict the opening to the larynx and the larynx itself is lifted; this prevents aspiration of food particles.
3. Irritant C-fibre nerve endings – stimulation of irritant receptors within the bronchi by inhalation of chemicals, particles or infective material produces a vagal reflex contraction of bronchial smooth muscle; this reduces the diameter of airways and increases mucus secretion, thus limiting the penetration of the offending material (see Wang et al. 1996).

Airway clearance

Cough reflex

Inhaled material and material brought up the bronchopulmonary tree to the trachea and larynx by mucociliary clearance can trigger a cough reflex. This is achieved by a

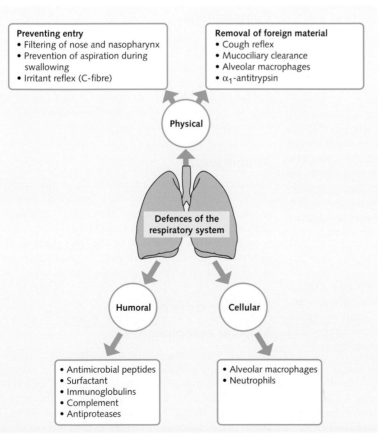

Fig. 2.17 Summary of defences of the respiratory system.

Preventing entry
- Filtering of nose and nasopharynx
- Prevention of aspiration during swallowing
- Irritant reflex (C-fibre)

Removal of foreign material
- Cough reflex
- Mucociliary clearance
- Alveolar macrophages
- α_1-antitrypsin

Physical

Defences of the respiratory system

Humoral

Cellular

- Antimicrobial peptides
- Surfactant
- Immunoglobulins
- Complement
- Antiproteases

- Alveolar macrophages
- Neutrophils

reflex deep inspiration that increases intrathoracic pressure whilst the larynx is closed. The larynx is suddenly opened, producing a high-velocity jet of air, which ejects unwanted material at high speed through the mouth.

Mucociliary clearance

Mucociliary clearance deals with a lot of the large particles trapped in the bronchi and bronchioles and debris brought up by alveolar macrophages. Respiratory epithelium is covered by a layer of mucus secreted by goblet cells and submucosal glands. Approximately 10–100 mL of mucus is secreted by the lung daily. The mucus film is divided into two layers:

1. Periciliary fluid layer about 6 μm deep, immediately adjacent to the surface of the epithelium. The mucus here is hydrated by epithelial cells. This reduces its viscosity and allows movement of the cilia.
2. Superficial gel layer about 5–10 μm deep. This is a relatively viscous layer forming a sticky blanket, which traps particles.

The cilia beat synchronously at 1000–1500 strokes per minute. Coordinated movement causes the superficial gel layer, together with trapped particles, to be continually transported towards the mouth at 1–3 cm/min. The mucus and particles reach the trachea and larynx where they are swallowed or expectorated. Importantly, mucociliary clearance is inhibited by:

- Tobacco smoke.
- Cold air.
- Drugs (e.g. general anaesthetics and atropine).
- Sulphur oxides.
- Nitrogen oxides.

The significance of mucociliary clearance is illustrated by cystic fibrosis (see Ch. 21), in which a defect in chloride channels throughout the body leads to hyperviscous secretions. In the lung, inadequate hydration causes excessive stickiness of the mucus lining the airways, preventing the action of the cilia in effecting mucociliary clearance. Failure to remove bacteria leads to repeated severe respiratory infections, which progressively worsen pulmonary function, ultimately leading to respiratory failure.

Humoral defences

Lung secretions contain a wide range of proteins which defend the lungs by various different mechanisms. Humoral and cellular aspects of the immune system are considered only briefly here; for more information see *Crash Course: Immunology and Haematology*.

Antimicrobial peptides

A number of proteins in lung fluid have antibacterial properties. These are generally low-molecular-weight proteins such as defensins, lysozyme and lactoferrin.

Surfactant

The alveoli are bathed in surfactant and this reduces surface tension and prevents the lungs from collapsing. Surfactant also contains proteins that play an important role in defence. Surfactant protein A (Sp-A) is the most abundant of these proteins and is hydrophilic. Sp-A has been shown to enhance the phagocytosis of microorganisms by alveolar macrophages. Sp-D, which is also hydrophilic, has a similar role to Sp-A with regard to immune defence.

Sp-B and Sp-C, which are hydrophobic in nature, have a more structural role in that they are involved in maintaining the surfactant monolayer and further reducing the surface tension. Surfactant deficiency in preterm babies is a major contributor to infant respiratory distress syndrome.

Immunoglobulins

Effector B lymphocytes (plasma cells) in the submucosa produce immunoglobulins. All classes of antibody are produced, but IgA production predominates. The immunoglobulins are contained within the mucus secretions in the respiratory tract and are directed against specific antigens.

Complement

Complement proteins are found in lung secretions, in particularly high concentrations during inflammation, and they play an important role in propagating the inflammatory response. Complement components can be secreted by alveolar macrophages (see below) and act as chemoattractants for the migration of cells such as neutrophils to the site of injury.

Antiproteases

Lung secretions contain a number of enzymes (antiproteases) that break down the destructive proteases released from dead bacteria, macrophages and neutrophils. One of the most important of these antiproteases is α_1-antitrypsin, produced in the liver. Genetic deficiency of α_1-antitrypsin leads to early-onset emphysema as a result of uninhibited protease activity in the lung.

Cellular defences

Alveolar macrophages

Alveolar macrophages are differentiated monocytes, and are both phagocytic and mobile. They normally reside in the lining of the alveoli where they ingest bacteria and debris, before transporting it to the bronchioles where it can be removed from the lungs by mucociliary clearance. Alveolar macrophages can also initiate and amplify the inflammatory response by secreting proteins that recruit other cells. These proteins include:

- Complement components.
- Cytokines (e.g. interleukin (IL)-1, IL-6) and chemokines.
- Growth factors.

Neutrophils

Neutrophils are the predominant cells recruited in the acute inflammatory response. Neutrophils emigrate from the intravascular space to the alveolar lumen, where intracellular killing of bacteria takes place by two mechanisms:

1. Oxidative – via reactive oxygen species.
2. Non-oxidative – via proteases.

Further reading

Wang, A.L., Blackford, T.L., Lee, L.Y., 1996. Vagal bronchopulmonary C-fibers and acute ventilatory response to inhaled irritants. Respir. Physiol. 104, 231–239.

Pulmonary circulation 3

Objectives

By the end of this chapter you should be able to:
- State the normal diastolic and systolic pressures in the pulmonary circulation.
- Describe recruitment and distension and how they affect pulmonary vascular resistance.
- Outline the factors that affect pulmonary blood flow and resistance of the pulmonary circulation.
- Describe the pattern of blood flow through the lungs in terms of three zones.
- Explain the term hypoxic vasoconstriction and its importance.
- Describe what is meant by the ventilation:perfusion ratio.

INTRODUCTION

This chapter will provide an overview of the pulmonary circulation, exploring the important concepts and factors that influence perfusion of the lungs. The pulmonary circulation is a highly specialized system which is adapted to accommodate the entire cardiac output both at rest and during exercise. The pulmonary circulation is able to do this because it is:

- A low-pressure, low-resistance system.
- Able to recruit more vessels with only a small increase in arterial pulmonary pressure.

Sufficient perfusion of the lungs is only one factor in ensuring that blood is aedequately oxygenated. The most important determinant is the way in which ventilation and perfusion are matched to each individual alveolus. Mismatching of ventilation:perfusion is a central fault in many common lung diseases.

BLOOD SUPPLY TO THE LUNGS

The lungs have a dual blood supply from the pulmonary and bronchial circulations. The bronchial circulation is part of the systemic circulation.

Pulmonary circulation

Function

The primary function of the pulmonary circulation is to allow the exchange of oxygen and carbon dioxide between the blood in the pulmonary capillaries and air in the alveoli. Oxygen is taken up into the blood whilst carbon dioxide is released from the blood into the alveoli.

Anatomy

Mixed-venous blood is pumped from the right ventricle through the pulmonary arteries and then through the pulmonary capillary network. The pulmonary capillary network is in contact with the respiratory surface (Fig. 3.1) and provides a huge gas-exchange area, approximately 50–100 m². Gaseous exchange occurs (carbon dioxide given up by the blood, oxygen taken up by the blood) and the oxygenated blood returns through the pulmonary venules and veins to the left atrium.

Bronchial circulation

The bronchial circulation is part of the systemic circulation; the bronchial arteries are branches of the descending aorta.

Function

The function of the bronchial circulation is to supply oxygen, water and nutrients to:

- Lung parenchyma.
- Airways – smooth muscle, mucosa and glands.
- Pulmonary arteries and veins.
- Pleurae.

An additional function of the bronchial circulation is in the conditioning (warming) of inspired air. The airways distal to the terminal bronchiole are supplied only by alveolar wall capillaries. For this reason, a pulmonary embolus may result in infarction of the tissues supplied by the alveolar wall capillaries, shown as a wedge-shaped opacity on the lung periphery of a chest X-ray.

Venous drainage

The lungs are drained by the pulmonary veins. These large veins carry oxygenated blood from the lungs into the left atrium of the heart.

Fig. 3.1 The pulmonary circulation. RA=right atrium; LA=left atrium; RV=right ventricle; LV=left ventricle.

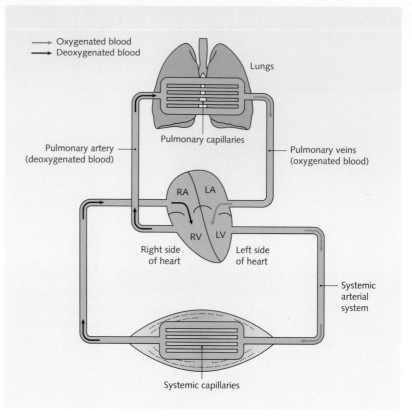

PULMONARY BLOOD FLOW

Mechanics of the circulation

Flow through the pulmonary artery is considered to be equal to cardiac output. However, in real terms the flow of blood through the pulmonary vasculature is actually slightly less than cardiac output. This is because a proportion of the coronary circulation from the aorta drains directly into the left ventricle and the bronchial circulation from the aorta drains into pulmonary veins, thus bypassing the lungs.

Pressures within the pulmonary circulation are much lower than in equivalent regions within the systemic circulation (Fig. 3.2). The volume of blood flowing through both circulations is approximately the same; therefore the pulmonary circulation must offer lower resistance than the systemic circulation.

Pulmonary capillaries and arterioles cause the main resistance to flow in the pulmonary circulation. Low resistance in the pulmonary circulation is achieved in two ways:

1. The large number of resistance vessels which exist are usually dilated; thus, the total area for flow is very large.

Fig. 3.2 Pressures within the pulmonary circulation

Site	Pressure (mmHg)	Pressure (cmH₂O)
Pulmonary artery systolic/diastolic pressure	24/9	33/11
Mean pressure	14	19
Arteriole (mean pressure)	12	16
Capillary (mean pressure)	10.5	14
Venule (mean pressure)	9.0	12
Left atrium (mean pressure)	8.0	11

2. Small muscular arteries contain much less smooth muscle than equivalent arteries in the systemic circulation, meaning they are more easily distended.

Many other factors affect pulmonary blood flow and pulmonary vascular resistance. These are discussed below.

Hydrostatic pressure

Hydrostatic pressure has three effects.

1. It distends blood vessels: as hydrostatic pressure rises, distension of the vessel increases.

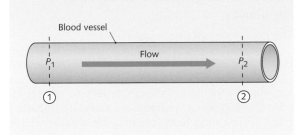

Fig. 3.3 Hydrostatic pressure in terms of driving force.

2. It is capable of opening previously closed capillaries (recruitment).
3. It causes flow to occur; in other words, a pressure difference (ΔP) between the arterial and venous ends of a vessel provides the driving force for flow (Fig. 3.3).

In situations where increased pulmonary flow is required (e.g. during exercise), the cardiac output is increased, which raises pulmonary vascular pressure. This causes recruitment of previously closed capillaries and distension of already open capillaries (Fig. 3.4), which reduces the pulmonary vascular resistance to flow. It is for this reason that resistance to flow through the pulmonary vasculature decreases with increasing pulmonary vascular pressure.

External pressure

Pressure outside a blood vessel will act to collapse the vessel if the pressure is positive, or aid distension of the vessel if the pressure is negative.

The tendency for a vessel to distend or collapse is also dependent on the pressure inside the lumen. Thus, it is the pressure difference across the wall (transmural pressure) which determines whether a vessel compresses or distends (Fig. 3.5).

Pulmonary vessels can be considered in two groups (Fig. 3.6): alveolar and extra-alveolar vessels.

Alveolar vessels

There is a dense network of capillaries in the alveolar wall; these are the alveolar vessels. The external pressure affecting these capillaries is alveolar pressure (normally atmospheric pressure). As the lungs expand, the capillaries are compressed. The diameter of the capillaries is dependent on the transmural pressure (i.e. the difference between hydrostatic pressure within the capillary lumen and pressure within the alveolus). If the alveolar pressure is greater than capillary hydrostatic pressure, the capillary will tend to collapse.

Vessels in the apex of the lung may collapse as the alveoli expand. This is more likely during diastole when venous (capillary) pressure falls below alveolar pressure (Fig. 3.5).

Extra-alveolar vessels

Extra-alveolar vessels are arteries and veins contained within the lung tissue. As the lungs expand, these vessels are distended by radial traction. The external pressure is similar to intrapleural pressure (subatmospheric, i.e. negative); therefore, transmural pressure tends to distend these vessels.

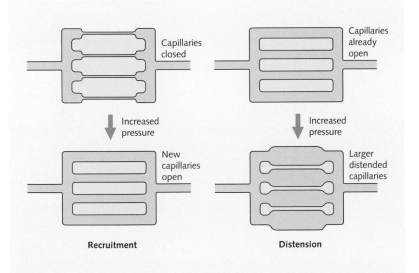

Fig. 3.4 Effect of increased pressure on pulmonary vasculature. In order to minimize pulmonary vascular resistance when pulmonary arterial pressure increases, new vessels are recruited and vessels that are already open are distended.

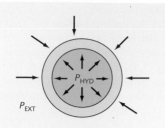

Fig. 3.5 Transmural pressure in pulmonary capillary. P_{EXT}, external pressure; P_{HYD}, hydrostatic pressure.

During inspiration, intrapleural pressure and thus the pressure outside the extra-alveolar vessels becomes even more negative, causing these vessels to distend even further, reducing vascular resistance and increasing pulmonary blood flow. At large lung volumes, the effect of radial traction is greater and the extra-alveolar vessels are distended more.

Effects of lung volume on alveolar capillaries

The capillary is affected in several ways.

Hydrostatic pressure within the capillaries is lowered during deep inspiration. This is caused by negative intrapleural pressure around the heart. This changes the transmural pressure and the capillaries tend to be compressed, increasing pulmonary vascular resistance (Fig. 3.7). At large lung volumes, the alveolar wall is stretched and becomes thinner, compressing the capillaries and increasing vascular resistance. This is a key mechanism in the development of pulmonary hypertension in patients with chronic obstructive pulmonary disease.

The factors affecting the capillary blood flow are:

- Hydrostatic pressure.
- Alveolar air pressure.
- Lung volume.

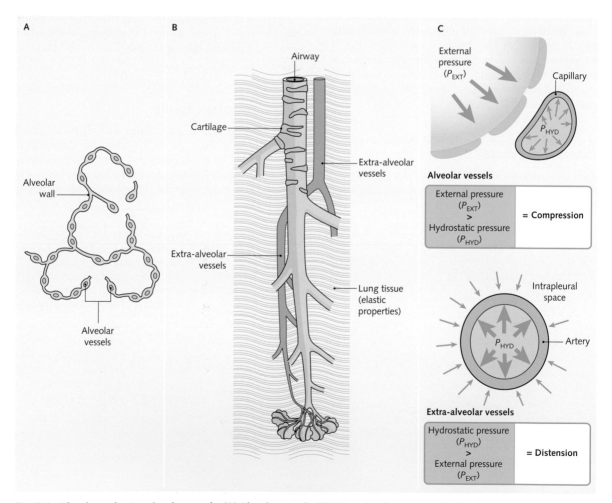

Fig. 3.6 Alveolar and extra-alveolar vessels. (A) Alveolar vessels. (B) Extra-alveolar vessels. (C) Alveolar vessels tend to collapse on deep inspiration, whereas extra-alveolar vessels distend by radial traction.

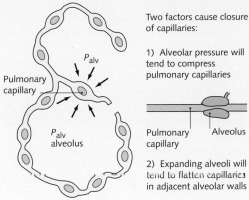

Fig. 3.7 Alveolar pressure and capillary compression.

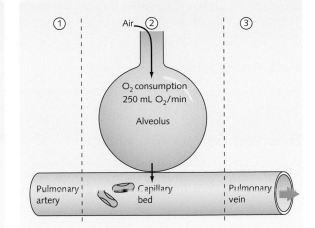

Fig. 3.8 Fick principle for measuring pulmonary blood flow. Fick theorized that the difference in oxygen content between pulmonary venous blood and pulmonary arterial blood must be due to uptake of oxygen in the pulmonary capillaries, and therefore the pulmonary blood flow can be calculated.

The factors affecting extra-alveolar vessels are:

- Hydrostatic pressure.
- Intrapleural pressure.
- Lung volume.
- Smooth-muscle tone.

Smooth muscle within the vascular wall

Smooth muscle in the walls of extra-alveolar vessels causes vasoconstriction, thus opposing the forces caused by radial traction and hydrostatic pressure within the lumen which are trying to distend these vessels. Drugs that cause contraction of smooth muscle therefore increase pulmonary vascular resistance.

Measurement of pulmonary blood flow

Pulmonary blood flow can be measured by three methods:

1. Fick principle (Fig. 3.8).
2. Indicator dilution method: a known amount of dye is injected into venous blood and its arterial concentration is measured.
3. Uptake of inhaled soluble gas (e.g. N_2O): the gas is inhaled and arterial blood values are measured.

Both the first and second methods give average blood flow, whereas the third method measures instantaneous flow. The third method relies upon N_2O transfer across the gas-exchange surface being perfusion-limited.

Fick theorized that, because of the laws of conservation of mass, the difference in oxygen concentration between mixed-venous blood returning to the pulmonary capillary bed $[O_2]_{pv}$ and arterial blood leaving the heart $[O_2]_{pa}$ must be caused by uptake of oxygen

within the lungs. This uptake must be equal to the body's consumption of oxygen (see Fig. 3.8).

Distribution of blood within the lung

Blood flow within the normal (upright) lung is not uniform. Blood flow at the base of the lung is greater than at the apex. This is due to the influence of gravity and therefore the pulmonary vessels at the lung base will have a greater hydrostatic pressure than vessels at the apex.

The hydrostatic pressure exerted by a vertical column of fluid is given by the relationship:

$$P = \rho \bullet g \bullet h$$

where ρ = density of the fluid, h = height of the column and g = acceleration due to gravity. From the equation above, it can be seen that:

- Vessels at the lung base are subjected to a higher hydrostatic pressure.
- The increase in hydrostatic pressure will distend these vessels, lowering the resistance to blood flow. Thus, pulmonary blood flow in the bases will be greater than in the apices.

In diastole, the hydrostatic pressure in the pulmonary artery is 11 cmH$_2$O. The apex of each lung is approximately 15 cm above the right ventricle, and the hydrostatic pressure within these vessels is lowered or even zero. Vessels at the apex of the lung are therefore narrower or even collapse because of the lower hydrostatic pressure within them.

Ventilation also increases from apex to base, but is less affected than blood flow because the density of air is much less than that of blood.

Pattern of blood flow

The distribution of blood flow within the lung can be described in three zones (Fig. 3.9).

Zone 1 (at the apex of the lung)

In zone 1, arterial pressure is less than alveolar pressure: capillaries collapse and no flow occurs. Note that, under normal conditions, there is no zone 1 because there is sufficient pressure to perfuse the apices.

Zone 2

In zone 2, arterial pressure is greater than alveolar pressure, which is greater than venous pressure. Postcapillary venules open and close depending on hydrostatic pressure (i.e. hydrostatic pressure difference in systole and diastole). Flow is determined by the arterial–alveolar pressure difference (transmural pressure).

Zone 3 (at the base of the lung)

In zone 3, arterial pressure is greater than venous pressure, which is greater than alveolar pressure. Blood flow is determined by arteriovenous pressure difference as in the systemic circulation.

Control of pulmonary blood flow

Pulmonary blood flow can be controlled by several local mechanisms in order to improve the efficiency of gaseous exchange, i.e.:

- Changes in hydrostatic pressure (as previously discussed).
- Local mediators (thromboxane, histamine and prostacylin), as in systemic circulation.
- Contraction and relaxation of smooth muscle within walls of arteries and arterioles.
- Hypoxic vasoconstriction (important mechanism in disease).

Hypoxic vasoconstriction

The aim of breathing is to oxygenate the blood sufficiently. This is achieved by efficient gaseous exchange between the alveoli and the bloodstream. If an area of lung is poorly ventilated and the alveolar partial pressure of oxygen (alveolar oxygen tension) is low, perfusion of this area with blood would lead to inefficient gaseous exchange. It would be more beneficial to perfuse an area that is well ventilated. This is the basis of hypoxic vasoconstriction.

Small pulmonary arteries and arterioles which are in close proximity to the gas-exchange surface and alveolar capillaries are surrounded by alveolar gas. Oxygen passes through the alveolar walls into the smooth muscle of the blood vessel by diffusion.

Fig. 3.9 Zones of pulmonary blood flow.

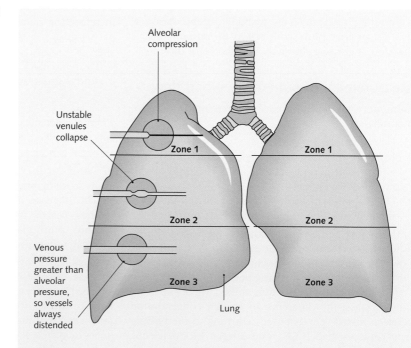

The high oxygen tension to which these smooth muscles are normally exposed acts to dilate the pulmonary vessels. In contrast, if the alveolar oxygen tension is low, pulmonary blood vessels are constricted, which leads to reduced blood flow in the area of lung which is poorly ventilated and diversion to other regions where alveolar oxygen tension is high.

It should be noted that it is the partial pressure of oxygen in the alveolus (P_AO_2) and not in the pulmonary artery (P_aO_2) that causes this response. The actual mechanism and the chemical mediators involved in hypoxic vasoconstriction are not known.

In summary:

- The aim of ventilation is to oxygenate blood and remove carbon dioxide.
- High levels of alveolar oxygen dilate pulmonary vessels.
- Low levels of alveolar oxygen constrict pulmonary blood vessels.
- This aims to produce efficient gaseous exchange.

Higher than normal alveolar carbon dioxide partial pressures also cause pulmonary blood vessels to constrict, thus reducing blood flow to an area that is not well ventilated.

Physiology, ventilation and gas exchange ④

● **Objectives**

By the end of this chapter you should be able to:
- Define all lung volumes and capacities, giving normal values, and understand the significance of each volume and capacity.
- Describe how breathing is brought about, naming the muscles involved and their actions.
- Understand the terms 'minute ventilation' and 'alveolar ventilation'.
- Define anatomical dead space and be able to describe methods of measuring anatomical dead space.
- Define lung compliance and explain what is meant by static and dynamic lung compliance.
- Describe the role of surfactant.
- Describe factors affecting the rate of diffusion across the blood–air interface.

INTRODUCTION

This chapter will provide an overview of the important principles that govern ventilation and gas exchange in the lungs. Ventilation is the flow of air in and out of the respiratory system (breathing); it is defined physiologically as the amount of air breathed in and out in a given time. The function of ventilation is to maintain blood gases at their optimum level, by delivering air to the alveoli where gas exchange can take place. The movement of air in and out of the lungs occurs due to pressure differences brought about by changes in lung volume. The respiratory muscles bring about these changes; however, the physical properties of the lungs (i.e. lung elasticity and airway resistance) also influence the effectiveness of ventilation. It is important to understand the priciples of ventilation, as many lung diseases affect the physical properties of the lung and therefore impair gas exchange by reducing the delivery of oxygen to the lungs.

Lung volumes

The gas held by the lungs can be thought of in terms of subdivisions, or specific lung volumes. Definitions of all the lung volumes and capacities (which are a combination of two or more volumes) are given in Figure 4.1. Lung volumes are important in clinical practice and are measured uring spirometry. A trace from a spirometer, showing key lung volumes, is reproduced in Figure 4.2. Other methods of measuring lung volumes, such as nitrogen washout, helium dilution and plethysmography, are used but are less relevant clinically (see Ch. 10).

Effect of disease on lung volumes

Understanding lung volumes is important because they are affected by disease. The residual volume (RV) and functional residual capacity (FRC) are particularly affected by common lung diseases such as asthma and chronic obstructive pulmonary disease (COPD) and these are considered in more detail below.

Residual volume and functional residual capacity

After breathing out, the lungs are not completely emptied of air. This is useful physiologically as a completely deflated lung requires significantly more energy to inflate it than one in which the alveoli have not completely collapsed. Even following a maximum respiratory effort (forced expiration), some air remains within the lungs. This occurs because, as the expiratory muscles contract during forced expiration, all the structures within the lungs (including the airways) are compressed by the positive intrapleural pressure. Consequently, the smaller airways collapse before the alveoli empty completely, meaning some air remains within the lungs; this is known as the residual volume.

During normal breathing (quiet breathing), the lung volume oscillates between inhalation and exhalation. In quiet breathing, after the tidal volume has been expired:

- Pressure outside the chest is equal to pressure inside the alveoli (i.e. atmospheric pressure).
- Elastic forces tending to collapse the lung are balanced by the elastic recoil trying to expand the chest.
- This creates a subatmospheric (negative) pressure in the intrapleural space.

Fig. 4.1 Descriptions of lung volumes and capacities

Air in lungs is divided into four volumes	
Tidal volume (TV)	Volume of air breathed in and out in a single breath: 0.5 L
Inspiratory reserve volume (IRV)	Volume of air breathed in by a maximum inspiration at the end of a normal inspiration: 3.3 L
Expiratory reserve volume (ERV)	Volume of air that can be expelled by a maximum effort at the end of a normal expiration: 1.0 L
Residual volume (RV)	Volume of air remaining in lungs at end of a maximum expiration: 1.2 L
Pulmonary capacities are combinations of two or more volumes	
Inspiratory capacity (IC) = TV + IRV	Volume of air breathed in by a maximum inspiration at the end of a normal expiration: 3.8 L
Functional residual capacity (FRC) = ERV + RV	Volume of air remaining in lungs at the end of a normal expiration. Acts as buffer against extreme changes in alveolar gas levels with each breath: 2.2 L
Vital capacity (VC) = IRV + TV + ERV	Volume of air that can be breathed in by a maximum inspiration following a maximum expiration: 4.8 L
Total lung capacity (TLC) = VC + RV	Only a fraction of TLC is used in normal breathing: 6.0 L
Most of these volumes can be measured with a spirometer (see Fig. 4.2)	

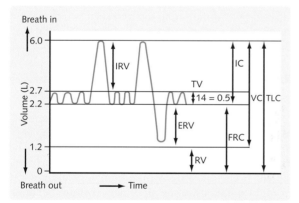

Fig. 4.2 Lung volumes and spirometry. IRV = inspiratory reserve volume; ERV = expiratory reserve volume; RV = residual volume; TV = tidal volume; FRC = functional residual capacity; IC = inspiratory capacity; VC = vital capacity; TLC = total lung capacity.

The lung volume at this point is known as functional residual capacity. Both RV and FRC can be measured using nitrogen washout, helium dilution and plethysmography (see Ch. 10).

Effects of disease on lung volumes

Disease affects lung volumes in specific patterns, depending on the pathological processes. Diseases can be classified as obstructive, restrictive or mixed, with each showing characteristic changes in lung volumes (Fig. 4.3).

Obstructive disorders

This group of disorders is characterized by obstruction of normal air flow due to airway narrowing, which, in general, leads to hyperinflation of the lungs as air is trapped behind closed airways. The RV is increased as gas that is trapped cannot leave the lung, and the RV:TLC (total lung capacity) ratio increases. In patients with severe obstruction, air trapping can be so extensive that vital capacity is decreased.

Restrictive disorders

Restrictive disorders result in stiffer lungs that cannot expand to normal volumes. All the subdivisions of volume are decreased and the RV:TLC ratio will be normal or increased (where vital capacity has decreased more quickly than RV).

MECHANICS OF BREATHING

In order to understand ventilation, we must also understand the mechanism by which it takes place, i.e. breathing. This section reviews the mechanics of breathing, including:

- The pressure differences that generate air flow.
- The respiratory muscles that effect these pressure differences.

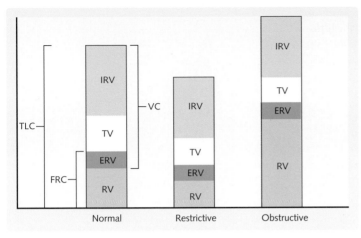

Fig. 4.3 Effect of disease on lung volumes. TLC = total lung capacity; FRC = functional residual capacity; IRV = inspiratory reserve volume; TV = tidal volume; ERV = expiratory reserve volume; RV = residual volume; VC = vital capacity.

Flow of air into the lungs

To achieve air flow into the lungs, we require a driving pressure (remember that air flows from high pressure to low pressure). Pressure at the entrance to the respiratory tract (i.e. at the nose and mouth) is atmospheric (P_{atm}). Pressure inside the lungs is alveolar pressure (P_A). Therefore:

- If $P_A = P_{atm}$, no air flow occurs (e.g. at FRC).
- If $P_A < P_{atm}$, air flows into the lungs.
- If $P_A > P_{atm}$, air flows out of the lungs.

As atmospheric pressure is constant, alveolar pressure must be altered to achieve air flow. If the volume inside the lungs is changed, Boyle's law (see box) predicts that pressure inside the lungs will also change. In the lungs, this is achieved by flattening of the diaphragm, which increases the thoracic volume and thus lowers intrapleural pressure, allowing air to flow into the lungs.

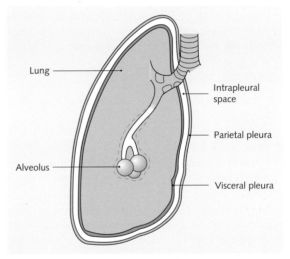

Fig. 4.4 Anatomy of the lungs.

In expiration, relaxation of the muscles of the chest wall allows the elastic recoil of the lungs to cause contraction of the lungs, reducing thoracic volume and increasing intrapleural pressure and thus expulsion of gas.

Intrapleural pressure

Intrapleural pressure plays an important role in generating air flow in and out of the lung during breathing. At FRC the elastic recoil of the lungs is exactly balanced by the elastic recoil of the chest wall (which acts to expand the chest). These two opposing forces create a subatmospheric (negative) pressure within the intrapleural space (Fig. 4.4). Because the alveoli communicate with the atmosphere, the pressure inside the lungs is higher than that of the intrapleural space. This creates a pressure gradient across the lungs, known as transmural pressure. It is transmural pressure (caused by the negative pressure in the pleural space) that ensures that the lungs are held partially expanded in the thorax. It effectively links the lungs (which are like suspended balloons) with the chest wall.

Intrapleural pressure fluctuates during breathing but is approximately 0.5 kPa at the end of quiet expiration. On inspiration, intrathoracic volume is increased; this lowers intrapleural pressure, making it more negative, causing the lungs to expand and air to enter. On expiration, the muscles of the chest wall relax and the lungs return to their original size by elastic recoil, with the expulsion of air.

During quiet breathing, intrapleural pressure is always negative; however, in forced expiration the intrapleural pressure becomes positive, forcing a reduction in lung volume with the expulsion of air.

Muscles of respiration

We have seen that the chest must be expanded in order to reduce intrapleural pressure and drive air into the lungs. This section describes how the muscles of respiration bring about this change in volume.

Thoracic wall

The thoracic wall is made up of (from superficial to deep):

- Skin and subcutaneous tissue.
- Ribs, thoracic vertebrae, sternum and manubrium.
- Intercostal muscles: external, internal and thoracis transversus.
- Parietal pleura.

Situated at the thoracic outlet is the diaphragm, which attaches to the costal margin, xyphoid process and lumbar vertebrae.

Intercostal muscles

The action of the intercostal muscles is to pull the ribs closer together. There are therefore two main actions:

1. External intercostal muscles pull the ribs upwards.
2. Internal intercostal muscles pull the ribs downwards.

External intercostal muscles

External intercostal muscles span the space between adjacent ribs, originating from the inferior border of the upper rib, and attaching to the superior border of the rib below. The muscle attaches along the length of the rib, from the tubercle to the costal–chondral junction, and its fibres run forward and downward (Fig. 4.5A).

Internal intercostal muscles

Internal intercostal muscles span the space between adjacent ribs, originating from the subcostal groove of the rib above, and attaching to the superior border of the rib below. The muscle attaches along the length

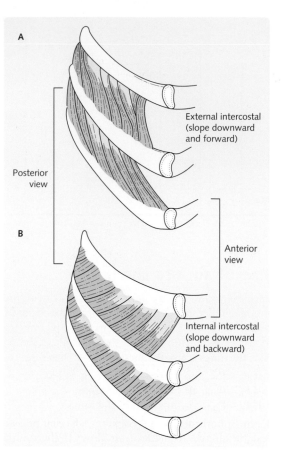

Fig. 4.5 Intercostal muscles. (A) External intercostal muscles; (B) internal intercostal muscles.

of the rib from the angle of the rib to the sternum, and its fibres run downward and backward (Fig. 4.5B).

Diaphragm

The diaphragm is the main muscle of respiration (Fig. 4.6). The central region of the diaphragm is tendinous; the outer margin is muscular, originating from the borders of the thoracic outlet.

The diaphragm has right and left domes. The right dome is higher than the left to accommodate the liver below. There is a central tendon that sits below the two domes, attaching to the xiphisternum anteriorly and the lumbar vertebrae posteriorly.

Several important structures pass through the diaphragm:

- The inferior vena cava passes through the right dome at the level of the eighth thoracic vertebra (T8).
- The oesophagus passes through a sling of muscular fibres from the right crus of the diaphragm at the level of T10.
- The aorta pierces the diaphragm anterior to T12.

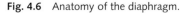

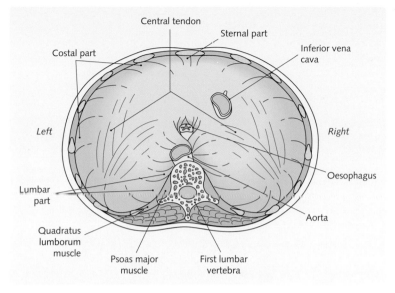

Fig. 4.6 Anatomy of the diaphragm.

The diaphragm attaches to the costal margin anteriorly and laterally. Posteriorly, it attaches to the lumbar vertebrae by the crura (left crus at L1 and L2, right crus at L1, L2 and L3). In addition, the position of the diaphragm changes relative to posture: it is lower when standing than sitting.

The motor and sensory nerve supply of the diaphragm is from the phrenic nerve. Blood supply of the diaphragm is from pericardiophrenic and musculophrenic branches of the internal thoracic artery.

> **HINTS AND TIPS**
>
> The phrenic nerve supplies the diaphragm (60% motor, 40% sensory). Remember, 'nerve roots 3, 4 and 5 keep the diaphragm alive'.

Function of the muscles of respiration

Breathing can be classified into inspiration and expiration, quiet or forced.

Quiet inspiration

In quiet inspiration, contraction of the diaphragm flattens its domes. This action increases the volume of the thorax, thus lowering intrapleural pressure and drawing air into the lungs. At the same time, the abdominal wall relaxes, allowing the abdominal contents to be displaced downwards as the diaphragm flattens.

The key muscle in quiet breathing is the diaphragm; however, the intercostal muscles are involved. With the first rib fixed, the intercostal muscles can expand the ribcage by two movements:

1. Forward movement of the lower end of the sternum.
2. Upward and outward movement of the ribs.

During quiet inspiration, these actions are small and the intercostal muscles mainly prevent deformation of the tissue between the ribs, which would otherwise lower the volume of the thoracic cage (Fig. 4.7).

> **HINTS AND TIPS**
>
> The change in intrathoracic volume is mainly caused by the movement of the diaphragm downwards. Contraction of the diaphragm comprises 75% of the energy expenditure during quiet breathing.

Quiet expiration

Quiet expiration is passive and there is no direct muscle action. During inspiration, the lungs are expanded against their elastic recoil. This recoil is sufficient to drive air out of the lungs in expiration. Thus, quiet expiration involves the controlled relaxation of the intercostal muscles and the diaphragm.

Forced inspiration

In addition to the action of the diaphragm:

- Scalene muscles and sternocleidomastoids raise the ribs anteroposteriorly, producing movement at the manubriosternal joint.
- Intercostal muscles are more active and raise the ribs to a far greater extent than in quiet inspiration.

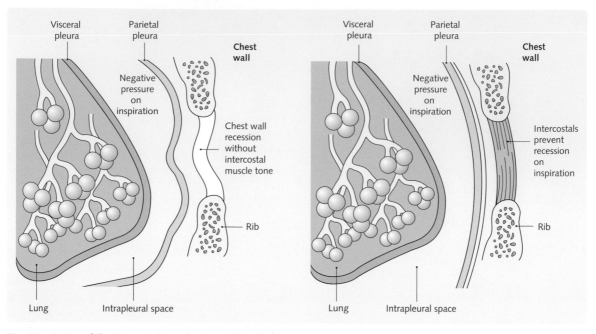

Fig. 4.7 Action of the intercostal muscles in quiet inspiration.

- The 12th rib, which is attached to quadratus lumborum, allows forcible downward movement of the diaphragm.
- Arching the back using erector spinae also increases thoracic volume.

During respiratory distress, the scapulae are fixed by trapezius muscles. The rhomboid muscles and levator scapulae, pectoralis minor and serratus anterior raise the ribs. The arms can be fixed (e.g. by holding the back of a chair), allowing the use of pectoralis major.

Forced expiration

Elastic recoil of the lungs is reinforced by contraction of the muscles of the abdominal wall. This forces the abdominal contents against the diaphragm, displacing the diaphragm upwards (Fig. 4.8).

HINTS AND TIPS

The features of forced inspiration/expiration are important clinically. It is vitally important to detect patients who are needing to use their accessory muscles in order to breathe. These patients are in respiratory distress and, as active respiration is energy-intensive, they will eventually tire. If you detect features of forced inspiration/expiration in a patient on the wards or in the emergency department, then urgent action is required and you should alert the medical team.

In addition, quadratus lumborum pulls the ribs down, adding to the force at which the abdominal contents are pushed against the diaphragm. Intercostal muscles prevent outward deformation of the tissue between the ribs.

Ventilation and dead space

Minute ventilation

Minute ventilation (V_E) is the volume of gas moved in and out of the lungs in 1 minute. In order to calculate (V_E) you need to know:

- The number of breaths per minute.
- The volume of air moved in and out with each breath (the tidal volume: V_T).

The normal frequency of breathing varies between 12 and 20 breaths per minute. Normal tidal volume is approximately 500 mL in quiet breathing. If a subject with a tidal volume of 500 mL took 12 breaths a minute, the minute ventilation would be $500 \times 12 = 6000$ mL/min.

Or, more generally:

$$V_E = V_T f$$

where V_E = minute ventilation, V_T = tidal volume and f = the respiratory rate (breaths/minute).

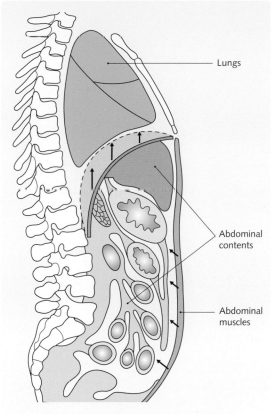

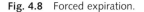

Abdominal contents pushing diaphragm upwards

Fig. 4.8 Forced expiration.

Alveolar ventilation

Not all inspired air reaches the alveoli; some stays within the trachea and other conducting airways (also known as dead space).

Therefore, two values of minute ventilation need to be considered:

1. Minute ventilation (V_E), as described above.
2. Minute alveolar ventilation (V_E), which is the amount of air that reaches the alveoli in 1 minute.

We can say that for one breath:

$$V_A = V_T - V_D$$

where V_A = the volume reaching the alveolus in one breath, and V_D = the volume of dead space. Hence, in 1 minute:

$$V_A = (V_T - V_D)f$$

Anatomical dead space

Not all of the air entering the respiratory system actually reaches the alveoli and takes part in gas exchange.

Anatomical dead space describes those areas of the airway not involved in gaseous exchange (i.e. the conducting zone). Included in this space are:

- Nose and mouth.
- Pharynx.
- Larynx.
- Trachea.
- Bronchi and bronchioles (including the terminal bronchioles).

The volume of the anatomical dead space (V_D) is approximately 150 mL (or 2 mL/kg of body weight). Anatomical dead space varies with the size of the subject and also increases with deep inspiration because greater expansion of the lungs also lengthens and widens the conducting airways.

Anatomical dead space can be measured using Fowler's method, which is based on the single-breath nitrogen test (Fig. 4.9). The patient makes a single inhalation of 100% O_2 and exhales through a gas analyser that measures N_2 concentration. On expiration, the nitrogen concentration is initially low as the patient breathes out the dead-space oxygen just inspired (100% O_2). The concentration of N_2 rises where the dead-space gas has mixed with alveolar gas (a mixture of nitrogen and oxygen). As pure alveolar gas is expired, nitrogen concentration reaches a plateau (the alveolar plateau).

If there were no mixing of alveolar and dead-space gas during expiration there would be a stepwise increase in nitrogen concentration when alveolar gas is exhaled (Fig. 4.9A). In reality, mixing does occur, which means that the nitrogen concentration increases slowly, then rises sharply. The dead-space volume is defined as the midpoint of this curve (where the two shaded areas are equal in Fig. 4.9B).

Physiological dead space

Anatomical dead space is not the only cause of 'wasted' ventilation, even in the healthy lung. The total dead space is known as physiological dead space and includes gas in the alveoli that does not participate in gas exchange.

Physiological dead space = anatomical dead space + alveolar dead space

Alveolar dead space comes about because gas exchange is suboptimal in some parts of the lung. If each acinus (or end respiratory unit) were perfect, the amount of air received by each alveolus would be matched by the flow of blood through the pulmonary capillaries. In reality:

- Some areas receive less ventilation than others.
- Some areas receive less blood flow than others.

Fig. 4.9 Measurement of anatomical dead space.

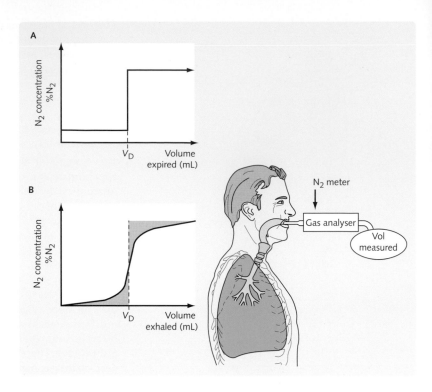

In a normal, healthy person, anatomical and physiological dead space are almost equal, alveolar dead space being very small (<5 mL). However, when lung disease alters ventilation:perfusion relationships the volume of alveolar dead space increases.

Physiological dead space can be measured using the Bohr equation. The method requires a sample of arterial blood and involves the analysis of carbon dioxide in expired air. Knowing that carbon dioxide is not exchanged in respiratory units that are not perfused, and that carbon dioxide in air is almost zero, it is possible to calculate the volume of physiological dead space.

Lung compliance and the role of surfactant

In order for ventilation to occur, the respiratory muscles must overcome the mechanical properties of the lungs and thorax, specifically the lung's tendency to elastic recoil.

The elastic properties of the lung are caused by:

- Elastic fibres and collagen in lung tissue.
- Surface tension forces in the lung created by the alveolar–liquid interface.

Compliance describes the distensibility or ease of stretch of lung tissue when an external force is applied to it. Elasticity (E) is the resistance to that stretch. Therefore:

$$C = 1/E$$

In respiratory physiology, we deal with:

- Compliance of the lung (C_L).
- Compliance of the chest wall (C_W).
- Total compliance (C_{TOT}) of the chest wall and lung together.

Lung compliance is the ease with which the lungs expand under pressure. The pressure to inflate arises from the transmural pressure (i.e. the difference between the intrapleural pressure and the intrapulmonary pressure); this is plotted against the change in volume on a pressure–volume curve (Fig. 4.10). Compliance represents the slope of the curve ($\Delta V : \Delta P$).

HINTS AND TIPS

Lung mechanics are often categorized as static or dynamic. Static mechanics do not change with time; lung statics help us to explore certain qualities of the lungs in isolation. In real life, air in the respiratory tree flows (i.e. it changes with time). Therefore lung dynamics give us a fuller picture of what actually happens during respiration.

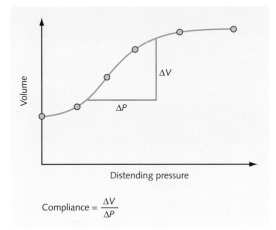

$$\text{Compliance} = \frac{\Delta V}{\Delta P}$$

Fig. 4.10 The pressure–volume curve.

Lung compliance varies with lung volume; compliance is greatest at the lower lung volumes and is smallest at higher lung volumes. For these reasons, lung compliance is sometimes quoted as specific lung compliance (sp.C_L).

$$\text{sp.}C_L = C_L/V_L$$

This change in lung compliance helps explain the difference in ventilation of the lung between apex and base. The lung volume in the base is less (because it is compressed) relative to the apex. Thus, the base of the lung has greater initial compliance than that of the apex. Because both base and apex are subject to intrapleural pressure changes of the same magnitude during inspiration, the base of the lung will therefore expand to a greater extent than the apex. This explains in part the regional difference of ventilation.

Chest wall compliance

The chest wall has elastic properties; at FRC these are equal and opposite to those in the lung (i.e. act to expand the chest). During inspiration, elastic forces (act to expand the chest wall) aid inflation; however, at approximately two-thirds of TLC, the chest wall has reached its resting position and any expansion beyond this point requires a positive pressure to stretch the chest wall.

Effect of disease on compliance

Emphysema and pulmonary fibrosis (Fig. 4.11) represent two extremes of lung compliance in disease. In emphysema the compliance of the lung is increased, i.e. the lung becomes more easily distended. This is due to the destruction of the normal lung architecture, including the elastic fibres and collagen. Impaired elastic recoil means that the lungs do not deflate adequately, contributing to air trapping.

In diseases that cause fibrosis, scar tissue replaces normal interstitial tissue. As a result, the lungs become stiffer and compliance decreases.

Structural changes in the thorax (e.g. kyphoscoliosis) can similarly alter compliance of the chest wall and reduce the ability of the chest wall to expand, thus producing a restrictive ventilatory defect.

Surface tension and surfactant

The elasticity, and therefore compliance of the lungs, is dependent on two factors:

1. Elastic fibres in lung tissue.
2. The surface tension of the alveolar lining (this lining is a thin film of liquid, the main component of which is surfactant).

Surface tension is a physical property of liquids that arises because fluid molecules have a stronger attraction to each other than to air molecules. Molecules on the surface of a liquid in contact with air are therefore pulled close together and act like a skin. When molecules of a liquid lie on a curved surface (e.g. in a bubble), surface tension acts to pull that surface inwards. If the bubble is to be prevented from collapsing there must be an equal and opposite force tending to expand it. This is provided by positive pressure within the bubble.

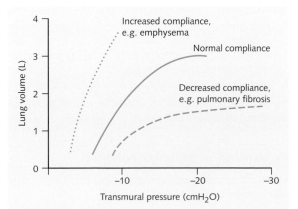

Fig. 4.11 Pressure–volume curves in disease.

Fig. 4.12 Law of Laplace

Laplace's law states that 'The pressure within a bubble is equal to twice the surface tension divided by the radius'

$$P = \frac{2T}{r}$$

where P = pressure within bubble
T = surface tension
r = radius

- The smaller a bubble (i.e. the more curved the surface), the larger the radial component.
- The larger the radial component, the greater the tendency to collapse.
- Smaller bubbles must have a greater internal pressure to keep them inflated.

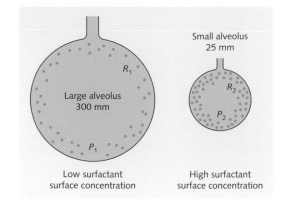

Fig. 4.13 Surface tension in the alveoli.

The alveoli are lined with liquid and are in contact with air. They can therefore be considered similar to tiny bubbles. Laplace's law (Fig. 4.12) tells us that the smaller a bubble, the greater the internal pressure needed to keep it inflated. If a bubble of about the same size as an alveolus was lined with interstitial fluid and filled with air it would require an internal pressure in the order of 3 kPa to prevent it from collapsing. The lungs would have a very low compliance and the forces involved in breathing would be extremely large. However, this is not the case because the alveoli are not lined with interstitial fluid, they are lined with surfactant.

Surfactant

Surfactant is manufactured by type II pneumocytes. It is first stored intracellularly as lamellar bodies and then released as tubular myelin (the storage form of active surfactant). Once in the alveolar air space, the tubular myelin unravels to form a thin layer of surfactant over type I and type II pneumocytes.

Surfactant is 90% lipid (mostly a phospholipid called dipalmitoyl phosphatidylcholine) and 10% protein. The three mechanical functions of surfactant are:

1. Prevention of alveolar collapse (gives alveolar stability).
2. Increase in lung compliance by reducing surface tension of alveolar lining fluid.
3. Prevention of transudation of fluid into alveoli.

Surfactant also has immunological functions, which are discussed in Chapter 2.

Prevention of alveolar collapse

There are two properties of surfactant that ensure alveolar stability:

1. The surface tension of the alveolar lining fluid varies with surface area. This is because surfactant reduces surface tension in proportion to its surface concentration. Surfactant is insoluble in water and floats on the surface of the alveolar lining fluid. In larger alveoli the surfactant is more dilute and thus the surface tension is higher (Fig. 4.13).
2. There is interaction between adjacent groups of alveoli. Therefore, collapsing alveoli pull on adjacent alveoli, preventing further collapse. This is termed alveolar interdependence.

Respiratory distress syndrome

Respiratory distress syndrome occurs in premature babies of less than 32 weeks' gestation; it is caused by a deficiency of surfactant production by type II pneumocytes. Difficulty in breathing occurs; breathing is rapid and laboured, often with an expiratory grunt. There is diffuse damage to alveoli with hyaline membrane formation. Treatment is with high-concentration oxygen therapy, which reverses the hypoxaemia.

Airway resistance

The previous section examined the elastic properties of the lungs (i.e. those caused by surface tension and tissue elasticity). However, in addition to overcoming the elastic properties of the lung during breathing, dynamic resistance to lung inflation must be overcome in order to provide effective ventilation.

The total pressure difference (P_{TOT}) required to inflate the lungs is the sum of the pressure to overcome lung compliance and the pressure to overcome dynamic resistance:

$$P_{TOT} = P_{COM} + P_{DYN}$$

where P_{COM} = pressure to overcome lung compliance and P_{DYN} = pressure to overcome the dynamic resistance.

Dynamic resistance itself comprises:

- Airway resistance.
- Resistance to tissues as they slide over each other – viscous tissue resistance.

$$P_{DYN} = P_{AR} + P_{VTR}$$

where P_{AR} = pressure to overcome airways resistance and P_{VTR} = pressure to overcome viscous tissue resistance.

Viscous tissue resistance comprises approximately 20% of the total dynamic resistance, i.e. the vast majority of the total resistance is provided by the airways.

Airway resistance is an important concept because it is increased in common diseases such as asthma and COPD. It is defined as the resistance to flow of gas within the airways of the lung.

Before we discuss airway resistance, it is important to outline pattern of flow.

Pattern of flow

The pattern of air flowing through a tube (e.g. an airway) varies with the velocity and physical properties of the airway (Fig. 4.14).

Turbulent flow

Turbulent flow is much more likely to occur with:

- High velocities (e.g. within the airways during exercise).
- Larger-diameter airways.
- Low-viscosity, high-density fluids.

Branching or irregular surfaces can also initiate turbulence.

Laminar flow

Laminar flow is described by Poiseuille's law (Fig. 4.15). In basic terms, Poiseuille's law means that the wider the tube, the lower the resistance to air flow. Importantly, the change in width is not directly proportional to the change in resistance: for a given reduction in the radius there is a 16-fold increase in resistance. Narrower or longer pipes have a higher resistance to flow and so flow rate is reduced.

Fig. 4.15 Poiseuille's law

Poiseuille's law states that, for a fluid under laminar flow conditions, the flow rate is directly related to the pressure drop between the two ends of a tube and the fourth power of the radius but inversely related to viscosity and length of pipe:

$$F = \frac{P\pi r^4}{8\eta L}$$

where F = flow rate
P = pressure drop
r = radius
η = viscosity
l = length of pipe
Remember, Poiseuille's law applies to laminar, not turbulent, flow.

Sites of airway resistance

When breathing through the nose, approximately one-half of the resistance to air flow occurs in the upper respiratory tract. This is significantly reduced when mouth breathing. Thus, approximately one-half of the resistance lies within the lower respiratory tract. Assuming laminar air flow, Poiseuille's law would predict that the major resistance to air flow would occur in the airways with a smaller radius. This is not the case because, although the individual diameter of each airway is small, the total cross-sectional area for flow increases (large number of small airways) further down the tracheobronchial tree.

HINTS AND TIPS

Remembering Poiseuille's law isn't drastically important, but understanding it is! So, remember that, in laminar flow, a small change in radius significantly affects either flow rate or pressure drop required to achieve the same flow. An example of this is bronchoconstriction in asthma.
- Flow varies directly with pressure drop.
- Flow varies inversely with viscosity.

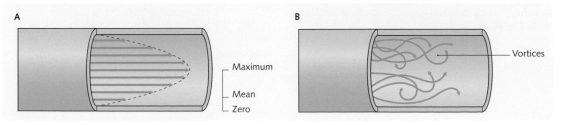

Fig. 4.14   (A) Laminar and (B) turbulent air flow.

In exercise, the airway resistance may increase significantly due to high air flows inducing turbulence. It is normal under these conditions to switch to mouth breathing to reduce airway resistance.

It is important to note that resistance of the smaller airways is difficult to measure. Thus, these small airways may be damaged by disease and it may be some time before this damage is detectable, thus representing a 'silent' zone.

Factors determining airway resistance

Factors affecting airway resistance are:

- Lung volume.
- Bronchial smooth-muscle tone.
- Altered airway calibre.
- Change in density and viscosity of inspired gas.

Lung volume

Airways are supported by radial traction of lung parenchyma and thus their diameter and resistance to flow are affected by lung volume:

- Low lung volumes tend to collapse and compress the airways, reducing their diameter and thus increasing resistance to flow.
- High lung volumes tend to increase radial traction, increasing the length and diameter of airways.

Bronchial smooth-muscle tone

Motor innervation of the smooth muscle of the airways is via the vagus nerve. The muscle has resting tone determined by the autonomic nervous system. This tone can be affected by a number of factors (Fig. 4.16).

Factors acting to decrease the airway diameter include:

- Irritant and cough receptors, C-fibre reflex.
- Pulmonary stretch receptors.
- Mediator release – inflammatory mediators (histamine, leukotrienes, etc.) cause bronchoconstriction.

Factors acting to increase the airway diameter include:

- Carbon dioxide.
- Catecholamine release.
- Other nerves – non-adrenergic, non-cholinergic nerves cause bronchodilatation.

> **HINTS AND TIPS**
>
> Increased smooth-muscle tone is very important in asthma. Inflammatory mediators act to narrow the airways and increase resistance to air flow.

> **HINTS AND TIPS**
>
> Things to remember:
> - The major site of airway resistance is medium-sized bronchi.
> - 80% of the resistance of the upper respiratory tract is presented by the trachea and bronchi.
> - Less than 20% of airway resistance is caused by airways less than 2 mm in diameter.

Effect of transmural pressure on airway resistance

Remember that the airways are not rigid tubes; they are affected by the pressures around them. The pressure difference between the gas in the airway and the pressure outside the airway is known as the transmural pressure difference. The pressure outside the airway reflects the intrapleural pressure (Fig. 4.17).

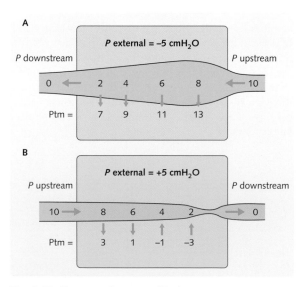

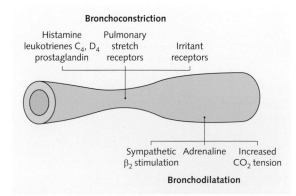

Fig. 4.16 Factors affecting bronchial smooth-muscle tone.

Fig. 4.17 Transmural pressure (Ptm).

During inspiration

The pressure within the pleural cavity is always negative and the alveolar pressure is greater than intrapleural pressure. The transmural pressure difference is always positive; thus the airway is distended (radial traction).

During expiration

The pressure within the alveolus is positive with respect to the intrapleural pressure; hence, the alveolus stays open. The transmural pressure difference, however, is dependent upon expiratory flow rate and intrapleural pressure.

During forced expiration, the positive intrapleural pressure is transmitted through the lungs to the external wall of the airways. In addition, there is a dynamic pressure drop from the alveolus to the airway caused by airway resistance. This is greater at high expiratory flow rates. Thus, the pressure in the lumen of the airway may be lower than the external wall pressure (negative transmural pressure), leading to collapse of the airways.

Thus, the harder the subject tries to exhale forcibly, the more the airways are compressed, so the rate of expiration does not rise as the increased pressure gradient (from alveoli to atmospheric pressure) is offset by the reduced calibre of the airways. This phenomenon is known as dynamic compression of airways.

Dynamic compression of airways is greater at lower lung volumes because the effect of radial traction holding the airways open is less. Thus it can be seen that, for a specific lung volume, there is a maximum expiratory flow rate caused by dynamic compression of the airways (Fig. 4.18). Any rate of expiration below this flow rate is dependent on how much effort is made to expel the air from the lungs and the flow is said to be effort-dependent. At maximum expiratory flow rate, any additional effort does not alter the expiratory flow rate (because of dynamic compression of airways) and the flow is said to be effort-independent.

Dynamic compression in disease

In patients with COPD, dynamic compression limits expiratory flow even in tidal breathing. The main reasons for this are:

- Loss of radial traction (due to destruction of the lung architecture) means the airways are more readily compressed.
- Increased lung compliance, leading to lower alveolar pressure and less force driving air out of the lungs.

The clinical consequences are airway collapse on expiration and air trapping in the alveoli. Patients sometimes demonstrate pursed-lip breathing as they attempt to increase pressure on expiration and reduce the amount of air trapped.

Measuring airway resistance

Airway resistance can be measured by plethysmography. In practice, estimates of airway resistance are made every day using simpler methods which rely on the relationship between resistance and air flow. Peak expiratory flow rate measures the maximum air flow achieved in a rapid, forced expiration. Spirometry measures the volume exhaled in a specified time (e.g. the forced expired volume in 1 second or FEV_1).

The work of breathing

The work of breathing is the work done by the respiratory muscles to overcome the forces described above, i.e. resistance to air flow and the elastic recoil of the lungs.

The work done (W) to change a volume (ΔV) of gas at constant pressure (P) is shown by the relationship below:

$$W = P\Delta V$$

Work done is measured in joules: a volume change of 10 L at a pressure of 1 $cmH_2O = 1$ J of energy.

Respiration normally represents just a small fraction of the total cost of metabolism (approximately 2%). However, the work required to inflate the lungs, along with this percentage, will rise if:

- Lungs are inflated to a larger volume (e.g. COPD and chronic severe asthma).
- Lung compliance decreases (e.g. fibrotic lungs).
- Airway resistance increases (e.g. COPD and asthma).
- Turbulence is induced in the airways (e.g. in high-flow rates experienced during strenuous exercise).

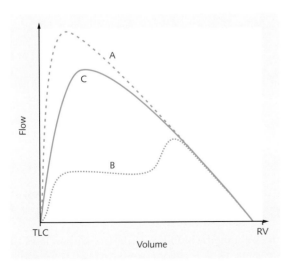

Fig. 4.18   Flow–volume curves made with spirometer. (A) Maximum inspiration and forced expiration. (B) Slow expiration initially, then forced. (C) Expiratory flow almost to maximum effort. TLC = total lung capacity; RV = residual volume.

In contrast, the work of breathing is reduced by bronchodilators, which act to decrease airway resistance.

The increased work requirement can be dramatic in patients with severe COPD; a great deal of energy is required just in order to breathe. This can also be understood in terms of the efficiency of ventilation (i.e. the amount of work done divided by energy expenditure). Efficiency of normal quiet breathing is low (about 10%) even in health. In COPD, efficiency decreases, and the work done increases, so that all the oxygen supplied from increasing ventilation is consumed by the respiratory muscles. The work of breathing can be illustrated by volume–pressure curves (Fig. 4.19).

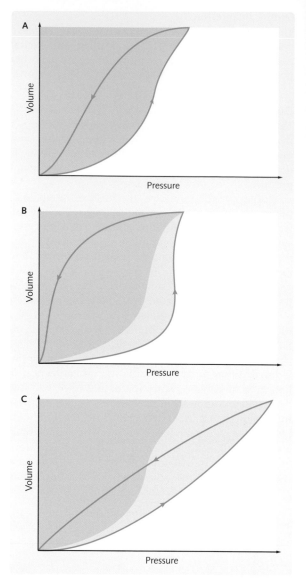

HINTS AND TIPS

Try to relate these concepts to respiratory failure. A patient with lung disease may be able to respond to impaired gas exchange by raising the ventilatory rate, leading to rapid, shallow breaths. This increases the work of breathing. If lung disease is severe, the work of breathing may become unsustainable. Respiratory muscles tire, ventilatory failure ensues and the patient must be mechanically ventilated, to reduce the work of breathing.

GASEOUS EXCHANGE IN THE LUNGS

This section discusses how gas is transferred from the alveoli to the bloodstream and from the bloodstream to the alveoli. A brief outline of how the laws of diffusion apply to the diffusion of gas from the airways to the circulation is given below. Time for diffusion and diffusion–perfusion limitations are also discussed.

Diffusion

Gas exchange between alveolar air and blood in the pulmonary capillaries takes place by diffusion.

- Diffusion occurs from an area of high concentration to an area of low concentration. Thus, the driving force for diffusion is concentration difference (ΔC).
- Diffusion will occur until the concentration in the two areas is equalized (i.e. net movement has ceased). Random movement of particles continues to occur and this is known as dynamic equilibrium.

Diffusion in the lungs occurs across a membrane and is therefore governed by Fick's law. Fick's law tells us that the rate of diffusion of a gas increases:

Fig. 4.19 The work of breathing. (A) Graph of normal lung volume against trans-lung pressure; (B) increased airway resistance (e.g. in asthma); (C) decreased compliance (e.g. in fibrotic lung disease).

- As the surface area of the membrane increases.
- The thinner the membrane.
- The greater the partial pressure gradient across the membrane.
- The more soluble the gas.

It is clear that the blood–gas interface with its large surface area of 50–100 m² and average thickness of 0.4 μm permits the high rate of diffusion required by the body.

The rate of diffusion across the alveoli is directly dependent upon the difference in partial pressures.

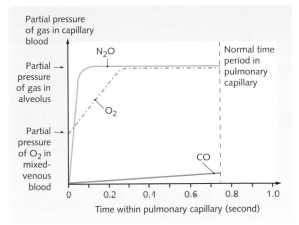

Fig. 4.21 Partial pressures of respiratory gases.

Perfusion and diffusion limitation

At the gas-exchange surface, gas transfer occurs through a membrane into a flowing liquid. There are two processes (Fig. 4.20) occurring:

- Diffusion across the alveolar capillary membrane.
- Perfusion of blood through pulmonary capillaries.

Uptake of a gas into the blood is dependent on its solubility and the chemical combination (e.g. with haemoglobin). If the chemical combination is strong, the gas is taken up by the blood with little rise in arterial partial pressure.

The solubility of nitrous oxide (N_2O) in the blood is low, and it does not undergo chemical combination with any component of the blood. Thus, rate of transfer of gas into the liquid phase is slow and partial pressure of the gas in the blood rises rapidly (Fig. 4.21). This reduces the partial pressure difference between alveolar gas and the blood and hence the driving force for diffusion. Nitrous oxide is, therefore, an example of a gas that is said to be perfusion-limited. Thus, the amount of nitrous oxide taken up by the blood is dependent almost solely upon the rate of blood flow through the pulmonary capillaries.

In the case of carbon monoxide (CO), the gas is taken up rapidly and bound tightly by haemoglobin; the arterial partial pressure rises slowly (Fig. 4.21). Thus, there is always a driving force (partial pressure difference) for diffusion (even at low perfusion rates) and the overall rate of transfer will be dependent on the rate of diffusion. This type of transfer is said to be diffusion-limited. Thus, the amount of carbon monoxide taken up by the blood is dependent on the rate of diffusion of carbon monoxide from the alveoli to the blood.

The transfer of oxygen is normally perfusion-limited because the arterial partial pressure of oxygen (P_aO_2) reaches equilibrium with the alveolar gas (P_AO_2) by about one-third of the way along the pulmonary capillary (Fig. 4.21); there is, therefore, no driving force for diffusion after this point. However, if the diffusion is slow because of emphysematous changes in the lung, then P_aO_2 may not reach equilibrium with the alveolar gas before the blood reaches the end of the capillary. Under these conditions, the transfer of oxygen is diffusion-limited.

Oxygen uptake in the capillary network

The time taken for the partial pressure of oxygen to reach its plateau is approximately 0.25 second. The pulmonary capillary volume under resting conditions is about 75 mL, which is approximately the same size as the stroke volume of the right ventricle. Pulmonary capillary blood is therefore replaced with every heart beat, approximately every 0.75 second. This far exceeds the time for transfer of oxygen into the bloodstream.

During exercise, however, the cardiac output increases and the flow rate through the pulmonary capillaries also increases. Because the lungs have the ability to recruit new capillaries and distend already

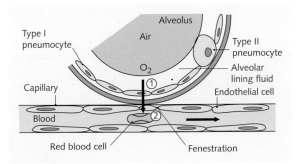

Fig. 4.20 Gas transfer across the alveolar capillary membrane. (1) Diffusion across membrane; (2) perfusion of blood through pulmonary capillaries.

open capillaries (see Ch. 3), the effect of increased blood flow rate on the time allowed for diffusion is not as great as one might expect. In strenuous exercise, the pulmonary capillary network volume may increase by up to 200 mL. This helps maintain the time allowed for diffusion, although it cannot keep it to the same value as at rest.

Carbon dioxide transfer

Diffusion rates of gas in blood are also of great importance in respiratory medicine. Diffusion in liquids is directly dependent upon the solubility of the gas, but inversely proportional to the square root of its molecular weight. Carbon monoxide diffuses 20 times more rapidly than oxygen, but has a similar molecular weight. Thus, the difference in rates of diffusion is caused by the much higher solubility of carbon dioxide.

Under normal conditions, the transfer of carbon dioxide is not diffusion-limited.

Measuring diffusion

Carbon monoxide is the gas most commonly used to study diffusing capacity. Because carbon monoxide is taken up into the liquid phase very quickly, the rate of perfusion of pulmonary capillaries does not significantly affect the partial pressure difference between alveolar gas and the bloodstream. In addition, carbon monoxide binds irreversibly to haemoglobin and is not taken up by the tissues.

In contrast, oxygen is not a good candidate for calculating diffusing capacity because it binds reversibly to haemoglobin; thus, mixed-venous partial pressure may not be the same as that of blood entering the pulmonary capillary bed. In addition, because oxygen is taken up less quickly than CO, perfusion has more of an effect.

HINTS AND TIPS

The terms diffusing capacity ($D_L CO$) and transfer factor ($T_L CO$) are interchangeable.

We therefore use the diffusing capacity of carbon monoxide ($D_L CO$) as a general measure of the diffusion properties of the lung.

One of the methods used to measure diffusion across the blood–gas interface is the single-breath method. A single breath of a mixture of carbon monoxide and air is taken. The breath is then held for approximately 10 seconds. The difference between inspiratory and expiratory concentrations of carbon monoxide is measured and therefore the amount of carbon monoxide taken up by the blood in 10 seconds is known. If the lung volume is also measured by the helium dilution method, it is possible to determine the transfer coefficient (KCO) or diffusion rate per unit of lung volume. This is a more useful measure of diffusion where lung volume has been lost: for example, after surgery or in pleural effusion. Because there can be many causes of a reduction in diffusing capacity, it is not a specific test for lung disease. It is, however, a sensitive test: it is able to demonstrate minor impediments to gas diffusion.

Factors that decrease the rate of diffusion include:

- Thickening of the alveolar capillary membrane (e.g. in fibrosing alveolitis).
- Oedema of the alveolar capillary walls.
- Increased lining fluid within the alveoli.
- Increased distance for gaseous diffusion (e.g. in emphysema).
- Reduced area of alveolar capillary membrane (e.g. in emphysema).
- Reduced flow of fresh air to the alveoli from terminal bronchioles.

Perfusion and gas transport (5)

Objectives

By the end of this chapter you should be able to:
- Describe what is meant by the ventilation:perfusion ratio.
- Describe the structure of haemoglobin and its ability to bind oxygen as well as draw and explain the oxygen dissociation curve for haemoglobin.
- Define hypoxia and know the four different types of hypoxia and their clinical importance.
- State the normal blood pH range and understand the difference between both acidotic and alkalis changes and respiratory and metabolic changes.

OVERVIEW

The pulmonary circulation is a highly specialized system adapted to accommodate the entire cardiac output, both at rest and during exercise, facilitated by its low pressure, low resistance and ability to recruit more vessels with only a slight increase in arterial pulmonary pressure.

However, good perfusion is not enough to ensure that the blood is adequately oxygenated. The most important determinant in arterial blood gas composition is the way in which ventilation and perfusion are matched to each alveolus. Mismatching of ventilation:perfusion is a central fault in many common lung diseases.

The ability of the lungs to change minute ventilation, and therefore alter the rate of excretion of CO_2, gives the respiratory system a key role in maintaining the body's acid–base status. This chapter therefore also reviews the fundamentals of acid–base balance and discusses the common acid–base disturbances.

THE VENTILATION–PERFUSION RELATIONSHIP

Basic concepts

To achieve efficient gaseous exchange, it is essential that the flow of gas (ventilation: V) and the flow of blood (perfusion: Q) are closely matched. The ideal situation would be where:

- All alveoli are ventilated equally with gas of identical composition and pressure.
- All pulmonary capillaries in the alveolar wall are perfused with equal amounts of mixed-venous blood.

Unfortunately, this is not the case as neither ventilation nor perfusion is uniform throughout the lung.

The partial pressure of oxygen in the alveoli determines the amount of oxygen transferred to the blood. Two factors affect the partial pressure of oxygen in the alveoli:

1. The amount of ventilation (i.e. the addition of oxygen to the alveolar compartment).
2. The perfusion of blood through pulmonary capillaries (i.e. the removal of oxygen from the alveolar compartment).

It is the ratio of ventilation to perfusion that determines the concentration of oxygen in the alveolar compartment.

Ventilation:perfusion ratio

By looking at the ventilation:perfusion ratio, we can see how well ventilation and perfusion are matched. By definition:

$$\text{Ventilation:perfusion ratio} = V_A/Q$$

where V_A = alveolar minute ventilation (usually about 4.2 L/min); Q = pulmonary blood flow (usually about 5.0 L/min). Thus, normal $V_A/Q = 0.84$ (i.e. approximately 1).

This is an average value across the lung. Different ventilation:perfusion ratios are present throughout the lung from apex to base.

Extremes of ventilation:perfusion ratio

Looking at the ventilation:perfusion ratio, it can be seen that there are two extremes to this relationship. These extremes were introduced in Chapter 1. Either there is:

1. No ventilation (a shunt): $V_A/Q = 0$.
2. No perfusion (dead space): $V_A/Q = \bullet$.

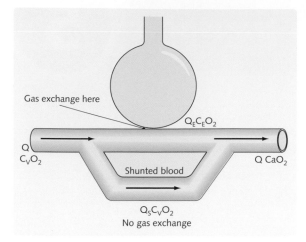

Fig. 5.1 Shunted blood. The shunted blood has a low oxygen concentration (i.e. of venous blood) and is known as the venous admixture.

Right-to-left shunt

A right-to-left shunt is described when the pulmonary circulation bypasses the ventilation process (Fig. 5.1), by either:

1. Bypassing the lungs completely (e.g. transposition of great vessels).
2. Perfusion of an area of lung that is not ventilated.

The shunted blood will not have been oxygenated or been able to given up its carbon dioxide; thus its levels of PO_2 and PCO_2 are those of venous blood. When added to the systemic circulation, this blood will proportionately decrease arterial PO_2; it is called the venous admixture.

In normal subjects, there is only a very small amount of shunting (about 1%). However, right-to-left shunting makes a significant contribution to abnormal gas exchange in some disease states, notably:

- Cyanotic congenital heart disease.
- Pulmonary oedema.
- Severe pneumonia.

Regional variation of ventilation and perfusion

Both ventilation and perfusion increase towards the lung base because of the effects of gravity.

Because the blood has a greater density than air, the gravitational effects on perfusion are much greater than on ventilation. This leads to a regional variation (Fig. 5.2) in the ventilation:perfusion ratio from lung apex (high V/Q) to lung base (low V/Q).

These regional variations in the ventilation:perfusion ratio are caused by the lung being upright; thus, changes in posture will alter the ventilation:perfusion ratio throughout the lung. For example, when lying down, the posterior area of the lung has a low ventilation:perfusion ratio and the anterior area has a high ventilation:perfusion ratio.

The effect of high and low ventilation:perfusion ratios on carbon dioxide and oxygen in the alveolus and blood is highlighted in Figure 5.3 and described below.

Fig. 5.2 Ventilation and perfusion at the lung apex, middle and base.

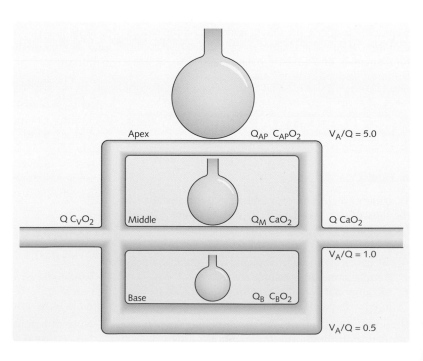

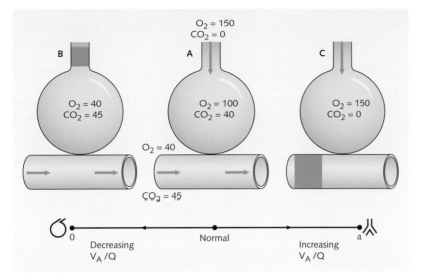

Fig. 5.3 The effect of altering the ventilation:perfusion ratio on the P_AO_2 and P_ACO_2 in a lung unit: (A) normal lung; (B) lung unit is not ventilated – O_2 falls and CO_2 rises within lung unit; (C) lung unit is not perfused – O_2 is not taken up and CO_2 does not diffuse into the alveolus.

At low ventilation:perfusion ratios (e.g. at the lung base)

Effect on carbon dioxide concentrations

Carbon dioxide diffuses from the blood to alveoli; however, because ventilation is low, carbon dioxide is not taken away as rapidly. Thus, carbon dioxide tends to accumulate in the alveolus until a new, higher steady-state P_ACO_2 is reached.

Assuming that the overall lung function is normal, this regional variation in P_ACO_2 will not affect overall P_vCO_2. Thus, reducing the ventilation:perfusion ratio will not increase P_aCO_2 above the mixed-venous value.

Effect on oxygen concentrations

Oxygen diffuses from the alveolus into the blood; however, because ventilation is low, oxygen taken up by the blood and metabolized is not replenished fully by new air entering the lungs. Oxygen in the alveolus is depleted until a new, lower steady-state P_AO_2 is reached. Because diffusion continues until equilibrium is achieved, the P_aO_2 of this unit will also be low (Fig. 5.4A).

At high ventilation:perfusion ratios (e.g. at the lung apex)

Effect on carbon dioxide concentrations

The carbon dioxide diffusing from the blood is nearly all removed; carbon dioxide in the alveolus is depleted until a new, lower steady-state P_ACO_2 is reached. Diffusion continues until equilibrium is achieved: P_aCO_2 will also be low.

Effect on oxygen concentrations

Oxygen diffusing from the alveolar gas is not taken away by the blood in such large amounts because the relative

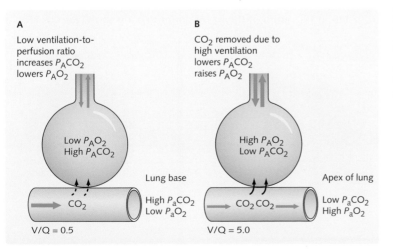

Fig. 5.4 Ventilation and perfusion at lung base (A) and apex (B). At the lung base perfusion is high and the V/Q ratio is low. This reduces alveolar O_2 and raises CO_2. At the apex the V/Q ratio is higher, leading to a high alveolar O_2 and more CO_2 blown off.

blood flow is reduced; in addition, oxygen is replenished with each breath. Thus, oxygen tends to accumulate in the alveolus until a new steady-state concentration is reached (Fig. 5.4B). Diffusion occurs until a new higher equilibrium is achieved; thus, P_aO_2 is also higher.

Measurement of ventilation and perfusion

Ventilation:perfusion scans

In clinical practice, ventilation:perfusion ratios are assessed primarily by means of radioisotope scans. Ventilation is detected by inhalation of a gas or aerosol labelled with the radioisotope ^{133}Xe. The distribution of pulmonary blood flow is tested with an intravenous injection of ^{99m}Tc-labelled macroaggregated albumin (MAA). These radioactive particles are larger than the diameter of the pulmonary capillaries and they remain lodged for several hours. A gamma camera is then used to detect the position of the MAA.

The two scans are then assessed together for 'filling defects' or areas where ventilation and perfusion are not matched. The technique is primarily used to detect pulmonary emboli. Spiral computed tomography scans are now superseding this technique. Figure 5.5 shows a lung scan following pulmonary embolism.

GAS TRANSPORT IN THE BLOOD

Oxygen transport

Oxygen is carried in the blood in two forms:

1. Dissolved in plasma.
2. Bound to haemoglobin.

Dissolved oxygen

To meet the metabolic demands of the body, large amounts of oxygen must be carried in the blood. We have seen that the amount of gas dissolved in solution is proportional to the partial pressure of the gas (Henry's law). Thus, with a normal arterial P_aO_2 (100 mmHg; 13.3 kPa), for each 100 mL of blood there is only 0.003 mL of dissolved oxygen or 15 mL of oxygen per minute based on a 5 L cardiac output. At rest, the body requires approximately 250 mL of oxygen per minute. Thus, if all the oxygen in the blood were carried in the dissolved form, cardiac output would meet only 6% of the demand.

Therefore most of the oxygen must be carried in chemical combination, not in simple solution. Oxygen is thus combined with haemoglobin.

Haemoglobin

Haemoglobin is found in red blood cells and is a conjugate protein molecule, containing iron within its structure. The molecule consists of four polypeptide subunits, two α and two β. Associated with each polypeptide chain is a haem group that acts as a binding site for oxygen. The haem group consists of a porphyrin ring containing iron and is responsible for binding of oxygen:

- Haemoglobin contains iron in a ferrous (Fe^{2+}) or ferric (Fe^{2+}) state.
- Only haemoglobin in the ferrous form can bind oxygen.
- Methaemoglobin (containing iron in a ferric state) cannot bind oxygen.

The quaternary structure of haemoglobin determines its ability to bind oxygen. In its deoxygenated state, haemoglobin (known as reduced haemoglobin) has a low affinity for oxygen. The binding of one oxygen molecule to haemoglobin causes a conformational change in its protein structure; this positive cooperativity allows easier access to the other oxygen-binding sites, thus increasing haemoglobin's affinity for further binding of oxygen. Haemoglobin is capable of binding up to four molecules of oxygen.

It should be noted that, during this reaction, the iron atom of the haem group remains in the ferrous (Fe^{2+})

Fig. 5.5 Ventilation:perfusion scan following pulmonary embolus. (Courtesy of Ivor Jones and the Nuclear Medicine staff, Derriford Hospital, Plymouth.)

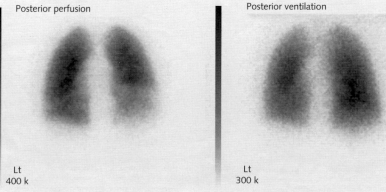

form. It is not oxidized to the ferric (Fe^{3+}) form. The interaction of oxygen with haemoglobin is oxygenation, not oxidation.

The main function of haemoglobin is to take up oxygen at the alveolar capillary membrane and to transport the oxygen within the blood and release it into the tissues. However, haemoglobin also has other functions:

- Buffering of H^+ ions.
- Transport of CO_2 as carbamino compounds.

Haemoglobin binding

Haemoglobin has four binding sites; the amount of oxygen carried by haemoglobin in the blood depends on how many of these binding sites are occupied. Therefore, the haemoglobin molecule can be said to be saturated or partially saturated:

- Saturated – all four binding sites are occupied by O_2.
- Partially saturated – some oxygen has bound to haemoglobin, but not all four sites are occupied.

If completely saturated, the maximum binding of oxygen to haemoglobin we could expect is:

$$150 \times 1.34 = 201 \text{ mL of oxygen per litre of blood}$$

In addition, there is approximately 10 mL of O_2 in solution. The total (210 mL) is called the oxygen capacity; the haemoglobin is said to be 100% saturated ($SO_2 = 100\%$). The actual amount of oxygen bonded to haemoglobin and dissolved in the blood at any one time is called the oxygen content.

The oxygen saturation (SO_2) of the blood is defined as the amount of oxygen carried in the blood, expressed as a percentage of oxygen capacity:

$$SO_2 = O_2 \text{ content}/O_2 \text{ capacity} \times 100$$

Cyanosis

Haemoglobin absorbs light of different wavelengths depending on whether it is in the reduced or oxygenated form. Oxyhaemoglobin appears bright red, whereas reduced haemoglobin appears purplish, giving a bluish pallor to skin. This is called cyanosis, which can be described as either central or peripheral. Cyanosis depends on the absolute amount of deoxygenated haemoglobin in the vessels, not the proportion of deoxygenated:oxygenated haemoglobin. In central cyanosis, there is more than 5 g/dL deoxygenated haemoglobin in the blood and this can be seen in the peripheral tissues (e.g. lips, tongue). Peripheral cyanosis is due to a local cause (e.g. vascular obstruction of a limb).

Oxygen dissociation curve

How much oxygen binds to haemoglobin is dependent upon the partial pressure of oxygen in the blood. This relationship is represented by the oxygen dissociation curve (Fig. 5.6A); this is an equilibrium curve at specific conditions:

- 150 g of haemoglobin per litre of blood.
- pH 7.4.
- Temperature 37° C.

Factors affecting the oxygen dissociation curve

The shape of the curve, and therefore oxygen delivery to the tissues, is affected by a number of factors, including:

- pH.
- CO_2.
- Temperature.
- Other forms of haemoglobin.

These factors shift the oxygen dissociation curve to the right or to the left:

- A shift to the right allows easier dissociation of oxygen (i.e. lower oxygen saturation at any particular PO_2) and increases the oxygen release from oxyhaemoglobin.
- A shift to the left makes oxygen binding easier (i.e. higher oxygen saturation at any particular PO_2) and increases the oxygen uptake by haemoglobin.

The following factors shift the curve to the right (Fig. 5.6B):

- Increased PCO_2 and decreased pH (increased hydrogen ion concentration), known as the Bohr shift.
- Increased temperature.
- Increase in 2,3-diphosphoglycerate (2,3-DPG), which binds to the β chains.

2,3-DPG is a product of anaerobic metabolism. Red blood cells possess no mitochondria and therefore carry out anaerobic metabolism to produce energy. 2,3-DPG binds more strongly to reduced haemoglobin than to oxyhaemoglobin. Concentrations of 2,3-DPG increase in chronic hypoxia, e.g. in patients with chronic lung disease, or at high altitude.

Other forms of haemoglobin

Fetal haemoglobin

Fetal haemoglobin differs from adult haemoglobin by having two γ chains instead of two β chains (Fig. 5.7).

Fetal haemoglobin has a higher affinity for oxygen because its γ chains bind 2,3-DPG less avidly than the β chains of adult haemoglobin and are therefore able to bind oxygen at lower partial pressures (maternal venous P_vO_2 is low: <40 mmHg).

Release of carbon dioxide from fetal haemoglobin causes a shift to the left of the fetal oxyhaemoglobin dissociation curve, thus increasing its affinity for oxygen.

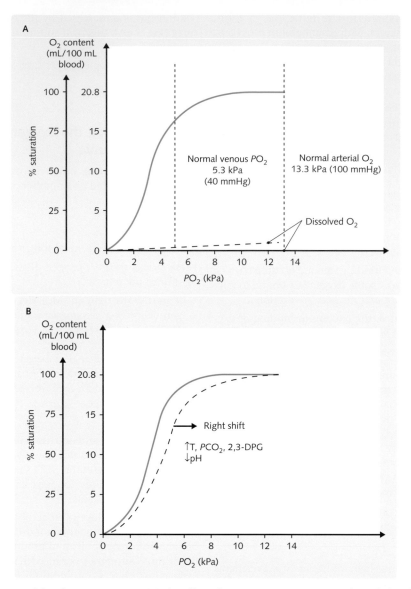

Fig. 5.6 (A) Oxyhaemoglobin dissociation curve. (B) The effect of temperature, PCO_2, pH and 2,3-diphosphoglycerate (2,3-DPG) on the oxyhaemoglobin dissociation curve.

This released carbon dioxide binds to maternal haemoglobin, causing a shift to the right of maternal haemoglobin, thus reducing the affinity of the latter for oxygen. Oxygen is therefore released by maternal haemoglobin and bound by fetal haemoglobin. This is known as the double Bohr shift.

Haemoglobin S

Haemoglobin S is a form of haemoglobin found in sickle cell anaemia. Sickle cell anaemia is an autosomal recessive disorder in which there is a defect in the β-globulin chain of the haemoglobin molecule.

There is a substitution of the amino acid valine for glutamine at position 6 of the β chain, forming haemoglobin S. The heterozygote has sickle cell trait and the homozygote sickle cell anaemia. The abnormal haemoglobin S molecules polymerize when deoxygenated and cause the red blood cells containing the abnormal haemoglobin to sickle. The fragile sickle cells haemolyse and may block vessels, leading to ischaemia and infarction.The heterozygous patient usually has an asymptomatic anaemia, and the homozygote has painful crises with bone and abdominal pain; there may also be intrapulmonary shunting.

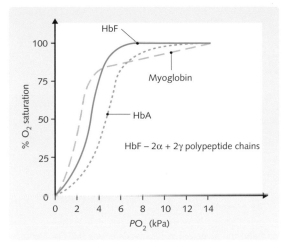

Fig. 5.7 Comparison of oxygen dissociation curves for myoglobin, fetal haemoglobin (HbF) and adult haemoglobin (HbA).

Thalassaemia

The thalassaemias are autosomal recessive disorders due to decreased production of either the α or the β chain of haemoglobin (Hb).There are two genes for the β chain and, depending on the number of normal genes, the thalassaemia is quoted as major or minor. There are four genes which code for the α chain, leading to various clinical disorders depending on the genetic defect. HbA$_2$ is present in a small amount in the normal population and consists of two α and two β chains. It is markedly raised in β-thalassaemia minor.

Full discussion of these disorders can be found in *Crash Course: Immunology and Haematology*.

Carboxyhaemoglobin (carbon monoxide poisoning)

Carbon monoxide (CO) displaces oxygen from oxy-haemoglobin because the affinity of haemoglobin for carbon monoxide is more than 200 times that for oxygen. This changes the shape of the oxyhaemoglobin dissociation curve. Figure 5.8 shows the effects of carbon monoxide poisoning:

- In this instance, oxygen capacity is 50% of normal (i.e. 50% HbO$_2$ and 50% HbCO). The actual value will depend on the partial pressure of CO (e.g. with a PCO of 16 mmHg, 75% of Hb will be in the form of HbCO).
- Saturation is achieved at a PO$_2$ of < 40 mmHg (below venous PO$_2$).
- HbCO causes a shift to the left for the oxygen dissociation curve (i.e. HbCO has a higher affinity for oxygen than normal HbO$_2$).
- Carbon monoxide binds to two of the four available haem groups.

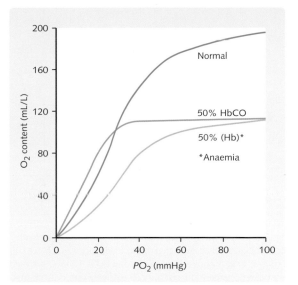

Fig. 5.8 Oxyhaemoglobin curve showing effects of anaemia and carbon monoxide poisoning (50% HbCO and anaemia compared with normal haemoglobin).

Carbon monoxide takes a long time to be cleared, but this can be speeded sped up or enhanced, not speeded. Up by ventilation with 100% oxygen. Additionally, the patient is not cyanosed because HbCO is cherry-red.

Carbon dioxide transport

There are three ways in which carbon dioxide can be transported in the blood:

1. Dissolved in plasma.
2. As bicarbonate ions.
3. As carbamino compounds.

Dissolved carbon dioxide

The solubility of carbon dioxide in the blood is much greater than that of oxygen (20 times greater); so, unlike oxygen, a significant amount (approximately 10%) of carbon dioxide is carried in solution.

Bicarbonate ions

Approximately 60% of carbon dioxide is transported as bicarbonate ions. Dissolved carbon dioxide interacts with water to form carbonic acid as follows:

$$CO_2 + H_2O \rightleftharpoons H_2CO_3 \qquad (1)$$

Carbonic acid rapidly dissociates into ions:

$$H_2CO_3 \rightleftharpoons H^+ + HCO_3^- \qquad (2)$$

The total reaction being:

$$CO_2 + H_2O \rightleftharpoons H_2CO_3 \rightleftharpoons H^+ + HCO_3^-$$

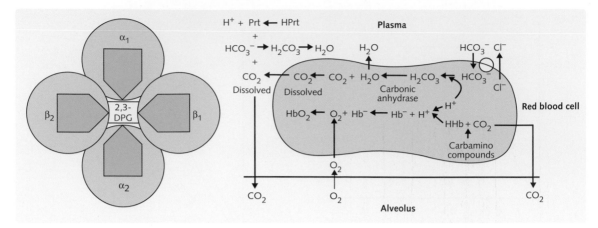

Fig. 5.9 The exchange of CO_2 and O_2 that occurs between the blood and the alveolar air. Bicarbonate ions (HCO_3^-) enter the red blood cell in exchange for chloride ions (which are transported out). Carbonic acid is formed once the O_2 is bound to Hb. Carbonic acid is converted to CO_2 and H_2O. The CO_2 is then excreted from the cell. CO_2 stored in carbamino compound form can be excreted from the cell passively without the involvement of an enzyme. 2,3-DPG = 2,3-diphosphoglycerate.

The first reaction is very slow in plasma, but within the red blood cell is dramatically speeded up by the enzyme carbonic anhydrase. Reaction 2 is very fast, but, if allowed to proceed alone, a large amount of H^+ would be formed, slowing down or halting the reaction. Haemoglobin has the property that it can bind H^+ ions and act as a buffer, thus allowing the reaction to go on rapidly.

$$H^+ + HbO_2^- \rightleftharpoons HHb + O_2$$
$$H^+ + Hb^- \rightleftharpoons HHb$$

The bicarbonate produced in the red blood cells diffuses down its concentration gradient into the plasma in exchange for chloride ions (Cl^-). This process is known as the chloride shift (Fig. 5.9).

Carbamino compounds

Carbon dioxide is capable of combining with proteins, interacting with their terminal amine groups to form carbamino compounds (Fig. 5.9). The most important protein involved is haemoglobin, as it is the most abundant in the blood. Approximately 30% of carbon dioxide is carried as carbamino compounds.

Haldane effect

Carriage of carbon dioxide is increased in deoxygenated blood because of two factors:

1. Reduced haemoglobin has a greater affinity for carbon dioxide than does oxyhaemoglobin.
2. Reduced haemoglobin is less acidic (i.e. a better proton acceptor: H^+ buffer) than oxyhaemoglobin.

The Haldane effect minimizes changes in pH of the blood when gaseous exchange occurs. The decrease in pH due to the oxygenation of haemoglobin is offset by the increase that results from the loss of CO_2 to the alveolar air. The reverse occurs in the tissues. This is an important effect because:

- In peripheral capillaries, the unloading of oxygen from haemoglobin aids the binding of carbon dioxide to haemoglobin.
- In pulmonary capillaries, the loading of oxygen on haemoglobin reduces the binding of carbon dioxide to haemoglobin.

This allows efficient gaseous exchange of carbon dioxide in the tissues and the lungs.

Carbon dioxide dissociation curve

The carriage of carbon dioxide is dependent upon the partial pressure of carbon dioxide in the blood. This relationship is described by the carbon dioxide dissociation curve. Compared with the oxygen dissociation curve:

- The carbon dioxide curve is more linear.
- The carbon dioxide curve is much steeper than the oxygen curve (between venous and arterial partial pressure of respiratory gases).
- The carbon dioxide curve varies according to oxygen saturation of haemoglobin.

Hypoventilation and hyperventilation

If P_aCO_2 is a measure of ventilation, it is appropriate in a review of carbon dioxide transport to consider two key concepts in respiratory medicine: hypoventilation and hyperventilation. For the body to function normally,

Fig. 5.10 Comparison of hyperventilation and hypoventilation

Hyperventilation	Hypoventilation
Causes	Causes
Anxiety Brainstem lesion Drugs	Obstruction: • Asthma • Chronic obstructive airways disease • Foreign body (e.g. peanut) Brainstem lesion Pneumothorax or lung collapse Trauma (e.g. fractured rib) Drugs, notably opioids
Consequences	Consequences
Ventilation too great for metabolic demand Too much CO_2 blown off from lungs $P_aCO_2 < 40$ mmHg	Ventilation is too low for metabolic demand Not enough CO_2 is blown off at the lungs $P_aCO_2 > 45$ mmHg

ventilation must meet the metabolic demand of the tissues (Fig. 5.10). Thus, metabolic tissue consumption of oxygen must be equal to the oxygen taken up in the blood from alveolar gas. Or, metabolic tissue production of carbon dioxide must be equal to the amount of carbon dioxide blown off at the alveoli.

Hypoventilation

The term 'hypoventilation' refers to a situation when ventilation is insufficient to meet metabolic demand.

Hyperventilation

The term 'hyperventilation' refers to a situation where ventilation is excessive to metabolic demand, thus blowing off carbon dioxide from the lungs.

Hypercapnia and hypocapnia

Hypercapnia

A high partial pressure (concentration) of carbon dioxide in the blood ($P_aCO_2 > 45$ mmHg) is termed 'hypercapnia'.

Hypocapnia

A low partial pressure of carbon dioxide in the blood ($P_aCO_2 < 40$ mmHg) is termed 'hypocapnia'.

Respiratory failure

Hypercapnia and hypocapnia are important concepts in the assessment of respiratory failure. Respiratory failure is defined as a $P_aO_2 < 8$ kPa (60 mmHg) and is divided into type I and type II, depending on the P_aCO_2.

In type I respiratory failure, $P_aCO_2 < 6.5$ kPa. P_aO_2 is low (hypoxaemic), but P_aCO_2 may be normal or low; this represents a ventilation:perfusion mismatch.

In type II respiratory failure, $P_aCO_2 > 6.5$ kPa. Both P_aO_2 and P_aCO_2 indicate that the lungs are not well ventilated.

The significance of this classification is that in type II respiratory failure, the patient may have developed tolerance to increased levels of P_aCO_2; in other words, the drive for respiration no longer relies on hypercapnic drive (high P_aCO_2) but on hypoxic drive (low P_aO_2). Thus, if the patient is given high-concentration oxygen therapy the hypoxic drive for ventilation may decrease and the patient may stop breathing.

Hypoxia

This is a condition in which the metabolic demand for oxygen cannot be met by the circulating blood.

Causes of hypoxia

Many cells can respire anaerobically; however, the neurons in the brain cannot and therefore need a constant supply of oxygen to maintain normal function. A severe shortage of oxygen to the brain can lead to unconsciousness and even death. Therefore, treatment of hypoxic patients is critically important. There are four principal types of hypoxia:

1. Hypoxic hypoxia.
2. Anaemic hypoxia.
3. Stagnant hypoxia (or static hypoxia).
4. Cytotoxic hypoxia (or histotoxic hypoxia).

Hypoxic hypoxia

This occurs when the arterial P_aO_2 is significantly reduced, so that haemoglobin in the blood exiting the lungs is not fully saturated with oxygen. Figure 5.11 highlights the main causes of hypoxic hypoxia.

The haemoglobin saturation is reduced in patients with hypoxic hypoxia. Most forms of hypoxic hypoxia can be corrected if patients are given hyperbaric oxygen to breathe. The high concentration of oxygen will increase the P_AO_2, and thus the P_aO_2, improving the oxygen saturation status of haemoglobin. In patients with right-to-left shunt, hyperbaric oxygen may not have any benefit, because the P_AO_2 will be normal, but since the blood is being shunted away from the alveoli the P_aO_2 will remain low.

Anaemic hypoxia

This occurs when there is a significant reduction in the concentration of haemoglobin, so the oxygen content of

Fig. 5.11 Causes of hypoxic hypoxia

Physiological
- At high altitude where there is a low oxygen tension in inspired air, the P_AO_2 and, accordingly, the P_aO_2 will fall

Pathological
- Hypoventilation:
  - Respiratory muscle weakness, e.g. chronic obstructive pulmonary disease, myasthenia gravis and poliomyelitis patients
  - Iatrogenic causes, e.g. general anaesthetics and analgesics (opiates) which act upon the respiratory centres in the medulla to decrease respiratory muscle activity
- Abnormal V/Q matching, e.g. airway obstruction, pulmonary embolism
- Impaired diffusing capacity, e.g. pulmonary oedema, as seen in left ventricular failure
- Right-to-left shunting, e.g. cyanotic congenital heart diseases, severe pneumonia

the arterial blood will be abnormally reduced. There are numerous causes of anaemia. It can be due to:

- Blood loss (e.g. large haemorrhage).
- Reduced synthesis of haemoglobin (e.g. vitamin B_{12} deficiency, folate deficiency).
- Abnormal haemoglobin synthesis due to a genetic defect (e.g. sickle cell anaemia).
- Carbon monoxide poisoning.

The P_AO_2 in anaemic patients is usually normal and the haemoglobin saturation is also normal. Patients become hypoxic because there is a reduction in the oxygen content in the blood as there is less haemoglobin than normal. Treating anaemic patients with hyperbaric oxygen will be of limited benefit because the blood leaving the lung will already be fully saturated. Anaemic patients will not appear to be cyanosed because the amount of deoxygenated blood leaving the respiring tissue will not be higher than normal.

Stagnant hypoxia

This is the result of a low blood flow, and hence a reduction in oxygen supply, to the tissues. This may occur with a reduced blood flow along an artery to a specific organ, with only that organ being affected; alternatively, reduced blood flow to all organs can occur if the cardiac output is significantly reduced (e.g. due to heart failure). There is usually nothing wrong with the lungs in terms of ventilation and perfusion in stagnant hypoxia, so the P_AO_2 and the P_aO_2 will be normal. Since the blood flow to the respiring tissues is slow, the tissues will try to extract as much available oxygen as possible from the arterial supply and so the venous PO_2 will be lowered and hence give rise to peripheral cyanosis.

Treatment with hyperbaric oxygen will not be beneficial to these patients as the blood leaving the lung will already be fully saturated. Only a slight rise in the level of oxygen dissolved within the blood plasma will occur.

Cytotoxic hypoxia

This occurs when the respiring cells within the tissues are unable to use oxygen, mainly due to poisoning of the oxidative enzymes of the cells. For example, in cyanide poisoning, cyanide combines with the cytochrome chain and prevents oxygen being used in oxidative phosphorylation.

In cytotoxic hypoxia both the P_AO_2 and the P_aO_2 are normal and so, again, treating these patients with oxygen will be of limited value. Since the oxygen is unable to be utilized by the tissues, the venous PO_2 will be abnormally high and cyanosis will not occur in these patients.

ACID–BASE BALANCE

Normal pH

The pH of the intracellular and extracellular compartments must be tightly controlled for the body to function efficiently, or at all. The normal arterial pH lies within a relatively narrow range: 7.35–7.45 ([H$^+$] range, 45–35 mmol/L). An acid–base disturbance arises when arterial pH lies outside this range. If the blood pH is less than 7.35, an acidosis is present; if pH is greater than 7.45, the term alkalosis is used. Although a larger variation in pH can be tolerated (pH 6.8–7.8) for a short time, recovery is often impossible if blood remains at pH 6.8 for long.

Such a tight control on blood pH is achieved by a combination of blood buffers and the respiratory and renal systems which make adjustments to return pH towards its normal levels.

Key concepts in acid–base balance

Metabolic production of acids

Products of metabolism (carbon dioxide, lactic acid, phosphate, sulphate, etc.) form acidic solutions, thus increasing the hydrogen ion concentration and reducing pH. We also have an intake of acids in our diet (approximately 50–100 mmol H$^+$ per day).We rely on three methods to control our internal hydrogen ion concentration:

1. Dilution of body fluids.
2. The physiological buffer system.
3. Excretion of volatile and non-volatile acids.

Buffers

A buffer is a substance that can either bind or release hydrogen ions, therefore keeping the pH relatively constant even when considerable quantities of acid or base are added. There are four buffers of the blood:

1. Haemoglobin.
2. Plasma proteins.
3. Phosphate.
4. Bicarbonate.

It is the bicarbonate system that acts as the principal buffer and which is of most interest in respiratory medicine.

We have already seen that CO_2 dissolves in water and reacts to form carbonic acid and that this dissociates to form bicarbonate and protons:

$$CO_2 + H_2O \rightleftharpoons H_2CO_3 \rightleftharpoons H^+ + HCO_3^-$$

This equilibrium tells us that changes in either CO_2 or HCO_3^- will have an effect on pH. For example, increasing CO_2 will drive the reaction to the right, increasing hydrogen ion concentration.

As changes in CO_2 and bicarbonate can alter pH, controlling these elements allows the system to control acid–base equilibrium. This is why the bicarbonate buffer system is so useful; the body has control over both elements:

- Carbon dioxide is regulated through changes in ventilation.
- Bicarbonate concentrations are determined by the kidneys.

Acid–base disturbances

As noted above, blood pH can either be higher than normal (alkalosis) or lower (acidosis). An acidosis can be caused by either:

- A rise in PCO_2.
- A fall in HCO_3^-.

Similarly, alkalosis can occur through:

- A fall in PCO_2.
- A rise in HCO_3^-.

Where the primary change is in CO_2 we term the disturbance 'respiratory', whereas a disturbance in bicarbonate is termed 'metabolic'. This allows us to classify four types of disturbance, outlined in Figure 5.12:

1. Respiratory alkalosis.
2. Respiratory acidosis.
3. Metabolic alkalosis.
4. Metabolic acidosis.

The disturbance was described as *primary* because the kidneys and lungs may try to return the acid–base disturbance towards normal values. This is called compensation and means that even in respiratory disturbances it may not be just CO_2 that is abnormal; bicarbonate may have altered too. Similarly, CO_2 may be abnormal in a metabolic disturbance. The ways in which the two systems compensate are:

- The respiratory system alters ventilation; this happens quickly.
- The kidney alters excretion of bicarbonate; this takes 2–3 days.

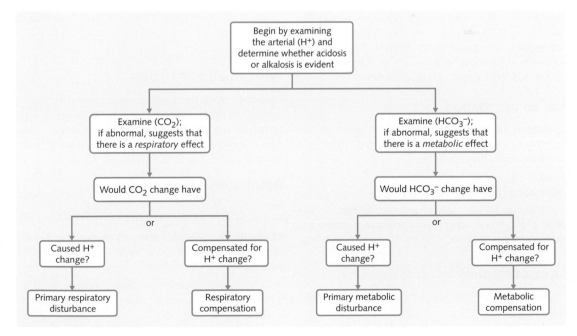

Fig. 5.12 Differentiating between acid–base disorders.

It is now clear that lung disease that affects gas exchange, and therefore PCO_2, will have major effects on the body's acid–base status. It is also clear that, whilst the respiratory system can act quickly to compensate for metabolic disturbances, it will take time for compensation to take place in respiratory disease; the renal system cannot act as quickly. We see this in clinical practice: a change in bicarbonate is characteristic of chronic lung disease, rather than acute lung disease.

Full details of assessment of acid–base status and interpretation of arterial blood gases can be found in Part 2 of this text.

Assessing acid–base disturbances

Assessing acid–base disorders is relatively simple if you approach the problem in stages.

1. Start with the pH: is it outside the normal range?
2. If there is an acidosis or alkalosis, can it be explained by a change in CO_2?
3. If so, then it is a primary disturbance due to a respiratory cause.
4. Now look at bicarbonate – has this changed to return the ratio to normal?
5. If so, it is a respiratory disorder with metabolic compensation.

Respiratory acidosis

Respiratory acidosis results from an increase in PCO_2 caused by:

- Hypoventilation (less CO_2 is blown off).
- Ventilation:perfusion mismatch.

From the Henderson–Hasselbalch equation, we see that an increase in PCO_2 causes an increase in hydrogen ion concentration (i.e. a reduction in pH). Thus, plasma bicarbonate concentration increases to compensate for the increased hydrogen ion concentration.

Renal compensation

The increase in hydrogen ion concentration in the blood results in increased filtration of hydrogen ions at the glomeruli, thus:

- Increasing HCO_3^- reabsorption.
- Increasing HCO_3^- production.

Thus, plasma HCO_3^- rises, compensating for the increased [H$^+$], i.e. renal compensation raises pH towards normal.

Causes of respiratory acidosis

Mechanisms reducing ventilation or causing V/Q mismatch include:

- Chronic obstructive pulmonary disease.
- Asthma.

- Blocked airway (by tumour or foreign body).
- Spontaneous lung collapse, brainstem lesion.
- Injury to the chest wall.

Drugs that reduce respiratory drive (ventilation) include morphine, barbiturates and general anaesthetics.

Respiratory alkalosis

Respiratory alkalosis results from a decrease in PCO_2 generally caused by alveolar hyperventilation (more carbon dioxide is blown off). This causes a decrease in hydrogen ion concentration and thus an increase in pH.

Renal compensation

The reduction in hydrogen ion concentration in the blood results in decreased hydrogen ion filtration at the glomeruli, thus:

- Reducing HCO_3^- reabsorption.
- Reducing HCO_3^- production.

Thus, plasma HCO_3^- falls, compensating for the reduced [H$^+$]; i.e. renal compensation reduces pH towards normal.

Causes of respiratory alkalosis

The causes of respiratory alkalosis include:

- Increased ventilation – caused by hypoxic drive in pneumonia, diffuse interstitial lung diseases, high altitude, mechanical ventilation, etc.
- Hyperventilation – brainstem damage, infection causing fever, drugs (e.g. aspirin), hysterical over-breathing.

Metabolic acidosis

Metabolic acidosis results from an excess of hydrogen ions in the body, which reduces bicarbonate concentration (shifting the equation below to the left). Respiration is unaffected; therefore, PCO_2 is initially normal.

Respiratory compensation

$$CO_2 + H_2O \rightleftharpoons H_2CO_3 \rightleftharpoons H^+ + HCO_3^-$$

The reduction in pH is detected by the peripheral chemoreceptors. This causes an increase in ventilation, which lowers PCO_2. Also:

- The above equation is driven further to the left, reducing hydrogen ion concentration and bicarbonate.
- The decrease in hydrogen ion concentration raises pH towards normal.

Respiratory compensation cannot fully correct the values of PCO_2, $[HCO_3{}^-]$ and $[H^+]$, as there is a limit to how far PCO_2 can fall with hyperventilation. Correction can be carried out only by removing the excess hydrogen ions from the body or restoring the lost bicarbonate (i.e. correcting the metabolic fault).

Causes of metabolic acidosis

Causes of metabolic acidosis are:

- Exogenous acid loading (e.g. aspirin overdose).
- Endogenous acid production (e.g. ketogenesis in diabetes).
- Loss of $HCO_3{}^-$ from the kidneys or gut (e.g. diarrhoea).
- Metabolic production of hydrogen ions. The kidneys may not be able to excrete the excess hydrogen ions immediately, or at all (as in renal failure).

Metabolic alkalosis

Metabolic alkalosis results from an increase in bicarbonate concentration or a fall in hydrogen ion concentration. Removing hydrogen ions from the right of the equation below drives the reaction to the right, increasing bicarbonate concentration. Decrease in hydrogen ion concentration raises pH; initially, PCO_2 is normal.

Respiratory compensation

$$CO_2 + H_2O \rightleftharpoons H_2CO_3 \rightleftharpoons H^+ + HCO_3{}^-$$

The increase in pH is detected by the peripheral chemoreceptors. This causes a decrease in ventilation which raises PCO_2. Also:

- The above equation is driven further to the right, increasing hydrogen ion and bicarbonate concentrations.
- The decrease in hydrogen ion concentration raises pH towards normal.

Respiratory compensation is through alveolar hypoventilation but ventilation cannot reduce enough to correct the disturbance. This can only be carried out by removing the problem either of reduced hydrogen ion concentration or increased bicarbonate concentration. This is done by reducing renal hydrogen ion secretion.

More bicarbonate is excreted because more is filtered at the glomerulus and less is reabsorbed in combination with hydrogen ions.

Causes of metabolic alkalosis

The causes of metabolic alkalosis include:

- Vomiting (hydrochloric acid loss from the stomach).
- Ingestion of alkaline substances.
- Potassium depletion (e.g. diuretic, excess aldosterone).

Control of respiratory function

Objectives

By the end of this chapter you should be able to:
- Understand the central control of breathing by the medulla.
- Describe the factors that stimulate central and peripheral chemoreceptors.
- Outline the responses of the respiratory system to changes in carbon dioxide concentration, oxygen concentration and pH.
- Discuss the mechanisms thought to influence the control of ventilation in exercise.

CONTROL OF VENTILATION

Control within the respiratory system

When considering control of breathing, the main control variable is P_aCO_2 (we try to control this value near to 40 mmHg or approximately 5.3 kPa). This can be carried out by adjusting the respiratory rate, the tidal volume, or both.

By controlling P_aCO_2 we are effectively controlling alveolar ventilation and thus P_ACO_2.

Although P_aCO_2 is the main control variable, P_aO_2 is also controlled, but normally to a much lesser extent than P_aCO_2. However, the P_aO_2 control system can take over and become the main controlling system when the P_aO_2 drops below 50 mmHg (~ 6.7 kPa).

Control can seem to be brought about by:

- Metabolic demands of the body (metabolic control)–tissue oxygen demand and acid–base balance. This acts in a feedback system whereby the brainstem looks at the measured level of P_aCO_2 and relates this to the desired level, adjusting it as necessary through methods such as increasing respiratory rate.
- Behavioural demands of the body (behavioural control) – singing, coughing, laughing (i.e. control is voluntary). This system will not be dealt with in this book.

Metabolic control of breathing

Metabolic control of breathing is a function of the brainstem (pons and medulla). The controller can be considered as specific groups of neurons (previously called respiratory centres).

Pontine neurons

The pontine respiratory group consist of expiratory and inspiratory neurons. Their role is to regulate (i.e. affect the activity of) the dorsal respiratory group and possibly the ventral respiratory group (neuron groups in the medulla).

Medullary neurons

It is believed that the medulla is responsible for respiratory rhythm.

Three groups of neurons associated with respiratory control have been identified in the medulla:

1. The dorsal respiratory group, situated in the nucleus tractus solitarius.
2. The ventral respiratory group, situated in the nucleus ambiguus and the nucleus retroambigualis.
3. The Bötzinger complex, situated rostral to the nucleus ambiguus.

These groups receive sensory information, which is compared with the desired value of control; adjustments are made to respiratory muscles to rectify any deviation from ideal.

- The dorsal respiratory group contains neuron bodies of inspiratory upper motor neurons. These inhibit the activity of expiratory neurons in the ventral respiratory group and have an excitatory effect on lower motor neurons to the respiratory muscles, increasing ventilation.
- Ventral respiratory group neurons contain inspiratory upper motor neurons which go on to supply through their lower motor neurons external intercostal muscles and accessory muscles.
- The Bötzinger complex contains only expiratory neurons. It works by inhibiting inspiratory neurons of the

dorsal and ventral respiratory groups and through excitation of expiratory neurons in the ventral respiratory group.

Effectors (muscles of respiration)

The major muscle groups involved are the diaphragm, internal and external intercostals and abdominal muscles.

The strength of contraction and coordination of these muscles is set by the central controller. If the muscles are not coordinated, this will result in abnormal breathing patterns.

Sensors (receptors)

Sensors report current values or discrepancies from ideal values for the various variables being controlled (e.g. P_aCO_2, P_aO_2 and pH) to the central controller. There are many types of sensors and receptors involved with respiratory control:

- Chemoreceptors – central and peripheral.
- Lung receptors – slowly adapting stretch receptors, rapidly adapting stretch receptors and C-fibres.
- Receptors in the chest wall – muscle spindles and Golgi tendon organs.
- Other receptors – nasal, tracheal and laryngeal receptors, arterial baroreceptors, pain receptors.

Chemoreceptors

Chemoreceptors monitor blood gas tensions, P_aCO_2, P_aO_2 and pH, and help keep minute volume appropriate to metabolic demands of the body. Therefore, chemoreceptors respond to:

- Hypercapnia.
- Hypoxia.
- Acidosis.

There are both central and peripheral chemoreceptors.

Central chemoreceptors

Central chemoreceptors are tonically active and vital for maintenance of respiration; 80% of the drive for ventilation is a result of stimulation of the central chemoreceptors. When they are inactivated, respiration ceases. These receptors are readily depressed by drugs (e.g. opiates and barbiturates).

The receptors are located in the brainstem on the ventrolateral surface of the medulla, close to the exit of cranial nerves IX and X. They are anatomically separate from the medullary respiratory control centre.

Central chemoreceptors respond to hydrogen ion concentration within the surrounding brain tissue and cerebrospinal fluid (CSF).

- Raised hydrogen ion concentration increases ventilation.
- Lowered hydrogen ion concentration decreases ventilation.

Diffusion of ions across the blood–brain barrier is poor. Blood levels of hydrogen ions and bicarbonate have little effect in the short term on the concentrations of hydrogen ions and bicarbonate in the CSF and thus have little effect on the central chemoreceptors.

Carbon dioxide, however, can pass freely by diffusion across the blood–brain barrier. On entering the CSF, the increase in carbon dioxide increases the free hydrogen ion concentration. This increase in hydrogen ion concentration stimulates the central chemoreceptors. Thus:

- Central chemoreceptors are sensitive to P_aCO_2, not arterial hydrogen ion concentration.
- Central chemoreceptors are not sensitive to P_aO_2.
- Because there is less protein in the CSF (<0.4 g/L) than in the plasma (60–80 g/L), a rise in P_aCO_2 has a larger effect on pH in the CSF than in the blood (CSF has lower buffering capacity).

Long-standing raised P_aCO_2 causes the pH of the CSF to return towards normal. This is because prolonged hypercapnia alters production of bicarbonate by the glial cells and allows bicarbonate to cross the blood–brain barrier. It can therefore diffuse freely into the CSF and alter the CSF pH. This is seen in patients with chronic respiratory failure, e.g. those with severe chronic obstructive pulmonary disease.

Peripheral chemoreceptors

Chemoreceptors are located around the carotid sinus and aortic arch. These are the carotid bodies and aortic bodies, respectively. Stimulation of peripheral chemoreceptors has both cardiovascular and respiratory effects. Of the two receptor groups, the carotid bodies have the greatest effect on respiration.

Carotid bodies

The carotid bodies contain two different types of cells. Type I cells are stimulated by hypoxia; they connect with afferent nerves to the brainstem. Type II cells are supportive (structural and metabolic), similar to glial cells of the central nervous system.

There is a rich blood supply to the carotid bodies (blood flow per mass of tissue far exceeds that to the brain); venous blood flow, therefore, remains saturated with oxygen.

The exact mechanism of action of the carotid bodies is not known. It is believed that type I (glomus) cells are activated by hypoxia and release transmitter substances that stimulate afferents to the brainstem.

Peripheral chemoreceptors are sensitive to:

- P_aO_2.
- P_aCO_2.
- pH.
- Blood flow.
- Temperature.

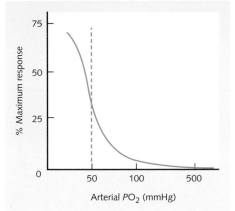

Fig. 6.1 Response of ventilation to P_aO_2. The response to a lowered P_aO_2 is small until the P_aO_2 falls below a value of 50 mmHg, after which point the response increases dramatically.

The carotid bodies are supplied by the autonomic nervous system, which appears to alter their sensitivity to hypoxia by regulating blood flow to the chemoreceptor:

- Sympathetic action vasoconstricts, increasing sensitivity to hypoxia.
- Parasympathetic action vasodilates, reducing sensitivity to hypoxia.

The relationship between P_aO_2 and the response from the carotid bodies is not a linear one. At a low P_aO_2 (<50 mmHg or 6.7 kPa), a further decrease in arterial oxygen tension significantly increases ventilation (Fig. 6.1). However, at levels of oxygen tension close to 100 mmHg, changes have little effect on ventilation. If P_aO_2 increases above 100 mmHg/13.3 kPa (achieved when breathing high-concentration oxygen), ventilation is only slightly reduced.

Unlike central chemoreceptors, peripheral chemoreceptors are directly stimulated by blood pH. Although peripheral chemoreceptors are stimulated by P_aCO_2, their response is much less than that of central chemoreceptors (less than 10% of the effect).

Receptors in the lung

Afferent impulses arising from receptors in the lung travel via the vagal nerve to the respiratory centres of the brain where they influence the control of breathing. There are three main types of afferent receptor:

1. Rapidly adapting receptors.
2. Slowly adapting receptors.
3. C-fibre receptors – formerly juxtapulmonary or J receptors.

Their characteristics are described in Figure 6.2 and their function discussed below.

Rapidly adapting receptors

Rapidly adapting receptors are involved in lung defence and form part of the cough reflex. This is reflected in their location in the upper airways. They produce only transitory responses and may be sensitized by inflammatory mediators, making them more sensitive to stimulation.

Slowly adapting receptors

Slowly adapting receptors are important in the control of breathing, not the cough reflex, and produce sustained responses. They are stimulated by inflation (which stretches the lungs):

- Inflation leads to decreased respiration (inflation reflex or Hering–Breuer reflex).
- Deflation leads to increased respiration (deflation reflex).

These reflexes are active in the first year of life, but are weak in adults. Therefore, they are not thought to determine the rate and depth of breathing in adults. However, these reflexes are seen to be more active if the tidal volume increases above 1.0 L and therefore might have a role in exercise.

Afferent fibres travel to the respiratory centres through the vagus nerve. The functions of these receptors are:

- The termination of inspiration.
- Regulation of the work of breathing.
- Reinforcement of respiratory rhythm in the first year of life.

However, if the nerve is blocked by anaesthesia there is no change seen in the rate and depth of breathing.

C-fibres

Stimulation of C-fibres results in:

- Closure of the larynx.
- Rapid, shallow breathing.
- Bradycardia.
- Hypotension.

C-fibres also contribute to the breathlessness of heart failure, and although they are afferent nerve endings, C-fibres are able to release inflammatory mediators (neurokinins and substance P).

Fig. 6.2 Characteristics of the three principal types of afferent receptors in the lung

Receptor type	Stretch receptors		C-fibre receptors
	Rapidly adapting stretch receptor (RAR)	**Slowly adapting stretch receptor (SAR)**	
Location in airway	Primarily upper airways – nasopharynx, larynx, trachea, carina	Trachea and main bronchus	Throughout airways
Location in airway wall	Just below epithelium	Airway smooth muscle	Alveolar wall and bronchial mucosa
Structure	Small myelinated fibres	Small myelinated fibres	Free nerve endings
Conduction speed	Fast	Fast	Slower
Stimuli	Mechanical deformation Chemical irritants and noxious gases Inflammatory stimuli	Inflation	Chemical mediators – histamine and capsaicin (an extract of chilli peppers and the 'C' that gives 'C-fibres' their name) Inflation and forced deflation Pulmonary vascular congestion Oedema – interstitial fluid in the alveolar wall

Receptors in the chest wall

Receptors in the chest wall consist of:

- Joint receptors – measure the velocity of rib movement.
- Golgi tendon organs – found within the muscles of respiration (e.g. diaphragm and intercostals) and detect the strength of muscle contraction.
- Muscle spindles – monitor the length of muscle fibres both statically and dynamically (i.e. detect muscle length and velocity).

These receptors help to minimize changes to ventilation imposed by an external load (e.g. lateral flexion of the trunk). They achieve this by modifying motor neuron output to the respiratory muscles. The aim is to achieve the most efficient respiration in terms of tidal volume and frequency. It is thought that stimulation of mechanoreceptors in the chest wall, along with hypercapnia and hypoxaemia, leads to increased respiratory effort in a patient with sleep apnoea. It is this sudden respiratory effort that then wakes the patient up.

Thus, reflexes from muscles and joints stabilize ventilation in the face of changing mechanical conditions.

Arterial baroreceptors

Hypertension stimulates arterial baroreceptors, which inhibit ventilation. Hypotension has the opposite effect.

Pain receptors

Stimulation of pain receptors causes a brief apnoea, followed by a period of hyperventilation.

COORDINATED RESPONSES OF THE RESPIRATORY SYSTEM

Response to carbon dioxide

Carbon dioxide is the most important factor in the control of ventilation. Under normal conditions P_aCO_2 is held within very tight limits and ventilatory response is very sensitive to small changes in P_aCO_2.

The response of ventilation to carbon dioxide has been measured by inhalation of mixtures of carbon dioxide, raising the P_aCO_2 and observing the increase in ventilation (Fig. 6.3).

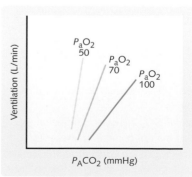

Fig. 6.3 The response of ventilation to CO_2. Note that at higher levels of P_aO_2 an increase in P_ACO_2 has less effect on ventilation (the curve is less steep).

Note that a small increase in P_aCO_2 causes a significant increase in ventilation. The response to P_aCO_2 is also dependent upon the arterial oxygen tension. At lower values of P_aO_2 the ventilatory response is more sensitive to changes in P_aCO_2 (steeper slope) and ventilation is greater for a given P_aCO_2. If the P_aCO_2 is reduced, this causes a significant reduction in ventilation.

Factors that affect ventilatory response to P_aCO_2 are:

- P_aO_2.
- Blood pH.
- Genetics.
- Age.
- Psychiatric state.
- Fitness.
- Drugs (e.g. opiates, such as morphine and diamorphine, reduce respiratory and cardiovascular drive).

Response to oxygen

As mentioned above, the response to reduced P_aO_2 is by stimulation of the peripheral chemoreceptors. This response, however, is not significant until the P_aO_2 drops to around 50 mmHg (6.7 kPa). The relationship between P_aO_2 and ventilation has been studied by measuring changes in ventilation while a subject breathes hypoxic mixtures (Fig. 6.4). It is assumed that end-expiratory P_AO_2 and P_ACO_2 are equivalent to arterial gas tensions.

The response to P_AO_2 is also seen to change with different levels of P_ACO_2.

- The greater the carbon dioxide tension, the earlier the response to low oxygen tension.
- Therefore, at high P_ACO_2, a decrease in oxygen tension below 100 mmHg (13.3 kPa) causes an increase in ventilation.

Under normal conditions, P_aO_2 does not fall to values of around 50 mmHg (6.7 kPa) and, therefore, daily control of ventilation does not rely on hypoxic drive. However, under conditions of severe lung disease, or at high altitude, hypoxic drive becomes increasingly important. A patient with COPD may rely almost entirely on hypoxic drive alone, having lost ventilatory response to carbon dioxide (described above). Central chemoreceptors have become unresponsive to carbon dioxide; in addition, ventilatory drive from the effects of reduced pH on peripheral chemoreceptors is lessened by renal compensation for the acid–base abnormality. Administration of high-concentration oxygen therapy (e.g. 100% O_2) may abolish any hypoxic drive that the patient was previously relying upon, depressing ventilation and worsening the patient's condition.

Response to pH

Remember that hydrogen ions do not cross the blood–brain barrier and therefore affect only peripheral chemoreceptors. It is difficult to separate the response from increased P_aCO_2 and decreased pH. Any change in pH may be compensated in the long term by the kidneys and therefore has less effect on ventilation than might be expected.

An example of how pH may drive ventilation is seen in the case of metabolic acidosis. The patient will try to achieve a reduction in hydrogen ion concentration by blowing off more carbon dioxide from the lungs. This is achieved by increasing ventilation.

Response to exercise

As human beings, we are capable of a huge increase in ventilation in response to exercise: approximately 15 times the resting level. In moderate exercise, the carbon dioxide output and oxygen uptake are well matched. Increases in respiratory rate and tidal volume do not cause hyperventilation, and the subject is said to be hyperpnoeic (i.e. have increased depth of breathing):

- P_aCO_2 does not increase, but may fall slightly.
- P_aO_2 does not decrease.
- In moderate exercise, arterial pH varies very little.

So where does the drive for ventilation come from? Many causes have been suggested for the increase in ventilation seen during exercise, but none is completely satisfactory:

- Carbon dioxide load within venous blood returning to the lungs affects ventilation.

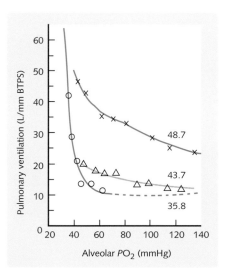

Fig. 6.4 The response of ventilation to P_AO_2 at three values of P_ACO_2. Lowered P_AO_2 has a much greater effect on ventilation when increased values of P_ACO_2 are present.

Fig. 6.5 Cyclical changes of P_aCO_2 with inspiration and expiration: (A) at rest; (B) during exercise. Larger oscillations are thought to alter ventilation.

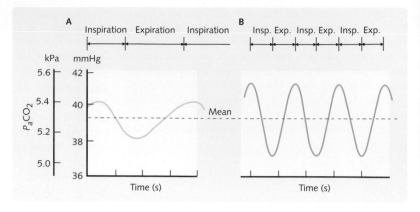

- There is a change in the pattern of oscillations of P_aCO_2 (Fig. 6.5).
- Central control of P_aCO_2 is reset to a lower value and held constant during exercise.
- Movement of limbs activates joint receptors, which contribute to increased ventilation.
- Increase in body temperature during exercise may also stimulate ventilation.
- The motor cortex stimulates respiratory centres.
- Adrenaline released in exercise also stimulates respiration.

The possible role of oscillations of P_aCO_2

It is suggested that there are cyclical changes of P_aCO_2, with inspiration and expiration. Although mean P_aCO_2 does not change during moderate exercise, the amplitude of these oscillations may increase, providing the stimulus for ventilation.

In heavy exercise, there can be measurable changes in P_aO_2 and P_aCO_2, which stimulate respiration. In addition, the pH falls because anaerobic metabolism leads to production of lactic acid (blood lactate levels increase 10-fold). This lactic acid is not oxidized because the oxygen supply cannot keep up with the demands of the exercising muscles (i.e. an 'oxygen debt' is incurred). Rises in potassium ion concentration and temperature may also contribute to the increase in ventilation.

When exercise stops, respiration does not immediately return to basal levels. It remains elevated to provide an increased supply of oxygen to the tissues to oxidize the products of anaerobic metabolism ('repaying the oxygen debt').

Abnormalities of ventilatory control

Cheyne–Stokes respiration

In Cheyne–Stokes respiration, ventilation alternates between progressively deeper breaths and then progressively shallower breaths, in a cyclical manner. Ventilatory control is not achieved and the respiratory system appears to become unstable:

- Arterial carbon dioxide and oxygen tensions vary significantly.
- Tidal volumes wax and wane (Fig. 6.6).
- There are short periods of apnoea separated by periods of hyperventilation.
- Cheyne–Stokes breathing is observed at various times:

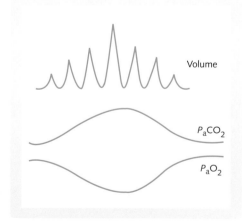

Fig. 6.6 Cheyne–Stokes respiration.

- At altitude – often when asleep.
- During sleep.
- During periods of hypoxia.
- After voluntary hyperventilation.
- During disease, particularly with combined right and left heart failure and uraemia.
- Secondary to brainstem lesions or compression.

RESPIRATORY RESPONSE TO EXTREME ENVIRONMENTS

Response to high altitude

At high altitude, the barometric pressure is much lower than at sea level. Hence, the partial pressure of oxygen is lower.

In addition, the partial pressure of water vapour is constant, because inspired air is saturated at body temperature. Therefore, the partial pressure of oxygen in the alveoli (and in the blood) is significantly lower than at sea level.

The carriage of oxygen in the blood is dependent on:

- Partial pressure of oxygen in the blood.
- Haemoglobin concentration.
- The oxyhaemoglobin dissociation curve.

At altitude the partial pressure of oxygen in the blood is lowered. This would tend to limit the amount of oxygen carriage. To combat this problem the body can:

- Hyperventilate in an attempt to decrease the partial pressure of carbon dioxide in the alveoli and therefore increase the partial pressure of oxygen.
- Increase the amount of haemoglobin in the blood, thereby increasing oxygen carriage (oxygen capacity).
- Shift the oxygen dissociation curve.
- Alter the circulation.
- Increase anaerobic metabolism in tissues, increase cytochrome oxidase activity and increase myoglobin in muscle tissue.

Basic pharmacology 7

By the end of this chapter you should be able to:
* Detail the mechanism of action of β-receptor agonists, anticholinergic drugs and glucocorticosteroids.
* Give examples of the indications and side-effects of the above drugs.
* Be aware of more specialist drugs such as theophyllines and sodium cromoglicate.
* Be familiar with delivery devices for respiratory drugs.

OVERVIEW

Many drugs are used to treat diseases of the respiratory system. Some are considered under the relevant diseases in Part 3; however, some important categories of drugs are introduced here. These categories are:

* Bronchodilators.
* Glucocorticosteroids.
* Mucolytics.
* Drugs used in smoking cessation.

BRONCHODILATORS

Bronchodilators are medications that reduce the resistance to air flow in the respiratory tract, thus increasing air flow to the lungs. They are most commonly used in asthma and chronic obstructive pulmonary disease (COPD) and can be grouped as follows:

* Short-acting β_2 agonists.
* Long-acting β_2 agonists.
* Short-acting anticholinergics.
* Long-acting anticholinergics.
* Theophyllines.

Short-acting β_2 agonists

Bronchial smooth muscle contains numerous β_2 receptors, which act through an adenylate cyclase/cAMP second-messenger system to cause smooth-muscle relaxation and hence bronchodilatation (Fig. 7.1). Examples of short-acting β_2 agonists are:

* Salbutamol.
* Terbutaline.

These drugs are usually inhaled as an aerosol, a powder or a nebulized solution but can also be given intravenously, intramuscularly and subcutaneously. They are used for acute symptoms and act within minutes, producing effects lasting 4–5 hours. When used in asthma they are commonly referred to as a 'reliever inhaler'.

The β_2 agonists are not completely specific and have some β_1 agonistic effects, especially in high doses:

* Tachycardia.
* Fine tremor.
* Nervous tension.
* Headache.

At the doses given by aerosol, these side-effects seldom occur. Tolerance may occur with high repeated doses.

Long-acting β_2 agonists

Like the short-acting β_2 agonists, these drugs also relax bronchial smooth muscle. They differ from the short-acting drugs in that:

* Their effects last for much longer (up to 12 hours).
* The full effect is only achieved after regular administration of several doses and, generally, less desensitization occurs.

For these reasons long-acting β_2 agonists should be used on a regular basis rather than to treat acute attacks. The main long-acting β_2 agonists are:

* Salmeterol (partial agonist).
* Formoterol (full agonist).
* Indacaterol.

Long-acting β_2 agonists are also available in a combined preparation with a corticosteroid. Combination inhalers are more convenient and there may also be pharmacological advantages when administered together. They are used in asthma and COPD. The main combination inhalers are:

* Salmeterol and fluticasone (Seretide).
* Formoterol and budesonide (Symbicort).
* Formoterol and beclometasone (Fostair).

Fig. 7.1 Mechanisms of action of β_2 agonists – relaxation of bronchial muscle (which leads to bronchodilatation) and inhibition of mast cell degranulation (β receptors on mast cell).

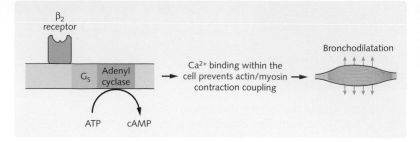

Due to the differing β agonist drug profiles, only combination inhalers containing a full, rather than a partial β agonist can be used as single maintenance and reliever therapy (SMART) for asthma. More details can be found in Part 3.

Anticholinergics

Anticholinergics are competitive antagonists of muscarinic acetylcholine receptors. They therefore block the vagal control of bronchial smooth-muscle tone in response to irritants and reduce reflex bronchoconstriction. Ipratropium bromide and oxitropium bromide are both anticholinergics; they have two mechanisms of action:

- Reduction of reflex bronchoconstriction (e.g. from dust or pollen) by antagonizing muscarinic receptors on bronchial smooth muscle.
- Reduction of mucous secretions by antagonizing muscarinic receptors on goblet cells.

Anticholinergics are available in short-acting forms, e.g. ipratropium, which reach their maximum effect within 60–90 minutes and act for 4–6 hours, and long-acting forms, e.g. tiotropium, which exert effects for around 18 hours. They are poorly absorbed orally and are therefore given by aerosol.

Anticholinergics are not the first-choice bronchodilator in asthma treatment because they only reduce the vagally mediated element of bronchoconstriction, having no effect on other important causes of bronchoconstriction such as inflammatory mediators. There is some evidence that anticholinergics are effective when given together with a β_2 agonist in severe asthma. Contrastingly, in COPD, cholinergic hyperactivity significantly contributes to bronchoconstriction and therefore anticholinergics are more effective bronchodilators. The main use of anticholinergics is in COPD, which does not respond as well to β_2 agonists.

Side-effects are rare, but include:

- Dry mouth.
- Urinary retention.
- Constipation.

Theophyllines

Theophyllines appear to work by inhibiting phosphodiesterase, thereby preventing the breakdown of cAMP (Fig. 7.2). The amount of cAMP within the bronchial smooth-muscle cells is therefore increased, which causes bronchodilatation in a similar way to β_2 agonists.

These drugs are metabolized in the liver and there is a considerable variation in half-life between individuals. This has important implications because there is a small therapeutic window, and blood levels must therefore be checked. Factors altering theophylline clearance are shown in Figure 7.3.

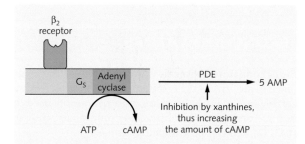

Fig. 7.2 Xanthines. The inhibition of phosphodiesterase (PDE) leads to an increase in cellular cyclic AMP (cAMP), which is believed to lead to bronchodilatation, as shown in Figure 7.1.

Fig. 7.3 Factors altering theophylline clearance	
Increased clearance	**Decreased clearance**
Smoking	Liver disease
Alcohol	Pneumonia
Rifampicin	Cimetidine
Childhood	Clarithromycin (erthromycin, etc.)
	Old age
i.e. P450 enzyme induction	i.e. P450 enzyme inhibition

Theophylline can be given intravenously in the form of aminophylline (theophylline with ethylenediamine), but must be administered very slowly (taking over 20 minutes to administer dose). Aminophylline is given in cases of severe asthma that do not respond to β_2 agonists.

GLUCOCORTICOSTEROIDS

Steroids reduce the formation, release and action of many different mediators involved in inflammation. Their mode of action is complex and involves gene modulation (Fig. 7.4) after binding to steroid receptors in the cytoplasm of cells and translocation of the active receptor into the nucleus. This has a number of effects, including:

- Downregulation of proinflammatory cytokines and mediators, e.g. phospholipase A_2.
- Production of anti-inflammatory proteins.

Steroids in respiratory treatment may be topical (inhaled) or systemic (oral or parenteral).

Inhaled steroids

These include:

- Beclometasone.
- Budesonide.
- Fluticasone.
- Ciclesonide.

Side-effects of inhaled steroids in adults are relatively minor (primarily, hoarseness and oral candidiasis). They may have a short-term effect on growth in children. Corticosteroid inhalers in asthma are commonly known as 'preventer inhalers'.

Oral steroids

The primary oral steroid is prednisolone. Side-effects of systemic steroids include:

- Adrenal suppression.
- Effects on bones (including growth retardation in children and osteoporosis in adults).
- Diabetes mellitus.
- Increased susceptibility to infection.
- Weight gain.
- Effects on skin (e.g. bruising and atrophy).
- Mood changes.

Because of these side-effects, regular oral steroids are avoided wherever possible.

Leukotriene receptor antagonists

Cysteinyl leukotrienes are eicosanoids that cause bronchoconstriction. Their proinflammatory actions centre on their ability to:

- Increase vascular permeability.
- Cause influx of eosinophils.

Leukotriene receptor antagonists (or 'leukotriene modifiers') therefore have anti-inflammatory and bronchodilatory effects.

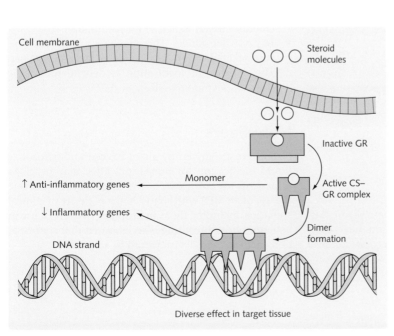

Fig. 7.4 Mechanism of action of steroids. Steroid molecules diffuse across cell membranes and bind to steroid receptors, forming CS–GR complexes. These complexes may bind to DNA as dimers and increase the expression of many different anti-inflammatory gene products. Alternatively, CS–GR monomers may block induction of inflammatory genes by exogenous stimuli.

The two key leukotriene receptor antagonists are montelukast and zafirlukast. Montelukast is used in prophylaxis of exercise-induced asthma and in patients with mild-to-moderate asthma whose symptoms are not well controlled by other asthma drugs.

Sodium cromoglicate

The mode of action of sodium cromoglicate is not completely understood. It is known to stabilize mast cells, possibly by blocking transport of calcium ions, and has no bronchodilator effect. It cannot be used to treat an acute attack, but is given for prophylaxis, especially in patients with atopy. The route of administration is by inhalation. Its mechanism of action is to:

- Prevent mast cell degranulation and hence mediator release.
- Reduce C-fibre response to irritants, therefore reducing bronchoconstriction.
- Inhibit platelet-activating factor-induced broncho-constriction.

In addition to its use in allergen-mediated asthma, sodium cromoglicate is effective in non-allergen-mediated bronchoconstriction (e.g. in exercise-induced asthma) and continued use results in reduced bronchial hyperactivity. It is often used in paediatrics. Nedocromil sodium is a drug with similar actions.

MUCOLYTICS

Mucolytics (e.g. carbocisteine and mecysteine hydrochloride) are designed to reduce the viscosity of sputum, thereby aiding expectoration. These drugs may be of benefit in treating acute exacerbations in COPD.

DRUGS USED IN SMOKING CESSATION

There are two main classes of drugs used in smoking cessation:

1. Nicotine replacement therapy (NRT).
2. Bupropion (amfebutamone).

NRT products (gums, patches and nasal sprays) are classified as over-the-counter medicines and have been shown to be effective in treating tobacco withdrawal and dependence. They should not be used in patients with severe cardiovascular disease (including immediately after myocardial infarction).

Bupropion is an antidepressant also licensed for use as an adjunct to smoking cessation. The main side-effects are a dry mouth and difficulty sleeping. The drug should not be used if there is a history of epilepsy or eating disorders.

In addition to pharmacological methods, a number of other interventions have been shown to be effective in helping smokers quit:

- Simple advice and/or brief counselling from GPs.
- Group counselling at smoking cessation clinics.
- Mass media campaigns (e.g. No Smoking Day).
- Helplines providing one-to-one telephone support.

DRUG DELIVERY DEVICES

Inhalers

These are devices used to deliver drugs to the lungs. There are several types and an appropriate choice should be made following consideration of the patient; for example, an elderly patient with arthritis will have difficulty using a non-breath-activated device.

- Metered dose inhaler (MDI). Medication is stored in a pressurized cannister with propellant. Classic MDIs require coordinated inspiration with depression of the medicated cannister. Newer devices can be primed and breath-activated, removing the need for complex coordination, e.g. Turbohaler and Twisthaler. Classic MDIs can be attached to an aerochamber to aid issues with coordination.
- Dry powder inhaler. These involve a powdered capsule of medication being loaded into the inhaler. The delivery of medication is dependent on the patient's inspiratory effort.

Nebulizers

Nebulizers are driven by air or oxygen and aerosolize liquid medication for inhalation. They may be given to patients for home use; however, guidelines advocate the use of an MDI with spacer in the majority of clinical scenarios, including those in hospital. They are of use in patients whose breathing is so laboured that coordination of an inhaler device would be impossible.

PART 2
CLINICAL ASSESSMENT

The respiratory patient – taking a history and exploring symptoms

8

● **Objectives**

By the end of this chapter you should be able to:
- Describe the most common presentations of respiratory disease.
- Give non-respiratory differential diagnoses for symptoms such as cough, chest pain and breathlessness.
- Identify the symptoms and signs which indicate serious pathology.
- Be comfortable with the structure and content of a respiratory history.

INTRODUCTION

The key to identifying and successfully treating the respiratory patient is to understand the pathophysiology and complex interplay between the principal symptoms of respiratory disease. These symptoms (breathlessness, sputum production, haemoptysis, wheeze and chest pain) are common to many different conditions. Clinical findings often overlap considerably and this can make diagnosis seem difficult. However, a good history focusing on the time course and progression of the illness will often reveal recognizable patterns of symptoms and enable you to narrow down the differential diagnoses. Indeed, the history should give you the diagnosis in between 50 and 80% of cases, and if not, at least a very short list of differential diagnoses.

The respiratory history follows the same format as the other systems, and this should be familiar to you. At every stage the goal is to be asking questions to either rule in or rule out diagnoses. Remember that common things are common and serious things are serious.

GENERAL STEPS

Ensure you are as prepared as possible for the patient encounter and have set distractions aside. Preferably find a quiet venue for the history; if things are busy on the ward consider taking the patient to the day room.

Select an appropriate time if possible – avoid drug rounds and meal times. A good history can take considerable time, especially when starting out or with complicated patients.

Introduce yourself to the patient and confirm the patient's name and date of birth. Explain what you wish to do and gain consent.

BREATHLESSNESS

Breathlessness or dyspnoea is a difficulty or distress in breathing and is a symptom of many different diseases. Breathlessness is a very common reason for referral to a respiratory clinic.

The patient may describe the symptom in a variety of ways. Common terms used are 'puffed', 'can't get enough air' and 'feeling suffocated'. A number of physiological factors (see end of this chapter) underlie this sensation and sometimes several mechanisms coexist to cause breathlessness. However, understanding the physiological basis of dyspnoea is of limited help clinically; it is a good history that is vital in diagnosing the underlying disease.

Key points to establish include the speed of onset of breathlessness, its progression and variability, exacerbating and relieving factors and response to any treatment. This can help to establish the severity of the underlying disease process: e.g. shortness of breath even at rest suggests much worse disease than that which only causes breathlessness on exercise. It is vital to question patients about the impact the breathlessness has on their quality of life, as severe lung disease can be debilitating, leading to depression and poorer outcomes. It is also important to ask specifically about breathlessness on lying flat (orthopnoea), which can occur in severe air flow obstruction or cardiac failure.

SPUTUM

Everybody produces airway secretions. In a healthy non-smoker, approximately 100–150 mL of mucus is produced every day. Normally, this mucus is transported up the airway's ciliary mucus escalator and swallowed. This process is not normally perceived. However, expectorating sputum is always abnormal, and is a sign that excess mucus has been generated. This can result from irritation of the respiratory tract (commonly caused by cigarette smoking or the common cold) or from infection. Sputum may be classified as:

- Mucoid: clear, grey or white.
- Serous: watery or frothy.
- Mucopurulent: a yellowish tinge.
- Purulent: dark green/yellow.

Always try to inspect the sputum and note its volume, colour, consistency and odour. These details can provide clues as to the underlying pathology. A yellow/green colour usually means infection and is due to myeloperoxidase produced by eosinophils or neutrophils. However, note that sputum in asthma contains high numbers of eosinophils and is often yellow or green without underlying infection.

Most bronchogenic carcinomas do not produce sputum. The exception is alveolar cell carcinoma, which produces copious amounts of mucoid sputum.

You may have to prompt the patient when investigating the volume of sputum. Is enough coughed up to fill a teaspoon/tablespoon/eggcup/sputum pot?

Chronic bronchitis is a particularly important cause of sputum production. This is defined as a cough productive of sputum for most days during at least 3 consecutive months, for more than 2 successive years. Detailed questioning about cough is needed in patients with chronic bronchitis. Useful questions include:

- Do you cough up sputum/spit/phlegm from your chest on most mornings?
- Would you say you cough up sputum on most days for as much as 3 months a year?
- Do you often need antibiotics from your GP in winter?
- Do you currently smoke or have you ever smoked? (chronic bronchitis is significantly more common in smokers)

Chronic bronchitis is a component of chronic obstructive pulmonary disease (COPD), which is a very common respiratory disease. It can be controlled well with smoking cessation and inhaled therapies; therefore it is important that the symptoms are detected early to give the patient the best possible outcome. A summary of the differences between cough in asthma and that in chronic bronchitis is shown in Figure 8.1.

HAEMOPTYSIS

Haemoptysis is coughing up blood; this needs to be differentiated from other sources of bleeding within the oral cavity and haematemesis (vomiting blood). This distinction is usually obvious from the history. Haemoptysis is not usually a solitary event and, so, if possible, the sputum sample should be inspected.

Fig. 8.1 Patterns of cough in asthma and chronic bronchitis

	Asthma	Chronic bronchitis
Timing	Worse at night	Worse in the morning
Nature	Dry (may be green sputum)	Productive
Chronicity	Intermittent	Persistent
Response to treatment	Associated wheeze is reversible	Associated wheeze is irreversible

Haemoptysis is a serious and often alarming symptom that requires immediate investigation. A chest radiograph is mandatory in a patient with haemoptysis, and the symptom should be treated as bronchogenic carcinoma until proved otherwise. Despite appropriate investigations, often no obvious cause can be found and the episode is attributed to a simple bronchial infection. Important respiratory causes of haemoptysis are:

- Bronchial carcinoma.
- Pulmonary embolism.
- Tuberculosis (TB).
- Pneumonia (particularly pneumococcal).
- Bronchiectasis.
- Acute/chronic bronchitis.

In investigating the cause of haemoptysis, ask about any preceding events, such as respiratory infection or a history of deep vein thrombosis, and establish the frequency and volume and whether it is fresh or altered blood.

You must also establish what, if any, risk factors the patient has for a particular differential diagnosis. Therefore it is important to ask about things such as smoking history (bronchial carcinoma), foreign travel (TB), recent immobilization due to a long-haul flight or surgery (pulmonary embolism) and a history of recurrent chest infections requiring treatment (bronchiectasis).

WHEEZE

Wheezing is a common complaint, complicating many different disease processes. Establish exactly what a patient means by 'wheeze'; used correctly, the term describes musical notes heard mainly on expiration caused by narrowed airways.

Wheezes are classified as either polyphonic (of many different notes) or monophonic (just one note). Polyphonic wheezes are common in widespread air flow obstruction; it is the characteristic wheeze heard in asthmatics. A localized monophonic wheeze suggests that a single airway is partially obstructed; this can also occur in asthma (e.g. by a mucus plug) but may be a sign of narrowing due to a tumour.

The symptom of wheezing is not diagnostic of asthma, although asthma and COPD are the commonest causes and they can be difficult to distinguish. You should establish whether the patient wheezes first thing in the morning (common in chronic bronchitis), at night (common in asthma) or on exercising.

Stridor is an audible inspiratory noise and indicates partial obstruction of the upper, larger airways, such as the larynx, trachea and main bronchus. It is very important that you differentiate between a wheeze and stridor because stridor is a serious sign requiring urgent investigation and can often be a medical emergency. Causes of obstruction include tumour, epiglottitis and inhalation of a foreign body.

CHEST PAIN

Pain can originate from most of the structures in the chest and can be classified as central or lateral. As with pain anywhere in the body, enquire about site, onset, character, radiation, associated factors, time, exacerbating/relieving factors and severity (SOCRATES). Make sure you ask specifically about the pain's relationship to breathing, coughing or movement; if it is made worse by these factors, it is likely to be pleural in origin. Pleural pain is sharp and stabbing in character and may be referred to the shoulder tip if the diaphragmatic pleura is involved. It can be very severe and often leads to shallow breathing, avoidance of movement and cough suppression. The commonest causes of pleural pain are pulmonary embolus or infection. Figure 8.2 summarizes the main causes of chest pain.

Respiratory causes of central, or retrosternal, chest pain include bronchitis and acute tracheitis. This pain is often made worse by coughing and may be relieved when the patient coughs up sputum.

OTHER ASSOCIATED SYMPTOMS

In addition to the principal presentations, there are several other symptoms that you should note.

Hoarseness

Ask if the patient's voice has changed at all in recent times, and if so, was there anything that preceded the change, e.g. overuse of the voice, thyroidectomy? There may be a simple, benign cause of hoarseness, such as:

- Cigarette smoking.
- Acute laryngitis as part of an acute upper respiratory tract infection.
- Use of inhaled steroids.

However, there may be a more sinister cause: like the bovine cough noted above, hoarseness may be a sign that a lung tumour is compressing the recurrent laryngeal nerve. Therefore, in a smoker any change in voice lasting longer than a few days should be investigated urgently to rule out malignancy.

Weight loss

Unintentional weight loss is always an important sign, raising suspicion of carcinoma. Establish how much weight the patient has lost, over what period, and whether there is any loss of appetite. Note, however, that it is common for patients with severe emphysema to lose weight.

Weight loss can also occur due to infection, particularly TB. Additional features to suggest TB as the underlying cause include chronic cough, night sweats and recent travel to/emigration from a country or region with a high prevalence of the disease, such as India and South Asia.

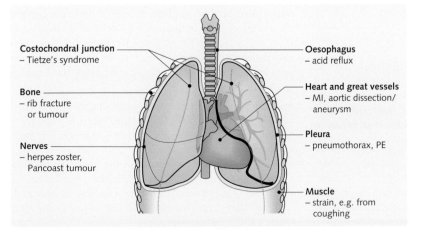

Fig. 8.2 Summary of causes of chest pain. PE = pulmonary embolism; MI = myocardial infarction.

Costochondral junction
– Tietze's syndrome

Bone
– rib fracture
or tumour

Nerves
– herpes zoster,
Pancoast tumour

Oesophagus
– acid reflux

Heart and great vessels
– MI, aortic dissection/
aneurysm

Pleura
– pneumothorax, PE

Muscle
– strain, e.g. from
coughing

Ankle swelling

Patients with COPD may comment that their ankles swell during acute exacerbations. Ask about this and check for oedema as part of your examination. It is an important sign of cor pulmonale, which is right-sided heart failure secondary to chronic lung disease.

Associated symptoms

Always ask about these additional features:

- Fevers and rigors, e.g. infection.
- Night sweats, e.g. malignancy or tuberculosis.
- Occupational factors, e.g. asbestos exposure and occupational asthma.
- Pets and travel history, e.g. allergic disease, malaria and tuberculosis.

PAST MEDICAL HISTORY

Ask about any illnesses and/or operations the patient has had in the past. Does the patient see the GP for anything regularly? For respiratory conditions ask especially about a history of asthma, recurrent infections or atopy, as well as the presence of diabetes and cardiac risk factors. Many patients with chronic disease also suffer with low mood and depression – ask questions around this.

Drug history

Get a comprehensive list of medications the patient is taking, along with doses. If the patient is unsure, then a quick call to the GP may be needed. Make sure to ask specifically about over-the-counter medications, and contraceptives in women. Also of note are any inhaler regimens, and whether these have changed recently.

Ensure patients know what each of their medications is for and that they can use an inhaler effectively if relevant.

Always ask about *allergies*!

Family history

A specific knowledge of respiratory disorders that run in the family can be useful in aiding diagnosis of atopic disorders such as asthma, but also rarer conditions such as cystic fibrosis and α_1-antitrypsin deficiency. More generally, a significant history of cardiac risk factors or death at a young age may be relevant.

Social history

This is an important area, especially for respiratory medicine. Occupational exposure to smoke, asbestos and particulate matter is important, as is a history of smoking, what was smoked and for how long. Information with regard to pets (both the patient's own and those of relatives or friends where significant time is spent) and travel history (from an infectious disease but also long-haul flight angle) are also significant.

Elucidate the effect the illness is having on the patient mentally and physically. For example, is the patient having issues at work or personally as a consequence of stress or having to take time off? Ask elderly patients if they are still able to make it to the shops and wash and dress themselves or whether they are limited by their symptoms.

Systems review

Next, conduct a full systems review to ensure things haven't been missed.

Closing gambit

Give the patient a last chance to flag things up that may have been prompted by your questions so far. Ask a question such as: 'Do you think there is anything I have missed?' or 'Is there anything else you think I should know?' It is also useful here to ask patients if they have any questions for you. This both empowers patients and gives you an idea as to which areas specifically they may be concerned about.

Summary

It is good practice to summarize things briefly back to the patient, cementing the story in your own mind as well as giving the patient a chance to correct unclear points or expand on any unresolved issues.

PATIENTS WITH KNOWN RESPIRATORY DISEASE

If a patient tells you he or she has a diagnosis of a respiratory disease then explore this. The patient's current presentation may or may not be related to this however. Patients may know considerably more than you about their condition; try not to let this disturb you and use it as a learning opportunity. Important things to clarify are:

- When and where were they diagnosed?
- Who do they see for follow-up?
- Have they ever been admitted to hospital before with their respiratory disease?
- If so, did they have to attend the intensive therapy unit, and if so, were they ventilated?
- If they have medication they can use as required, have they been using more recently, e.g. inhalers or COPD rescue packs?

- If they do use inhalers, check their inhaler technique.
- Have they had to have oral steroids in the past, or are they currently on them?

History taking requires considerable practice to perfect. Come up with a set order in which you are comfortable asking the questions you need and stick to it so things are not forgotten. As good practice, always come up with a list of differential diagnoses for all the patients you see, and do not look in the notes until after you have presented your history to someone and had feedback.

By the end of this chapter you should be able to:
- Understand the principles of respiratory examination.
- Understand and describe the clinical features of respiratory distress on general inspection.
- Describe the examination findings for common lung diseases, including pneumonia, asthma and chronic obstructive pulmonary disease (COPD).
- Understand how pleural effusion, pneumothorax and consolidation can be distinguished on clinical examination.
- Describe the features of lung fibrosis on examination.

INTRODUCTION

As with any examination, it is important that you:

- Introduce yourself to the patient.
- Explain to the patient the purpose of the examination and gain consent.
- Wash your hands before you begin and when you finish the examination.

For a respiratory examination, patients should be fully exposed to the waist, comfortable and sitting at 45°, with their hands by their sides. The structure of the respiratory examination is always:

- Inspection.
- Palpation.
- Percussion.
- Auscultation.

GENERAL INSPECTION

The purpose of general inspection is to gain as much information about the patient as possible before you begin examining him or her. It is an important skill to learn as a doctor, as you will often decide how sick a patient is purely on the basis of your initial observations and this will then guide whether you do a thorough history and examination or begin emergency management (see Ch. 12).

General inspection is hugely important in respiratory examination as a large amount of information can be learnt about the patient by simply observing from the bedside. When inspecting the patient you should ask yourself the following questions:

- Is this patient in respiratory distress (Fig. 9.1)?
- What is the patient's respiratory rate (Fig. 9.2)?

- Can the patient talk to me in full sentences without becoming breathless?
- Is the patient's breathing noisy (is there wheeze or stridor?)?
- What is the patient's pattern of breathing (Fig. 9.3)?
- Are there inhalers, sputum pots or oxygen around the bedside?
- Is there any hint as to the underlying cause of the respiratory disease – i.e cachexia in lung cancer or classic features of scleroderma in lung fibrosis?
- Is there any evidence of potential side-effects of respiratory medications – i.e. steroids (Fig. 9.4) or tremor with salbutamol excess?

Hands

Examination of the hands is a key stage in the respiratory examination as there are many important peripheral manifestations of respiratory disease. Ask patients to place their hands in front of them and carefully inspect for the following features:

- Tar staining.
- Clubbing.
- Peripheral cyanosis.
- CO_2 retention.
- Tremor.
- Muscle wasting.
- Rheumatoid arthritis.

Tar staining

Tar staining is an important clinical feature to note as smoking is an important risk factor for many lung diseases, including COPD and lung cancer. Tar staining is a yellow discoloration of the fingers and is usually most notable around the fingertips (Fig. 9.5).

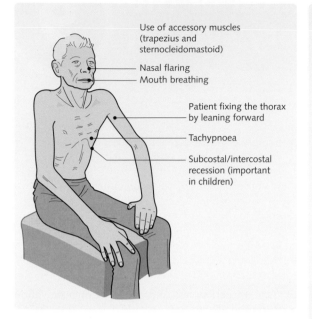

Use of accessory muscles (trapezius and sternocleidomastoid)

Nasal flaring
Mouth breathing

Patient fixing the thorax by leaning forward

Tachypnoea

Subcostal/intercostal recession (important in children)

Fig. 9.1 Features of respiratory distress. These clinical findings are important signs of respiratory distress. With these features the patient will require urgent attention.

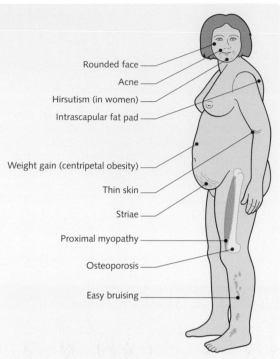

Rounded face
Acne
Hirsutism (in women)
Intrascapular fat pad

Weight gain (centripetal obesity)

Thin skin

Striae

Proximal myopathy

Osteoporosis

Easy bruising

Fig. 9.4 Side-effects of long-term steroid treatment.

Fig. 9.2	Respiratory rate
Normal respiratory rate	12–20 breaths/min
Tachypnoea	>20 breaths/min
Bradypnoea	<12 breaths/min

Fig. 9.3	Abnormal breathing patterns
Breathing pattern	**Causes**
Kussmaul's respiration (hyperventilation with deep sighing respirations)	Diabetic ketoacidosis Aspirin overdose Acute massive pulmonary embolism
Cheyne–Stokes respiration (increased rate and volume of respiration followed by periods of apnoea)	Terminal disease Increased intracranial pressure
Prolongation of expiration	Air flow limitation
Pursed-lip breathing	Air trapping

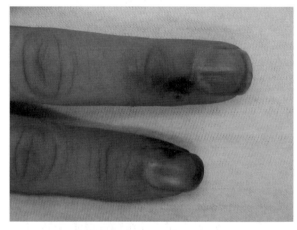

Fig. 9.5 Tar staining.

Clubbing

Clubbing is a painless, bulbous enlargement of the distal fingers, which is accompanied by softening of the nail bed and loss of nail bed angle (Fig. 9.6). One method of detecting clubbing is to look for Shamroth's sign (Fig. 9.7). The respiratory causes of clubbing include the following.

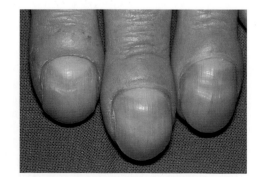

Fig. 9.6 Clubbing.

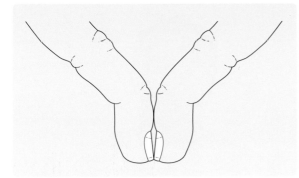

Fig 9 7 Shamroth's sign (finger clubbing)

- Congenital
  - Cystic fibrosis.
- Malignant
  - Bronchial carcinoma.
  - Mesothelioma.
- Suppurative
  - Empyema.
  - Bronchiectasis.
- Lung fibrosis

There are other non-respiratory causes, which include inflammatory bowel disease, liver cirrhosis, congenital cyanotic heart disease, infective endocarditis and hyperthyroidism.

Peripheral cyanosis

Peripheral cyanosis is bluish discoloration of the skin and represents >5 g/dL of haemoglobin in its reduced form. In lung disease this is caused by inaedequate oxygenation, i.e. in asthma, COPD and pulmonary embolism.

CO_2 retention

There are several signs of CO_2 retention that can be detected in the hands:

- Warm, well-perfused hands.
- Palmar erythema (reddening of the palms).
- Bounding radial pulse.
- CO_2 retention flap.

The CO_2 retention flap is elicited by asking patients to hold their arms outstretched and to extend their wrists fully. Patients should remain in this position for 30 seconds; in the presence of CO_2 retention they will develop a coarse, irregular tremor (so-called CO_2 retention flap).

Tremor

It is common for respiratory patients using β_2 agonists (i.e. salbutamol) to develop a fine resting tremor. This tremor is again assessed by asking patients to hold their arms outstretched. Unlike CO_2 retention, this tremor is very fine and regular and can be exaggerated by laying a piece of paper over the patient's hands.

Muscle wasting and bony deformities of the hands

These signs are often indirectly related to lung disease and thus are not essential to detect in the respiratory examination. However, if they are detected, they can provide useful information as to the underlying pathology of lung disease. Unilateral muscle wasting of the hands (particularly in T1 distribution) may hint at the presence of a Pancoast's tumour. Patients with rheumatoid arthritis have classical hand deformities (Fig. 9.8): this autoimmune condition is also associated with lung fibrosis.

Radial pulse

A normal resting pulse in an adult is 60–100 bpm. Bradycardia is defined as a pulse rate of less than 60 bpm.

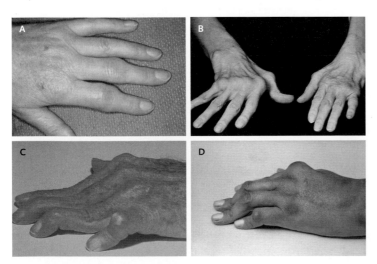

Fig. 9.8 Rheumatoid hands showing (A–D) swan neck, boutonnière, ulnar deviation and Z thumbs.

Fig. 9.9	Radial pulse
Rate <100 bpm	Normal
Rate >100 bpm (tachycardia)	Pain Shock Infection Thyrotoxicosis Sarcoidosis Pulmonary embolism Drugs, e.g. salbutamol Iatrogenic causes
Full, exaggerated arterial pulsation (bounding pulse)	CO_2 retention Thyrotoxicosis Fever Anaemia Hyperkinetic states

and tachycardia of greater than 100 bpm. Palpate the radial pulse and count for 15 seconds, then multiply by four to give a rate per minute. Is the pulse regular (Fig. 9.9)?

The radial pulse can also be assessed for the presence of pulsus paradoxus. In normal individuals the pulse decreases slightly in volume on inspiration and systolic blood pressure falls by 3–5 mmHg. In severe obstructive diseases (e.g. severe asthma) the contractile force of respiratory muscles is so great that there is a marked fall in systolic pressure on inspiration. A fall of greater than 10 mmHg is pathological.

HINTS AND TIPS

You will gain marks if your examination looks fluent and professional. It is easy to move smoothly from introducing yourself and shaking the patient's hand, to examination of the hands, to testing the radial pulse. Then you can discreetly test for respiratory rate without patients realising and altering their breathing.

Head and neck

Examination of the face

First, observe the face generally. You may notice:

- Signs of superior vena cava obstruction (Fig. 9.10).
- Cushingoid features (Fig. 9.4).

Look at the mouth for signs of:

- *Candida* infection – white coating on tongue, often seen after steroids or antibiotics.
- Central cyanosis.

Central cyanosis is blue discoloration of the mucous membranes of the mouth and represents >5 g/dL of haemoglobin in its reduced form. In lung disease this is caused by inadequate oxygenation, i.e. in asthma, COPD or pulmonary embolism.

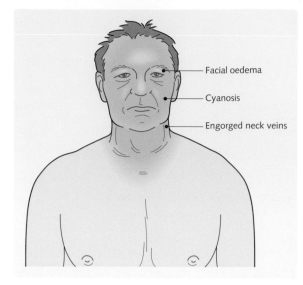

Fig. 9.10 Superior vena cava (SVC) obstruction. Can occur in patients with an apical lung tumour.

Eyes

Examine the eyes for evidence of anaemia by asking the patient to look up whilst pulling down (gently) the lower eyelid. A pale conjunctiva is indicative of anaemia.

Examine the eyes carefully, looking for evidence of Horner's syndrome (Fig. 9.11), which is characterized by:

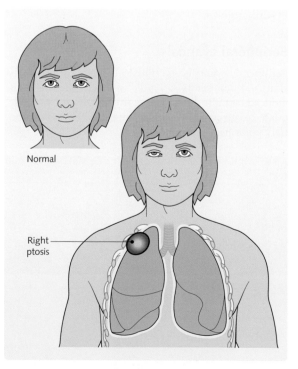

Fig. 9.11 Horner's syndrome.

- Partial ptosis (drooping of the eyelid).
- Miosis (small pupil).
- Anhydrosis (lack of sweating).

In respiratory medicine Horner's syndrome can be caused by a Pancoast's tumour (see Ch.19), which is an apical lung tumour. This tumour can press on the sympathetic chain as it ascends in the neck, causing Horner's syndrome.

Examination of the neck

In the neck it is important to examine;

- Trachea (Fig. 9.12) and cricosternal distance (Fig. 9.13).
- Jugular venous pressure (JVP).
- Lymph nodes (Fig. 9.14).

When examining the JVP ensure the patient is at 45° and ask the patient to turn the head to the left (Fig. 9.15). A normal JVP is visible just above the clavicle in between the two heads of sternocleidomastoid. The JVP can be difficult to see and so it can be accentuated by the hepatojugular reflux (i.e. press down gently over the liver; this increases venous return to the heart and thus increases the JVP). Once found, the height of the JVP should be measured from the sternal notch. If this is >4 cm the JVP is said to be raised (Fig. 9.16).

Develop a set system of palpating the lymph nodes of the neck. Sit the patient up and examine from behind with both hands (Fig. 9.15).

The chest

General inspection of the chest

When undertaking a close inspection of the chest it is important to pay specific attention to:

- Chest wall deformities (Fig. 9.17).
- Abnormalities of the spine (Fig. 9.18).
- Surgical thoracic incisions (Fig. 9.19).
- Radiotherapy tattoos.

Deformities of the chest wall and spine are important clinically as they can restrict the ventilatory capacity of the lungs.

Palpation

Palpation in the respiratory examination primarily involves assessing chest expansion both anteroposteriorly (AP) and laterally (Fig. 9.20). When testing chest expansion in the AP direction, place the palms of both hands on the pectoral region and ask the patient to take a deep breath. The chest should expand symetrically. Any asymmetry suggests pathology on the side that fails to expand adequately. Testing lateral expansion of the chest involves gripping the chest (Fig. 9.20) between both hands and then asking the patient to take a deep

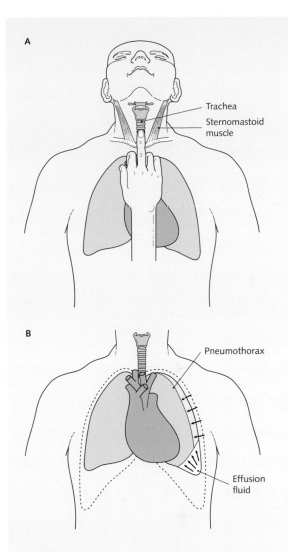

Fig. 9.12 Tracheal deviation. (A) Tracheal deviation is measured by placing the index and ring fingers on either head of the clavicle. The middle finger is then placed gently on the trachea. In normal patients the trachea will be equidistant between the two heads of the clavicle, i.e. your middle finger will be the same distance from index and ring fingers. (B) In the presence of a tension pneumothorax on the left, the pressure of air in the pleural space causes the trachea to shift to the right. On clinical examinaton the trachea would be closer to the right clavicular head than the left.

breath whilst observing the movement of your own thumbs. Again, the movement of your thumbs should be symmetrical and any asymmetry suggests pathology on the side of the chest that does not expand fully.

Next, examine for the position of the apex beat by moving your hand inwards from the lateral chest until you feel the pulsation. The apex beat should be in the fifth intercostal space at the midclavicular line.

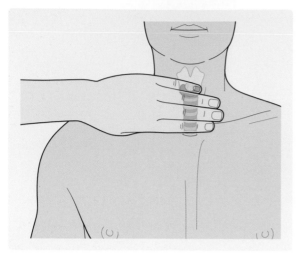

Fig. 9.13 Cricosternal distance. Measure the distance (using your fingers) between the sternal notch and the cricoid cartilage. This distance is normally 3–4 fingers. Less than 3 fingers is indicative of air flow limitation (common in chronic obstructive pulmonary disease).

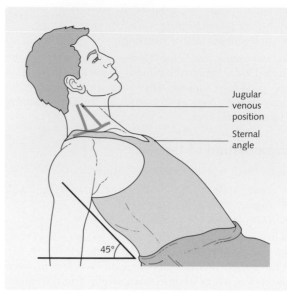

Fig. 9.15 Jugular venous pressure (JVP).

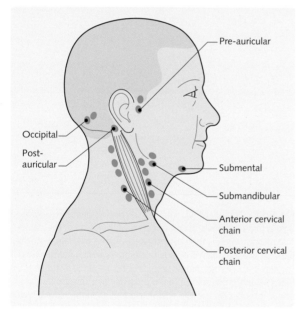

Fig. 9.14 Anatomy of cervical lymph nodes.

Fig. 9.16 Abnormalities of the jugular venous pressure (JVP)

Abnormality of JVP	Cause
Raised with normal waveform	Cor pulmonale Fluid overload
Raised with absent waveform	Superior vena cava obstruction
Absent	Dehydration, shock

Displacement of the apex beat normally signifies cardiomegaly but other respiratory conditions may cause the apex beat to become displaced, including:

- Pulmonary fibrosis.
- Bronchiectasis.
- Pleural effusions.
- Pneumothoraces.

Finally, in palpation you may find it useful to perform tactile vocal fremitus by placing the ulnar edge of your hand on the chest wall whilst asking the patient to say '99' repeatedly. This is repeated throughout the chest both front and back, comparing opposite zones. The vibrations produced by this manoeuvre are transmitted through the lung parenchyma and felt by the hand. Tactile vocal fremitus is increased by consolidation of the lungs and decreased by pleural effusions and pleural thickening.

Percussion

Percussion is an extremely useful tool in the respiratory examination, as the percussion note provides information about the consistency of the lung matter underlying the chest wall, i.e. whether it is air, fluid or solid.

Percussion is performed by placing the middle finger of your non-dominant hand on the chest wall palm downwards in an intercostal space. You then strike this finger with the terminal phalanx (fingertip) of the middle finger of your dominant hand. In order to achieve a good percussion note, the striking finger should be partially flexed and struck at right angles to the other finger.

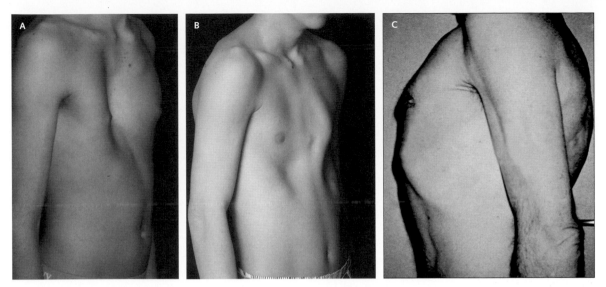

Fig. 9.17 Chest wall deformities. (A) Pectus excavatum: a benign condition whereby the sternum is depressed in relation to the ribs. (B) Pectus carinatum (pigeon chest): the sternum is more prominent in comparison to the ribs – often caused by severe childhood asthma. (C) Barrel chest: the anteroposterior diameter of the chest is greater than the lateral diameter. Caused by hyperinflation of the lungs.

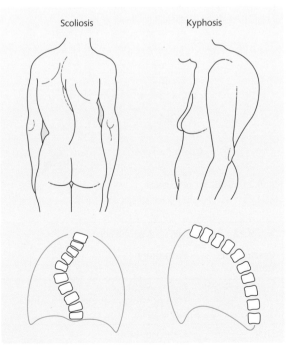

Fig. 9.18 Spinal deformities. Scoliosis increased lateral curvature of the spine. Kyphosis increased forward curvature of the spine (osteoporosis/ankylosing spondylitis). Both cause ventilatory defects and can cause respiratory failure.

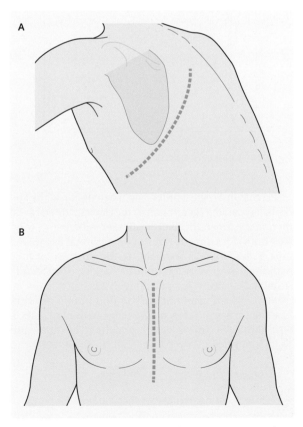

Fig. 9.19 Common thoracic surgical incisions. (A) Lateral thoracotomy; (B) Midline stenotomy.

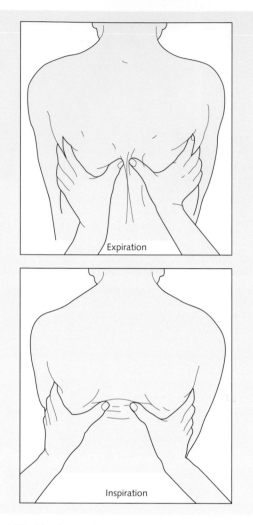

Fig. 9.20 Chest expansion.

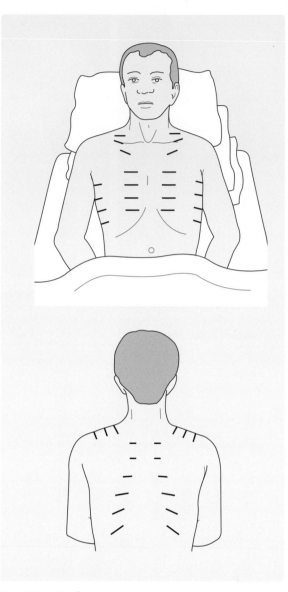

Fig. 9.21 Sites for percussion.

Percuss in a logical order. Begin percussion at the apices by percussing (gently) on to the clavicles directly and then move down the chest wall, remembering to compare both sides directly (Fig. 9.21). A normal percussion note is described as resonant; in the presence of lung pathology the percussion note may be described as dull, stony dull or hyperresonant (Fig. 9.22).

Map out any abnormality you find but do not confuse the cardiac borders or liver edge with lung pathology; they will sound dull normally. The note also sounds muffled in a very muscular or obese patient.

HINTS AND TIPS

When percussing, remember that the upper lobe predominates anteriorly and the lower lobe predominates posteriorly.

Fig. 9.22	Abnormalities of percussion
Percussion note	**Pathology**
Hyperresonant	Pneumothorax Also possible in emphysema with large bullae
Dull	Consolidation Fibrosis Pleural thickening Collapse Infection
Stony dull	Pleural effusion

Fig. 9.23 Abnormal breath sounds

Abnormality	Definition	Associated with:
Breath sounds		
Diminished vesicular breath sounds	Reduced breath sounds	• Airway obstruction • Asthma • COPD
Bronchial breathing	Harsh breath sounds whereby inspiration and expiration are of equal duration	• Consolidation • Pneumonia • Empyema
Added sounds		
Monophonic wheeze	Prolonged musical sound (expiratory)	Large-airway obstruction
Polyphonic wheeze	Prolonged musical sound – many notes (expiratory)	Small-airway obstruction • Asthma
Coarse crackles	Non-musical uninterrupted sounds (inspiratory)	• Consolidation • COPD
Fine crackles	Non-musical uninterrupted sounds (inspiratory) like Velcro	Early inspiration • Pulmonary oedema Late inspiration • Fibrosis
Pleural rub		• Pneumonia • Pulmonary embolism • Pleurisy

COPD, chronic obstructive pulmonary disease.

Auscultation

Normal breath sounds are described as vesicular and have a rustling quality heard in inspiration and the first part of expiration. Listen to the patient's chest:

- Using the bell of the stethoscope in the apices (supraclavicular area).
- Using the diaphragm of the stethoscope elsewhere on the chest.

Auscultate in a logical order, comparing the two sides (as for percussion) and ask the patient to breathe through an open mouth.

You should be listening for:

- Diminished breath sounds.
- Bronchial breathing.
- Added sounds, such as wheezes or stridor, crackles or pleural rubs.

It is important to remember that added sounds that disappear when the patient coughs are not significant (Fig. 9.23).

Vocal resonance

Vocal resonance is the auscultatory equivalent of tactile vocal fremitus. It is performed using the diaphragm of the stethoscope on the chest and asking the patient to say '99'. Vocal resonance is increased by consolidation and reduced by conditions such as pleural effusion and pneumothoraces.

Whispering pectoriloquy

Whispering pectoriloquy is a variation of vocal resonance that can be used to confirm the presence of consolidation. The patient is asked to whisper '99'. In normal lung this cannot be heard by auscultation. However, solid lung conducts sound better than normal aerated lung and thus in patients with areas of consolidation the words are clear and seem to be spoken into the examiner's ear.

Summary

Once you have finished your examination, sum up the positive findings in a clear and concise manner. Normally, to complete the respiratory examination you would inform the examiner that you would like to:

- Examine a sputum pot.
- Take a peak flow reading.
- Examine the patient's temperature and oxygen saturations.

Figure 9.24 summarizes the common clinical findings for the most common respiratory conditions.

Fig. 9.24 Summary of signs found on examination of the respiratory system

	Consolidation	Pneumothorax	Pleural effusion	Lobar collapse	Pleural thickening
Chest radiograph	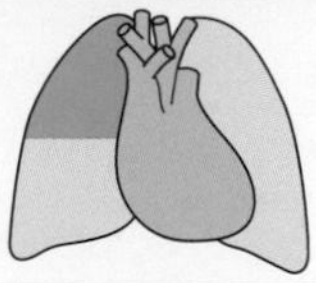	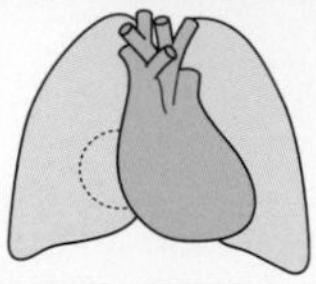	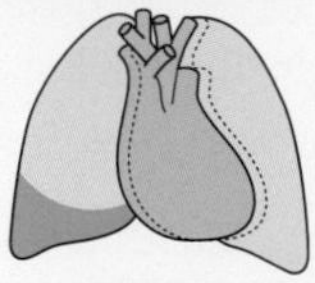	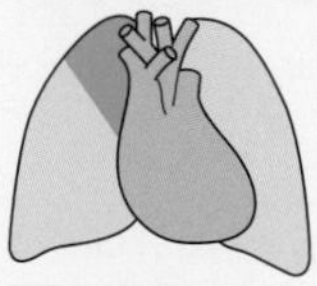	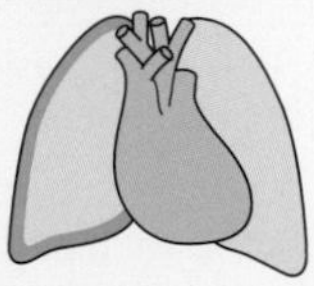
Mediastinal shift and trachea	None	None (simple), away (tension)	None or away	Towards the affected side	None
Chest wall excursion	Normal or decreased on the affected side	Normal or decreased on the affected side	Decreased on the affected side	Decreased	Decreased
Percussion note	Dull	Hyper-resonant	Stony dull	Dull	Dull
Breath sounds	Increased (bronchial)	Decreased	Decreased	Decreased	Decreased
Added sounds	Crackles	Click (occasional)	Rub (occasional)	None	None
Tactile vocal fremitus or vocal resonance	Increased	Decreased	Decreased	Decreased	Decreased

The respiratory patient: clinical investigations

By the end of this chapter you should be able to:
- Summarise the basic blood tests performed.
- Describe the key information provided by arterial blood gas analysis.
- Describe what tests can be performed on a sputum sample.
- Describe the indications for bronchoscopy, the reasons for biopsy and bronchoalveolar lavage and histopathology in diagnosing respiratory disease.
- Describe how to perform a peak exploratory flow rate test accurately and its limitations.
- Describe the importance of spirometry in differentiating obstructive from restrictive disorders.
- Discuss the implications of an abnormal transfer factor test.
- Understand and interpret flow–volume loops and describe how airway compliance and resistance can be calculated.
- Describe the use of exhaled nitric oxide in respiratory disease.
- List indications for exercise testing and describe the different types, including the shuttle test and 6-minute walk test.

INTRODUCTION

There are a large number of investigations in respiratory medicine, ranging from basic bedside tests to more invasive procedures such as bronchoscopy. As you read this chapter, you should bear in mind that some of the investigations below are performed only rarely in specialized pulmonary laboratories whilst others are performed by patients at home every day. The investigations that are most commonly performed, and which you should have a thorough knowledge of, include:

- Arterial blood gas analysis.
- Sputum examination.
- Basic tests of pulmonary function.
- Bronchoscopy.
- Chest radiographs (chest X-rays).

Other, less commonly performed investigations will be discussed in less detail in this chapter.

ROUTINE INVESTIGATIONS

Blood tests

In the associated figures, you will find some of the commonly performed haematological tests:

- Full blood count (Fig. 10.1).
- Differential white blood cell count (Fig. 10.2).
- Other haematological tests (Fig. 10.3).

Clinical chemistry

The commonly performed biochemical tests are shown in Figure 10.4.

If malignancy is suspected, you should also perform liver function tests and test alkaline phosphatase as an indicator of metastases. In addition, endocrine tests should be performed for paraneoplastic manifestations, such as syndrome of inappropriate antidiuretic hormone (see Ch. 19 for more detail).

Tests of blood gases

Arterial blood gas analysis

Blood gas analysis of an arterial blood sample is mandatory in all acute pulmonary conditions. The analysis should always be performed initially on room air and then repeated soon after starting oxygen therapy to assess response to treatment.

A heparinized sample of arterial blood is tested using a standard automated machine, which measures:

- P_aO_2.
- P_aCO_2.
- Oxygen saturation.

Blood pH, standard bicarbonate and base excess are either given on the standard readout or can be calculated. The patient's results are compared with the normal ranges (Figs 10.5 and 10.6) and assessed in two parts:

- Degree of arterial oxygenation – is the patient hypoxic?
- Acid–base balance disturbances.

Fig. 10.1 Full blood count

Test	Normal values	Diagnostic inference	
		Increased values	Decreased values
Haemoglobin (g/dL)	Male: 13–18 Female: 11.5–16.5	Increased in chronic respiratory disease such as COPD, as part of a secondary polycythaemia due to long-standing hypoxia	Decreased in anaemia (look at MCV for further information); a normal MCV (i.e. normocytic anaemia) is common in chronic disease
Mean cell volume (MCV: fL)	76–98	Macrocytosis (vitamin B_{12} or folate deficiency, etc.)	Microcytosis (common in iron-deficiency anaemia and thalassaemias)
Red blood cells ($\times 10^9$/L)	Male: 4.5–6.5 Female: 3.8–5.8	Polycythaemia; may be secondary to chronic lung disease, smoking, altitude	

Fig. 10.2 Differential white blood cell count

Cell type	Normal values	Diagnostic inference	
		Increased values	Decreased values
White blood cell	$4–11 \times 10^9$/L	Bacterial infections Malignancy Pregnancy Long term steroids	Viral infections Drugs Systemic lupus erythematosus Overwhelming bacterial infection
Neutrophil	$2.5–7.5 \times 10^9$/L 60–70%	Bacterial infections Malignancy Pregnancy Steroid treatment	Viral infections Drugs Systemic lupus erythematosus Overwhelming bacterial infection
Eosinophil	$0.04–0.44 \times 10^9$/L 1–4%	Allergic reactions Asthma Sarcoidosis Pneumonia Eosinophilic granulomatosus	Steroid therapy
Monocyte	$0.2–0.8 \times 10^9$/L 5–10%	Tuberculosis	Chronic infection
Lymphocyte	$1.5–4.0 \times 10^9$/L 25–30%	Infection Cytomegalovirus infection Toxoplasmosis Tuberculosis	Tuberculosis

Fig. 10.3 Other haematological tests

Test performed	Normal values	Diagnostic inference	
		Increased values	Decreased values
C-reactive protein (CRP)	Normal <4 mg/L Changes more rapidly than erythrocyte sedimentation rate	Acute infection, inflammation; same as erythrocyte sedimentation rate	Levels often normal in malignancy
Anti-streptolysin O (ASO) titre	Normal <200 IU/mL	Confirms recent streptococcal infection	

Before accurate interpretation of the results, a detailed history of the patient, including a detailed drug history, is needed. However, the arterial blood gas results can then help you identify the underlying abnormality, as well as its severity. Different underlying pathologies will cause different patterns on the arterial blood gas. It is also important to remember that a metabolic disturbance (such as high lactate from shock) can be partially or completely compensated for by the respiratory system, which may be seen clinically as an increased

Fig. 10.4 Biochemical blood tests

Test performed	Normal values	Diagnostic inference	
		Increased values	Decreased values
Potassium	3.5–5.0 mmol/L		Adrenocorticotrophic hormone (ACTH) secreting tumour β agonists
Angiotensin-converting enzyme (ACE)	10–70 U/L	Sarcoidosis	
Calcium	2.12–2.65 mmol/L	Malignancy Sarcoidosis Squamous cell carcinoma of the lung	
Glucose	3.5–5.5 mmol/L	Adrenocorticotrophic hormone (ACTH) secreting tumour Long-term steroid use Pancreatic dysfunction	

Fig. 10.5 Arterial blood gases

Test performed	Normal values	Diagnostic inference	
		Increased values	Decreased values
pH	7.35–7.45	Alkalosis hyperventilation	Acidosis CO_2 retention
P_aO_2	>10.6 kPa		Hypoxic
P_aCO_2	4.7–6.0 kPa	Respiratory acidosis (if pH decreased)	Respiratory alkalosis (if pH increased)
Base excess	±2 mmol/L	Metabolic alkalosis	Metabolic acidosis
Standardized bicarbonate	22–25 mmol/L	Metabolic alkalosis	Metabolic acidosis

Fig. 10.6 Summary of arterial blood gas findings and possible underlying pathologies

pH	P_aO_2	P_aCO_2	Summary	Causes
Normal	Normal	Normal	Normal	N/A
Increased	Normal/increased	Low	Respiratory alkalosis	Hyperventilation
Increased or normal	Normal/low	Increased	Metabolic alkalosis with respiratory compensation	Vomiting Drugs Burns
Decreased	Decreased	Increased	Respiratory acidosis	Asthma Chronic obstructive pulmonary disease Neuromuscular disease
Decreased or normal	Increased	Low/normal	Metabolic acidosis with respiratory compensation Respiratory acidosis	Diabetic ketoacidosis Sepsis Drugs Type 1 respiratory failure

respiratory rate and will be demonstrated in the arterial blood gas result.

Pulse oximetry

This is a simple, non-invasive method of monitoring the percentage of haemoglobin that is saturated with oxygen. The patient wears a probe on a finger or earlobe and this is linked to a unit which displays the readings. The unit can be set to sound an alarm when saturation drops below a certain level (usually 90%). The pulse oximeter works by calculating the absorption of light by haemoglobin, which alters depending on whether it is saturated with oxygen or desaturated. A number of factors may lead to inaccurate oximeter readings. These include:

- Poor peripheral perfusion, such as in hypothermia or Raynaud's disease.
- Carbon monoxide poisoning.
- Skin pigmentation.
- Nail varnish.
- Dirty hands.

A more accurate assessment of oxygen saturation, if necessary, can be obtained by arterial blood gas analysis.

Microbiology

Microbiological examination is possible with samples of sputum, bronchial aspirate, pleural aspirate, throat swabs and blood. The aim of examination is to identify bacteria, viruses or fungi.

Tests to request are microscopy, culture and antibiotic sensitivity. The microbiological findings should be interpreted in view of the whole clinical picture.

Bacteriology

Sputum

Testing of sputum for the presence of bacteria is the most common microbiological test performed in respiratory medicine. Obtain the sample, preferably of induced sputum, before antibiotic treatment is started. Collect in a sterile container, inspect the sample and send it to the laboratory.

Request Gram stain, Ziehl–Neelsen stain (for tuberculosis) and anaerobic cultures. Culture on Löwenstein–Jensen medium to detect tuberculosis. A sputum sample is valuable in diagnosing suspected pneumonia, tuberculosis and aspergillosis, or if the patient presents with an unusual clinical picture.

Failure to isolate an organism from the sputum is not uncommon.

Resistance to commonly used antibiotics is often found in bacteria responsible for respiratory tract infections; therefore, antibiotic sensitivity testing is vital.

More modern techniques can be used in the laboratory for quicker results. This is particularly useful in the identification of tuberculosis, which can take several weeks to grow on conventional media. The ELISPOT assay (enzyme-linked immunosorbent spot) works by detecting cytokine production (interferon-γ) in response to specific antibodies on the plate. Interferon-γ release assays (such as QuantiFERON) can also be used to identify *Mycobacterium tuberculosis* quickly so that treatment can be commenced before the cultures are back.

Blood culture

A blood culture should always be performed in patients with fever and lower respiratory tract infection. Collect a large volume of blood and divide it equally into two bottles of nutrient media, one for aerobic and the other for anaerobic bacteria. Collect two or three cultures over 24 hours.

Blood cultures identify systemic bacterial and fungal infections. Results may be positive while sputum culture is negative. Again, it is important to collect an initial set of cultures before starting antibiotic therapy.

Upper respiratory specimens

Microscopy is generally unhelpful because of the abundant commensals of the upper respiratory tract which contaminate samples.

Throat specimens can be collected using a Dacron or calcium alginate swab. The tonsils, posterior pharynx and any ulcerated areas are sampled. Avoid contact with the tongue and saliva, as this can inhibit identification of group A streptococci. In the modern hospital setting, nose swabs are routinely used to identify patients colonized with meticillin-resistant *Staphylococcus aureus* (MRSA). However, this can often be a commensal organism and not the underlying cause of symptoms.

A sinus specimen is collected with a needle and syringe. The specimen is cultured for aerobic and anaerobic bacteria. Common pathogens of sinuses are *Streptococcus pneumoniae, Haemophilus influenzae, Moraxella catarrhalis, Staphylococcus aureus* and anaerobes.

Coxiella burnetii, Mycoplasma pneumoniae and *Legionella* are difficult to culture; therefore, results of serology must be used.

Lower respiratory specimens

Techniques used to collect samples include expectoration, cough induction with saline, bronchoscopy, bronchial alveolar lavage, transtracheal aspiration and direct aspiration through the chest wall. Some of these techniques are considered below under the more invasive procedures.

Viral testing

Because of the small size of viral particles, light microscopy provides little information: it is able to visualize viral inclusions and cytopathic effects of viral infection.

Viral serology

Viral serology is the most important group of tests in virology. Serological diagnoses are obtained when viruses are difficult to isolate and grow in cell culture.

Specimens should be collected early in the acute phase because viral shedding for respiratory viruses lasts 3–7 days; however, symptoms commonly persist for longer. A repeated sample should be collected 10 days later.

Viral serology also identifies the virus and its strain or serotype, and is able to evaluate the course of infection. Viral serology is not commonly used in clinical practice as antiviral therapies are relatively ineffective and not commonly used to treat viral respiratory tract infections. However, they can be useful from an epidemiological perspective, such as in the identification of different strains of the influenza virus for the development of vaccines.

Cell culture

Specimens for cell cultures are obtained from nasal washings, throat swabs, nasal swabs and sputum. Viruses cannot be cultured without living cells.

Fungal testing

Fungal infections may be serious, especially in immunocompromised patients, where they can cause systemic infection; invasive fungal infections require blood culture. Repeated specimens from the site need to be taken to rule out contaminants in cultures.

Common fungal infections are *Candida* and *Aspergillus*. Microscopic identification may be difficult for *Aspergillus* because it is common in the environment. Culture is rarely helpful in identifying *Aspergillus*; the *Aspergillus* precipitins test is of more use.

It is important to remember that fungal infections are uncommon in healthy individuals. Therefore, if a young, previously healthy person is found to have a fungal infection, you should also investigate for an underlying cause of that person's immune compromise, such as malignancy, diabetes or human immunodeficiency virus (HIV).

MORE INVASIVE PROCEDURES

Bronchoscopy

Bronchoscopy allows the visualization of the trachea and larger bronchi and can be used to sample tissues via brushings, lavage or biopsy. Two types of bronchoscope are used:
- Flexible fibreoptic bronchoscope.
- Rigid bronchoscope (under general anaesthetic).

In practice, the flexible bronchoscope is used in most instances. Patients may be lightly sedated to reduce anxiety and suppress the cough mechanism. Topical lidocaine is used to anaesthetize the pharynx and vocal cords.

The main indications for bronchoscopy are:
- Diagnosis of lung cancer (e.g. after an abnormal chest X-ray or haemoptysis).
- Staging of lung cancer.
- Diagnosis of diffuse lung disease.
- Diagnosis of infections (especially in immunocompromised hosts).

Bronchoalveolar lavage

Sterile saline (usually around 100 mL) is infused down the flexible bronchoscope and then aspirated. This technique is commonly used to look for evidence of neoplasms or opportunistic infections in immunocompromised patients. If this is done in the acute setting and the patient is unwell, a smaller volume of saline is used to avoid airway compromise, known as bronchial washing.

Transbronchial biopsy

Transbronchial biopsy provides samples from outside the airways, e.g. of alveolar tissue. The technique is performed using biopsy forceps attached to a flexible bronchoscope. The bronchoscopist cannot directly visualize the biopsy site and may be assisted by fluoroscopic imaging. Complications include pneumothorax or haemorrhage.

Percutaneous fine-needle aspiration

This technique is used to sample peripheral lesions under the guidance of radiography.

Open and thoracoscopic lung biopsy

In some cases of diffuse lung disease, or where a lesion cannot easily be reached, more extensive lung biopsy is required for diagnosis. Open-lung biopsy is performed through a thoracotomy with the patient under general anaesthesia. However, video-assisted thorascopic techniques are increasingly used as a less invasive alternative.

Endobronchial USS (EBUS)

Endobronchial ultrasound is a new technique whereby an ultrasound probe is placed down the bronchoscope, allowing visualization of deeper structures such as lymph nodes, which can then be biopsied.

Pleural tap (thoracocentesis)

This is the drainage of a small amount of fluid from a pleural effusion. This can be done blind or under ultrasound or computed tomography guidance. It is an important investigation to identify the underlying cause of an effusion. The sample can appear serous, bloody (haemothorax, usually after trauma) or pus-filled (empyema). Any sample extracted can be analysed in several different ways to help identify the pathology. This includes microscopy, cytopathology, culture and biochemical analysis of its contents. The biochemical analysis can determine whether the effusion is a transudate or exudate using Light's criteria, which in turn points towards possible underlying causes (Fig. 10.7).

HISTOPATHOLOGY

Histopathology is the investigation and diagnosis of disease from the examination of tissues.

Fig. 10.7	Pleural tap analysis	
	Transudate	**Exudate**
Appearance	Clear fluid	Cloudy
Pleural fluid/ serum protein ratio	<0.5	>0.5
Pleural fluid/ serum lactate dehydrogenase ratio	<0.6	>0.6
Pleural fluid lactate dehydrogenase	<2/3 upper limit of normal for serum	>2/3 upper limit of normal for serum
Causes	Heart failure Liver failure Nephrotic syndrome	Pneumonia Lung cancer and other malignancies (including breast and lymphoma) Pulmonary embolism

Light's criteria from Light et al. (1972).

Histopathological examination of biopsy material

The histopathological examination is a vital test in cases of suspected malignancy, allowing a definitive diagnosis to be made. Biopsy material is obtained by the techniques described above, in addition to:

- Pleural biopsy.
- Lymph node biopsy.

Histological features of malignant neoplasms are:

- Loss of cellular differentiation.
- Abundant cells undergoing mitosis, many of which are abnormal.
- High nuclear:cytoplasm ratio.
- Cells or nuclei varying in shape and size.

Other uses of histopathology include diagnosing interstitial lung diseases such as cryptogenic fibrosing alveolitis.

Cytological examination of sputum

Cytological examination is useful in diagnosing bronchial carcinoma and has the advantage of being a non-invasive, quick test; however, it is dependent upon adequate sputum production. Sputum is obtained by:

- Induction/inhalation of nebulized hypertonic saline.
- Transtracheal aspiration.
- Bronchoscopy.
- Bronchial washings or bronchoalveolar lavage

Exfoliated cells (in the sputum, pleural fluid, bronchial brushings or washings or fine-needle aspirate of lymph nodes and lesions) are examined, primarily for signs of malignancy.

INVESTIGATIONS OF PULMONARY FUNCTION

Tests of pulmonary function are used in:

- Diagnosis of lung disease.
- Monitoring disease progression.
- Assessing patient response to treatment.

Tests of ventilation

Ventilation can be impaired in two basic ways:

- The airways become narrowed (obstructive disorders).
- Expansion of the lungs is reduced (restrictive disorders).

These two types of disorder have characteristic patterns of lung function which can be measured using the tests below.

Forced expiration

Peak expiratory flow rate (PEFR) is a simple and cheap test that uses a peak flow meter (Fig. 10.8) to measure the maximum expiratory rate in the first 10 ms of expiration. Peak flow meters can be issued on prescription and used at home by patients to monitor their lung function.

Before measuring PEFR (Fig. 10.9), the practitioner should instruct the patient to:

- Take a full inspiration to maximum lung capacity.
- Seal the lips tightly around the mouthpiece.
- Blow out forcefully into the peak flow meter, which is held horizontally.

The best of three measurements is recorded and plotted on the appropriate graph. Normal PEFR is 400–650 L/min in healthy adults. At least two recordings per day are required to obtain an accurate pattern. A patient would normally be asked to do this for a couple of weeks in order to obtain a peak flow diary, which could then be analysed to look at the type of airways disease.

PEFR is reduced in conditions that cause airway obstruction:

- Asthma, where there is wide diurnal variation in PEFR, known as 'morning dipping' (Fig. 10.10).
- Chronic obstructive pulmonary disease (COPD).
- Upper-airway tumours.

Other causes of reduced PEFR include expiratory muscle weakness, inadequate effort and poor technique. PEFR

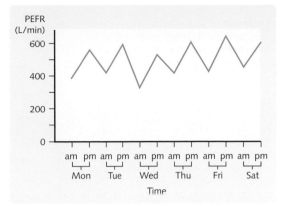

Fig. 10.10 Typical peak expiratory flow rate (PEFR) graph for an asthmatic patient.

is not a good measure of air flow limitation because it measures only initial expiration; it is best used to monitor progression of disease and response to treatment.

In asthma, regular monitoring of PEFR with a home device can be useful at predicting the onset of an exacerbation and the severity. Asthma patients can be given an information sheet telling them what to do if their peak flow is lower than normal, depending on how severe the reduction is. This can help reduce the severity and length of exacerbations (by starting treatment earlier) and also ensure that the sickest patients seek medical help sooner.

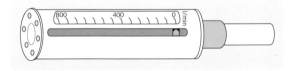

Fig. 10.8 Peak flow meter.

> **HINTS AND TIPS**
>
> Alex, a 9-year-old boy, was becoming wheezy and short of breath after mild exertion. His GP asked him to keep a peak flow diary, which showed diurnal variation with morning dipping. As this was suggestive of asthma, the GP prescribed bronchodilators which Alex used about three times a week to control his symptoms.

Forced expiratory volume and forced vital capacity

The forced expiratory volume in 1 second (FEV_1) and the forced vital capacity (FVC) are measured using a spirometer. The spirometer works by converting volumes of inspiration and expiration into a single line trace. The subject is connected by a mouthpiece to a sealed chamber (Fig. 10.11). Each time the subject breathes, the volume inspired or expired is converted into the vertical position of a float. The position of the float is recorded on a rotating drum by means of a pen attachment. Electronic devices are becoming increasingly available.

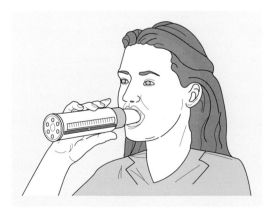

Fig. 10.9 Patient performing peak expiratory flow rate test.

Fig. 10.11 Spirometry. The measurement of lung volume by displacement of a float within a sealed chamber is recorded on a paper roll by a pen.

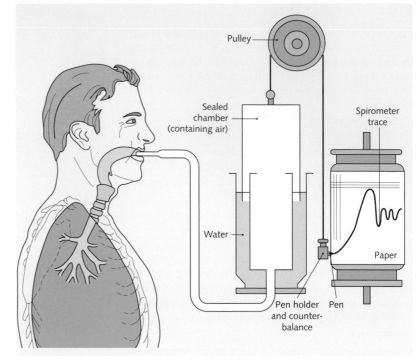

FEV$_1$ and FVC

FEV_1 and FVC are related to height, age and sex of the patient. FEV_1 is the volume of air expelled in the first second of a forced expiration, starting from full inspiration. FVC is a measure of total lung volume exhaled; the patient is asked to exhale with maximal effort after a full inspiration.

FEV$_1$:FVC ratio

The FEV_1:FVC ratio is a more useful measurement than FEV_1 or FVC alone. FEV_1 is 80% of FVC in normal subjects. The FEV_1:FVC ratio is an excellent measure of airway limitation and allows us to differentiate obstructive from restrictive lung disease.

In restrictive disease:

- Both FEV_1 and FVC are reduced, often in proportion to each other.
- FEV_1:FVC ratio is normal or increased (>80%).

Whereas in obstructive diseases:

- High intrathoracic pressures generated by forced expiration cause premature closure of the airways with trapping of air in the chest.
- FEV_1 is reduced much more than FVC.
- FEV_1:FVC ratio is reduced (<80%).

Flow–volume loops

Flow–volume loops are graphs constructed from maximal expiratory and inspiratory manoeuvres performed on a spirometer. The loop is made up of two halves: above the x-axis is the flow of air out of the mouth on expiration, and below the x-axis, flow into the mouth on inspiration. The loop shape can identify the type and distribution of airway obstruction. After a small amount of gas has been exhaled, flow is limited by:

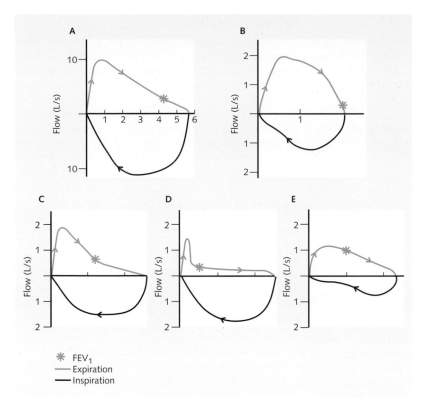

* FEV_1
— Expiration
— Inspiration

- Elastic recoil force of the lung.
- Resistance of airways upstream of collapse.

When looking at flow–volume loops, look for a normal-shaped loop (Fig. 10.12A): a triangular expiratory curve created by an initially fast expiration of air, slowing down as total lung capacity (TLC) is reached, and a semicircular inspiratory curve. Any deviation away from this triangle and semicircle pattern suggests pathology. Additionally, read off the FEV_1 (marked by a star) from the x-axis. Reduced FEV_1 suggests an obstructive airway disease.

Flow–volume loops are useful in diagnosing upper-airway obstruction (Fig. 10.12B), restrictive and obstructive disease.

In restrictive diseases:

- Maximum flow rate is reduced (read from y-axis).
- Total volume exhaled is reduced (read from x-axis).
- Flow rate is high during the latter part of expiration because of increased lung recoil.

In obstructive diseases:

- Flow rate is low in relation to lung volume.
- Expiration ends prematurely because of early airway closure, most easily spotted by a scooped-out appearance after the point of maximum flow rather than the triangular-shaped expiratory curve seen in healthy lungs.

Tests of lung volumes

The amount of gas in the lungs can be thought of as being split into subdivisions, with disease processes altering these volumes in specific ways. In measuring tidal volume and vital capacity, we use spirometry; alternative techniques are needed for the other volumes.

Residual volume (RV) and functional residual capacity (FRC)

One important lung volume, RV, is not measured in simple spirometry, because gas remains in the lungs at the end of each breath (otherwise the lungs would collapse). Without a measure for RV, we cannot calculate FRC or TLC.

RV is a useful measure in assessing obstructive disease. In a healthy subject, RV is approximately 30% of TLC. In obstructive diseases such as COPD, the lungs are hyperinflated with 'air trapping' so that RV is greatly increased and the ratio of RV:TLC is also increased. There are three methods of measuring RV: helium dilution, plethysmography and nitrogen washout.

Helium dilution

The patient is connected to a spirometer containing a mixture of 10% helium in air. Helium does not cross the alveolar–capillary membrane into the bloodstream and so, after several breaths, the helium concentration in the spirometer and lung becomes equal. TLC can be calculated from the difference in helium concentration at the start of the test and at equilibrium; then RV can be calculated by subtracting vital capacity from TLC.

This method only measures gas that is in communication with the airways.

Body plethysmography

Plethysmography determines changes in lung volume by recording changes in pressure. The patient sits in a large airtight box and breathes through a mouthpiece (Fig. 10.13). At the end of a normal expiration, a shutter closes the mouthpiece and the patient is asked to make respiratory efforts. As the patient tries to inhale, box pressure increases. Using Boyle's law, lung volume can be calculated.

In contrast to the helium dilution method, body plethysmography measures all intrathoracic gas, including cysts, bullae and pneumothoraces, i.e. non-communicating air spaces. This is important in emphysematous subjects with bullae, in whom helium dilution underestimates RV.

This technique tends to be done in specialized respiratory centres in respiratory function laboratories.

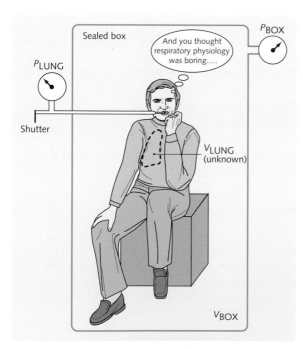

Fig. 10.13 Plethysmography. This assumes pressure at the mouth is the pressure within the lung.

Nitrogen washout

Following a normal expiration, the patient breathes 100% oxygen. This 'washes out' the nitrogen in the lungs. The gas exhaled subsequently is collected and its total volume and the concentration of nitrogen are measured. The concentration of nitrogen in the lung before washout is 80%. The concentration of nitrogen left in the lung can be measured by a nitrogen meter at the lips, measuring end-expiration gas. Assuming no net change in the amount of nitrogen (it does not participate in gas exchange), it is possible to estimate the FRC.

Tests of diffusion

Oxygen and carbon dioxide pass by diffusion between the alveoli and pulmonary capillary blood. The diffusing capacity of carbon monoxide measures the ability of gas to diffuse from inspired air to capillary blood, and also reflects the uptake of oxygen from the alveolus into the red blood cells. Carbon monoxide is used because:

- It is highly soluble.
- It combines rapidly with haemoglobin.
- The single-breath test is the test most commonly used to determine diffusing capacity.

Single-breath test

The patient takes a single breath from RV to TLC. The inhaled gas contains 0.28% carbon monoxide and 13.5% helium. The patient is instructed to hold the breath for 10 seconds before expiring. The concentration of helium and carbon monoxide in the final part of the expired gas mixture is measured and the diffusing capacity of carbon monoxide is calculated. You need to know the haemoglobin level before the test.

In practice, the transfer factor is used in preference to the diffusing capacity. In the normal lung, the transfer factor accurately measures the diffusing capacity of the lungs, whereas in diseased lung diffusing capacity also depends on:

- Area and thickness of alveolar membrane.
- Ventilation:perfusion relationship.

Transfer factor

Transfer factor (T_LCO) is defined as the amount of carbon monoxide transferred per minute, corrected for the concentration gradient of carbon monoxide across the alveolar capillary membrane (Fig. 10.14).

The transfer factor is reduced in conditions where there are:

- Fewer alveolar capillaries.
- Ventilation:perfusion mismatches.
- Reduced accessible lung volumes.

Fig. 10.14	Conditions that affect the transfer factor	
	Decreased transfer factor	**Increased transfer factor**
Pulmonary causes	Emphysema; loss of lung tissue; diffuse infiltration	Pulmonary haemorrhage
Cardiovascular causes	Low cardiac output, pulmonary oedema	Thyrotoxicosis
Other causes	Anaemia	Polycythaemia

Gas transfer is a relatively sensitive but non-specific test, useful for detecting early disease in lung parenchyma; transfer coefficient is a better test. The transfer coefficient (KCO) is corrected for lung volumes and is useful in distinguishing causes of low T_LCO due to loss of lung volume:

- T_LCO and KCO are low in emphysema and fibrosing alveolitis.
- T_LCO is low, but KCO is normal, in pleural effusions and consolidation.

Testing lung mechanics

Lung compliance

Compliance is a measure of distensibility. It is defined as the volume change per unit of pressure across the lung. Lung compliance increases in emphysema, as the lung architecture is destroyed. In contrast, pulmonary fibrosis stiffens alveolar walls and decreases compliance (Fig. 10.15).

Lung compliance is measured by introducing a balloon into the oesophagus to estimate intrapleural pressure and then asking the patient to breathe out from TLC into a spirometer. This produces a pressure–volume curve. A lung of high compliance expands to a greater extent than one of low compliance when both are exposed to the same transpulmonary pressure.

Airway resistance

Airway resistance is defined as the pressure difference between the alveolus and mouth required to produce air flow of 1 L/s. Airway resistance is predominantly created by the upper respiratory tract but can be increased by asthma, COPD and endobronchial obstruction (e.g. tumour or foreign body).

Airway resistance can be measured by plethysmography. The patient is instructed to pant, causing pressure within the plethysmograph to increase during inspiration and decrease during expiration. The greater the airway resistance, the greater are the pressure swings in the chest and plethysmograph.

Closing volume

As lung volumes decrease on expiration, there is a point at which smaller airways begin to close; this is known as the closing volume of the lungs (Fig. 10.16). Closing volume is usually expressed as a percentage of vital capacity. In young subjects, closing volume is approximately 10% of vital capacity and increases with age, being approximately 40% of vital capacity at 65 years of age.

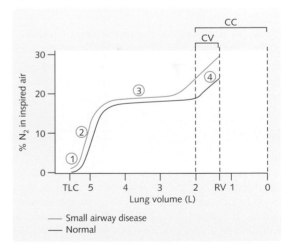

— Small airway disease
— Normal

Fig. 10.16 Closing volume. Airways in lower lung zones close at low lung volumes and only those alveoli at the top of the lungs continue to empty. Because concentration of nitrogen in alveoli of upper zones is higher, the slope of the curve abruptly increases (phase 4). Phase 4 begins at larger lung volumes in individuals with even minor degrees of airway obstruction, increasing closing volume. CV = closing volume; CC = closing capacity; TLC = total lung capacity. (Courtesy of The Ciba Collection of Medical Illustrations, illustrated by Frank H Netter, 1979.)

Fig. 10.15	Causes of altered lung compliance
Reduced compliance	**Increased compliance**
Pulmonary venous pressure increased	Old age
Alveolar oedema	Emphysema
Fibrosis	Bronchoalveolar drugs
Airway closure	

In diseases such as asthma or COPD the smaller airways close earlier, i.e. at a higher lung volume. An increase in closing volume against predicted values is a sensitive measure of early lung disease and may even show changes caused by cigarette smoking before the patient is symptomatic.

The test uses the single-breath nitrogen method, as described above.

Exercise testing

Exercise testing is primarily used to:

- Diagnose unexplained breathlessness which is minimal at rest.
- Assess the extent of lung disease, by stressing the system.
- Determine the level of impairment in disability testing.
- Assist in differential diagnosis (e.g. when it is not known whether a patient is limited by cardiac or lung disease).
- Test the effects of therapy on exercise capacity.
- Prescribe a safe and effective exercise regime.

There are a number of established tests, including the shuttle test, and a progressive exercise test, which is commonly performed on a cycle ergometer.

Shuttle test

This is a standardized test in which the patient walks up and down a 10-metre course, marked by cones, in a set time interval. The time intervals are indicated by bleeps played from a tape recorder and become progressively shorter. The test is stopped if patients become too breathless or if they cannot reach the cone in the time

Fig. 10.17	Medical Reseach Council dyspnoea scale
Grade	Degree of breathlessness related to activities
1	Not troubled by breathlessness except on strenuous exercise
2	Short of breath when hurrying or walking up a slight hill
3	Walks slower than contemporaries on level ground because of breathlessness, or has to stop for breath when walking at own pace
4	Stops for breath after walking about 100 metres or after a few minutes on level ground
5	Too breathless to leave the house, or breathless when dressing or undressing

allowed. Usually, oxygen saturations, heart rate and breathlessness (using the Medical Research Council dyspnoea scale: Fig. 10.17) are measured at the beginning and the end to provide objective and subjective measures of the level of dyspnoea.

Cardiopulmonary exercise testing

This is performed in a laboratory and stresses the patient to a predetermined level based on heart rate. It is useful for preoperative assessment to assess suitability for anaesthetic. A number of tests are made as the patient exercises, including:

- Electrocardiograph.
- Volume of gas exhaled.
- Concentration of oxygen and carbon dioxide in exhaled gas.

The volume of gas exhaled per minute (V_E L/min), oxygen consumption (VO_2 L/min) and carbon dioxide output (VCO_2 L/min) are then calculated. The test indicates whether exercise tolerance is limited by the cardiovascular or respiratory system and assesses increases in heart rate and ventilation against a known oxygen uptake.

Further reading

Light, R., Macgregor, M., Luchsinger, P., et al., 1972. Pleural effusions: the diagnostic separation of transudates and exudates. Ann. Intern. Med. 77, 507–513.

The respiratory patient: imaging investigations

Objectives

By the end of this chapter you should be able to:
- Describe how to read a posteroanterior (PA) plain film chest radiograph.
- Describe the differences between collapse and consolidation.
- List indications for ultrasound in respiratory medicine.
- Understand other respiratory imaging techniques, such as computed tomography (CT) and magnetic resonance imaging (MRI) and discuss the pros and cons of V/Q scanning versus CT pulmonary angiogram (CTPA) in the diagnosis of pulmonary emboli.

PLAIN RADIOGRAPHY

The plain film radiograph is of paramount importance in the evaluation of pulmonary disease. The standard radiographic examinations of the chest are described below.

Posteroanterior erect radiograph (PA chest)

In the PA erect radiograph, X-rays travel from the posterior of the patient to the film, which is held against the front of the patient (Fig. 11.1). The scapula can be rotated out of the way, and accurate assessment of cardiac size is possible. The radiograph is performed in the erect position because:

- Gas passes upwards, making the detection of pneumothorax easier.
- Fluid passes downwards, making pleural effusions easier to diagnose.
- Blood vessels in mediastinum and lung are represented accurately.

Lateral radiograph

Lateral views help to localize lesions seen in PA views; they also give good views of the mediastinum and thoracic vertebrae (Fig. 11.2). Valuable information can be obtained by comparison with older films, if available.

In women of reproductive age, radiography should be performed within 28 days of last menstruation.

Reporting a chest X-ray

Always view chest radiographs on a viewing box and follow a set routine for reporting plain films. If possible, compare with the patient's previous films.

Clinical data

Take down the following details:
- Patient's name.
- Age and sex.
- Clinical problem.
- Date of radiography.

Technical qualities

Note that radiographs contain right- or left-side markers.

With good penetration of X-rays, you should just be able to see the vertebral bodies through the cardiac shadow. In overpenetration, the lung fields appear too black. Conversely, in underpenetration, the lung fields appear too white.

Note the projection (anteroposterior (AP), PA or lateral; erect or supine). This can give a good indication of the overall health of the patient, e.g. an erect PA film suggests the patient was able to sit or stand unaided, whereas a supine AP film suggests the patient was too unwell to move at all. To deduce whether the patient was straight or rotated, compare the sternal ends of both clavicles.

With adequate inspiration, you should be able to count six ribs anterior to the diaphragm. Make sure that the whole-lung field is included.

Also note any foreign bodies, such as endotracheal tubes, electrocardiograph leads or pacemakers. These can point towards the overall state of the patient, as well as possible comorbidities.

Lungs

The lung fields should look symmetrical, with fine lung markings throughout. It is easiest when describing an abnormality to divide the lung into approximate upper,

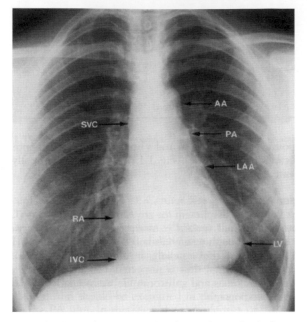

Fig. 11.1 Normal posteroanterior chest radiograph. The lungs are equally transradiant; the pulmonary vascular pattern is symmetrical. AA=aortic arch; SVC=superior vena cava; PA=pulmonary artery; LAA=left atrial appendage; RA=right atrium; LV=left ventricle; IVC=inferior vena cava. (Courtesy of Dr D Sutton and Dr JWR Young.)

middle and lower zones, rather than trying to guess a lobe (often impossible without a lateral film). If the lung fields are asymmetrical, combine with clinical findings to determine which is the abnormal side. If the lung fields look symmetrical, but abnormal, think of a pathology that would affect both lungs.

Some examples of common findings include:

- Reduced lung markings in one lung only – you should always rule out a pneumothorax. Look for a lung edge and tracheal deviation away from the affected side.
- Reduced lung markings in both lungs – think of destructive parenchymal disease such as emphysema.
- Patchy change in one lung – most likely an infectious process, such as bacterial pneumonia. If it is in the apex, consider tuberculosis.
- Patchy change in both lungs – consider parenchymal disease such as pulmonary fibrosis. Also consider non-respiratory causes, such as pulmonary oedema. This would be made more likely by a large heart shadow.
- Dense shadowing on one or both sides with a meniscus (air–fluid level) – likely a pleural effusion.
- Dense shadowing on one or both sides without a meniscus – could be consolidation, secondary to infection. If there is a complete 'white-out' of one lung, consider severe infection. Also check the history and make sure the patient hasn't had a pneumonectomy!
- Well-demarcated, round patches of shadowing – the most important thing to rule out here is malignancy. Further imaging and, if possible, a biopsy are needed. If the clinical findings are suggestive of infection, it could be an abscess – look for an air–fluid level.

Heart and mediastinum

When examining the cardiac shadow, observe the position, size and shape of the heart. It is important to note that, due to the projection of the X-rays in an AP film, you cannot accurately assess heart size, as it will always look bigger than it actually is. This can only be done on a PA film. A normal-size heart should be less than 50% of the width of the whole thorax. You must also assess if the cardiac borders are clearly visible. If they are not, this may indicate consolidation of the lung immediately next to them, which will be of similar density and will blur the border.

Note whether the trachea is central or deviated to either side. This information should be combined with findings in the lung fields. If the trachea is moving away from a lung field which has very few lung markings and looks very dark, think of a pneumothorax. If it is moving

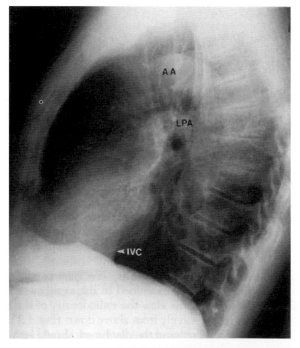

Fig. 11.2 Normal lateral chest radiograph. AA=aortic arch; LPA=left pulmonary artery; IVC=inferior vena cava. (Courtesy of Dr D Sutton and Dr JWR Young.)

towards a lung field which has increased lung markings and shadowing, consider lobar collapse. Identify blood vessels and each hilum. Very prominent blood vessels may be a sign of pulmonary hypertension.

Other

Note the following points:

- Diaphragm – visible behind the heart; costophrenic angles are acute and sharp. An erect chest X-ray can also be used by surgeons to rule out bowel perforation. If this is the case, air can be seen under the diaphragm (pneumoperitoneum).
- Bones – ribs, clavicles, sternum, thoracic vertebrae.
- Finally, recheck the apices, behind the heart, and hilar and retrodiaphragmatic regions.

Lateral radiograph

On a lateral radiograph, note the following:

- Diaphragm – right hemidiaphragm seen passing through the heart border.
- Lungs – divide lungs into area in front, behind and above the heart.
- Retrosternal space – an anterior mass will cause this space to be white.
- Fissures – horizontal fissure (faint white line that passes from midpoint of hilum to anterior chest wall); oblique fissure (passes from T4/5 through hilum to the anterior third of the diaphragm).
- Hilum.
- Bones – check vertebral bodies for shape, size and density; check sternum.

Interpreting abnormalities

Once you have completed your overall review of the film, return to any areas of abnormal lucency or opacity and assess them according to:

- Number – single or multiple.
- Position and distribution (lobar, etc.).
- Size, shape and contour.
- Texture (homogeneous, calcified, etc.).

The radiological features of common lung conditions are described below.

Collapse

Atelectasis (collapse) is loss of volume of a lung, lobe or segment for any cause. The most important mechanism is obstruction of a major bronchus by tumour, foreign body or bronchial plug.

PA and lateral radiographs are required. Compare with old films where available. The silhouette sign can help localize the lesion (Fig. 11.3).

Fig. 11.3 The silhouette sign	
Non-aerated area of lung	**Border that is obscured**
Right upper lobe	Right border of ascending aorta
Right middle lobe	Right heart border
Right lower lobe	Right diaphragm
Left upper lobe	Aortic knuckle and upper left cardiac border
Lingula of left lung	Left heart border
Left lower lobe	Left diaphragm

HINTS AND TIPS

The lateral borders of the mediastinum are silhouetted against the air-filled lung that lies underneath. This silhouette is lost if there is consolidation in the underlying lung.

Signs of lobar collapse

Signs of lobar collapse are:

- Decreased lung volume.
- Displacement of pulmonary fissures.
- Compensatory hyperinflation of remaining part of the ipsilateral lung.
- Elevation of hemidiaphragm on ipsilateral side.
- Mediastinal and hilar displacement; trachea pulled to side of collapse.
- Radiopacity (white lung).
- Absence of air bronchogram.

Some signs are specific to lobe involvement.

In upper-lobe collapse of the right lung, a PA film is most valuable in making the diagnosis; the collapsed lobe lies adjacent to the mediastinum (Fig. 11.4A).

In the left lung, a lateral film is most valuable in making the diagnosis; the lobe collapses superomedially and anteriorly (Fig. 11.4B).

Lower-lobe collapse causes rotation and visualization of the oblique fissure on PA film.

A lateral film is most valuable in diagnosing middle-lobe collapse. A thin, wedge-shaped opacity between horizontal and oblique fissures is seen.

Consolidation

Consolidation is seen as an area of white lung and represents fluid or cellular matter where there would normally be air (Figs 11.5 and 11.6). There are many causes of consolidation, including:

- Pneumonia.
- Pulmonary oedema.

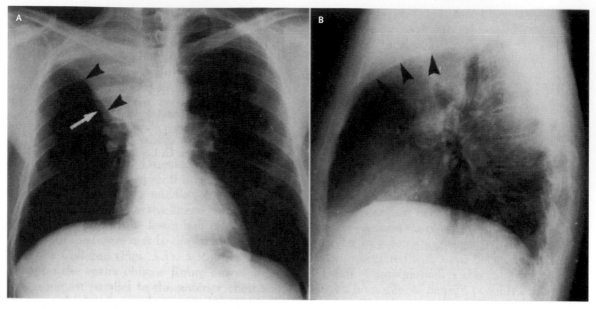

Fig. 11.4 (A and B) Right upper-lobe collapse. The horizontal and oblique fissures (black arrowheads) are displaced. There is a mass (white arrow) at the right hilum. (Courtesy of Dr D Sutton and Dr JWR Young.)

Fig. 11.5 Radiological distribution of alveolar processes		
	Bat-wing pattern	
Segmental pattern	**Acute**	**Chronic**
Pneumonia	Pulmonary oedema	Atypical pneumonia
Pulmonary infarct	Pneumonia	Lymphoma
Segmental collapse	Pulmonary haemorrhage	Sarcoidosis
Alveolar cell carcinoma		Pulmonary alveolar proteinosis
		Alveolar cell carcinoma

In contrast to collapse:

- The shadowing is typically heterogeneous (i.e. not uniform).
- The border is ill defined.
- Fissures retain their normal position.

There are two patterns of distribution:

- Segmental or lobar distribution.
- Bat-wing distribution.

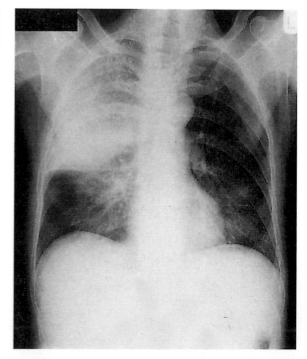

Fig. 11.6 Consolidation of the right upper lobe. (Courtesy of Professor CD Forbes and Dr WF Jackson.)

106

Peripheral lung fields may be spared (e.g. in pulmonary oedema). Air bronchograms may be seen, because they are delineated by surrounding consolidated lung.

Interstitial patterns

Three types of interstitial pattern exist (linear, nodular and honeycomb), and overlap may occur.

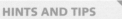

> **HINTS AND TIPS**
>
> An elderly woman presented to her GP with fever, a productive cough and general malaise. A chest X-ray showed left lower-lobe consolidation with air bronchograms. Air bronchograms are mostly seen in infection, when consolidated alveoli are lying adjacent to air-filled small and medium bronchioles. These radiographic features suggested a left lower-lobe pneumonia, for which she was treated accordingly.

Linear pattern

A linear pattern is seen as a network of fine lines running throughout the lungs. These lines represent thickened connective tissue and are termed Kerley A and B lines:

> **HINTS AND TIPS**
>
> Kerley B lines can help to limit the possible diagnoses. They are caused by increased fluid between alveoli, in the interlobular septa. They are seen in pulmonary oedema and malignant lymphatic infiltration.

Nodular pattern

This pattern is seen as numerous well-defined small nodules (1–5 mm) evenly distributed throughout the lung. Causes include miliary tuberculosis and chickenpox pneumonia.

Honeycomb pattern

A honeycomb pattern indicates extensive destruction of lung tissue, with lung parenchyma replaced by thin-walled cysts. Pneumothorax may be present. Normal pulmonary vasculature is absent. Pulmonary fibrosis leads to a honeycomb pattern. This must be quite severe to be seen on chest X-ray. It is more commonly identified on CT scan.

Pulmonary nodules

Solitary nodules

The finding of a solitary pulmonary nodule on a plain chest radiograph is not an uncommon event. The nodule, which is commonly referred to as a coin lesion, is usually well circumscribed, less than 6 cm in diameter, lying within the lung. The rest of the lung appears normal and the patient is often asymptomatic.

A solitary nodule on a chest X-ray may be an artefact or it may be due to:

* Malignant tumour – bronchial carcinoma or secondary deposits
* Infection – tuberculosis (Fig. 11.7) or pneumonia.
* Benign tumour – hamartoma.

If the patient is older than 35 years of age, then malignancy should be at the top of the list of possible differential diagnoses. If the lesion is static for a long period of time, as determined by reviewing previous radiographs, then it is likely to be a benign lesion. However, a slow-growing nodule in an elderly patient is likely to be malignant.

It is important to take into account clinical history and compare with a past chest radiograph if available. You should be able to distinguish carcinoma from other causes:

* Size of lesion – if lesion is > 4 cm diameter, be suspicious of malignancy.
* Margin – an ill-defined margin suggests malignancy.
* Cavitation indicates infection or malignancy.

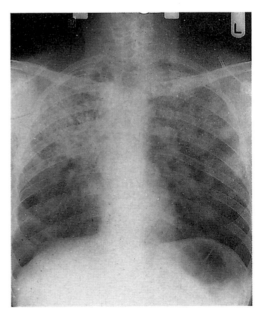

Fig. 11.7 Tuberculosis in a Greek immigrant to the UK. This film shows multiple areas of shadowing, especially in the upper lobes, and several lesions have started to cavitate. (Courtesy of Professor CD Forbes and Dr WF Jackson.)

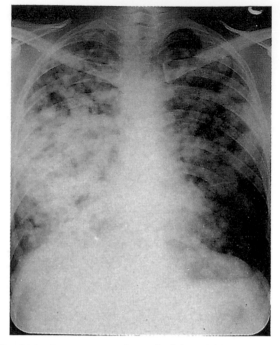

Fig. 11.8 Snowstorm mottling in both lung fields. In this case, the underlying diagnosis was testicular seminoma, with disseminated haematogenous metastases. (Courtesy of Professor CD Forbes and Dr WF Jackson.)

- Calcification – unlikely to be malignancy.
- Presence of air bronchogram – sign of consolidation, not malignancy.

Multiple nodules

Metastases are usually seen as well-defined nodules varying in size, which are more common at the periphery of lower lobes (Fig. 11.8) – they are also known as cannonball metastases; cavitation may be present. Abscesses are cavitated with a thick and irregular wall. Cysts are often large.

Other nodules include:

- Rheumatoid nodules.
- Wegener's granulomatosis.
- Multiple arteriovenous malformations.

Hilar masses

Normal hilar complex includes:

- Proximal pulmonary arteries and bifurcations.
- Bronchus.
- Pulmonary veins.
- Lymph nodes, not seen unless enlarged.

Hilar size varies from person to person, so enlargement is difficult to diagnose (Fig. 11.9). Radiological features of the hilum are:

- Concave lateral margin.

Fig. 11.9	Causes of hilar enlargement	
	Bilateral enlargement	
Unilateral enlargement	**Enlarged lymph nodes**	**Enlarged vessels**
Bronchial carcinoma	Lymphomas	Left-to-right cardiac shunts
Metastatic malignancy	Sarcoidosis	Pulmonary arterial hypertension
Lymphomas	Cystic fibrosis	Chronic obstructive pulmonary disease
Primary tuberculosis	Infectious mononucleosis	Left heart failure
Sarcoidosis	Leukaemia	Pulmonary embolism
Pulmonary embolus		
Pulmonary valve stenosis		

- Equal radiopacity.
- Left hilum lies higher than right.

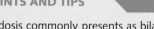
HINTS AND TIPS

Sarcoidosis commonly presents as bilateral lymphadenopathy.

PA films are most valuable in assessing hilar shadow, but you must always consult the lateral film. Technical qualities of the film need to be adequately assessed before conclusions can be made because patient rotation commonly mimics hilar enlargement.

Mediastinal masses

A mediastinal mass typically has a sharp, concave margin, visible due to the silhouette sign. Lateral films may be particularly useful. Mediastinal masses are frequently asymptomatic and are grouped according to their anatomical position (Fig. 11.10). CT is advised where there is a doubt as to the nature of the lesion.

Anterior mediastinal masses

Characteristics of anterior mediastinal masses are:

- Hilar structures still visible.
- Mass merges with the cardiac border.
- A mass passing into the neck is not seen above the clavicles.
- Small anterior mediastinal masses are difficult to see on PA films.

Fig. 11.10	Mediastinal masses	
Anterior masses	Middle masses	Posterior masses
Retrosternal thyroid	Bronchial carcinoma	Neurogenic tumour
Thymic mass	Lymphoma	Paravertebral abscess
Dermoid cyst	Sarcoidosis	Oesophageal lesions
Lymphomas	Primary tuberculosis	Aortic aneurysm
Aortic aneurysm	Bronchogenic cyst	

Middle mediastinal masses

- A middle mediastinal mass merges with hila and cardiac border.
- The majority are caused by enlarged lymph nodes.

Posterior mediastinal masses

In posterior mediastinal masses the cardiac border and hila are seen but the posterior aorta is obscured. Vertebral changes may be present.

HINTS AND TIPS

Tension pneumothorax is seen as a displacement of the mediastinum and trachea to the contralateral side, depressed ipsilateral diaphragm and increased space between the ribs.

Pleural lesions

Pneumothorax

Pneumothorax is usually obvious on normal inspiratory PA films. Look carefully at upper zones, because air accumulates first here; you will see an area devoid of lung markings (black lung), with the lung edge outlined by air in the pleural space. Small pneumothoraces can be identified on the expiratory film and may be missed in the supine film.

Tension pneumothorax

Tension pneumothorax is a medical emergency. You should never see a chest X-ray of a tension pneumothorax, as it is life-threatening. If you suspect your patient has one and he or she is increasingly dyspnoeic, you must treat the condition immediately.

Pleural effusions

PA erect radiography is performed. Classically, there is a radiopaque mass at the base of the lung and blunting of the costophrenic angle, with the pleural meniscus higher laterally than medially. Large effusions can displace the mediastinum contralaterally.

A horizontal upper border implies that a pneumothorax is also present. An effusion has a more homogeneous texture than consolidation and air bronchograms are absent.

Mesothelioma

Mesothelioma is a malignant tumour of the pleura, which may present as discrete pleural deposits or as a localized lesion.

On chest X-ray, thickened pleura is seen; in 50% of cases the pleural plaques lie on the medial pleura, causing the medial margin to be irregular. Pleural effusions are common, usually containing blood (Fig. 11.11). Rib destruction is uncommon.

Vascular patterns

Normal vascular pattern

Lung markings are vascular in nature. Arteries branch vertically to upper and lower lobes. On erect films, upper-lobe vessels are smaller than lower-lobe vessels. It is difficult to see vessels in the peripheral one-third of lung fields.

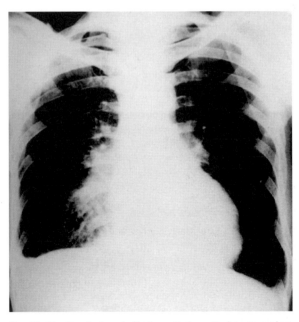

Fig. 11.11 Small pleural effusions. Both costophrenic angles are blunted. (Courtesy of Dr D Sutton and Dr JWR Young.)

Pulmonary venous hypertension

On erect films, upper-lobe vessels are larger than lower-lobe vessels. Pulmonary venous hypertension is associated with oedema and pleural effusions.

Pulmonary arterial hypertension

Pulmonary arterial hypertension is seen as bilateral hilar enlargement associated with long-standing pulmonary disease.

Testing patterns of ventilation

Ventilation:perfusion relationships

Ventilation:perfusion relationships are measured by means of isotope scans (also known as *V/Q* scans); these are described below.

Ventilation scans

Ventilation is detected by inhalation of a gas or aerosol labelled with the radioisotope Xe. The patient breathes and rebreathes the gas until it comes into equilibrium with other gases in the lung.

Inequality of ventilation

In diseases such as asthma or chronic obstructive pulmonary disease (COPD) the lungs may be unevenly ventilated. Inequality of ventilation is measured using the single-breath nitrogen test, similar to the method for measuring anatomical dead space, described above.

Perfusion scans

Radioactive particles larger than the diameter of the pulmonary capillaries are injected intravenously, where they remain for several hours. ^{99m}Tc-labelled macro-aggregated albumin (MAA) is used. A gamma camera is then used to detect the position of the MAA particles. The pattern indicates the distribution of pulmonary blood flow.

Inequality of perfusion

This occurs in conditions such as a pulmonary embolus, where there is good ventilation of the lung but poor perfusion due to venous thrombosis. This can be detected using a *V/Q* scan or, more commonly nowadays, with a specialized CT scan focusing on the pulmonary vasculature.

Ventilation:perfusion scans

Ventilation:perfusion scans are primarily used to detect pulmonary emboli. The principle is that a pulmonary embolus produces a defect on the perfusion scan (a filling defect) which is not matched by a defect on the ventilation scan, i.e. there is an area of the lung that is ventilated but not perfused.

Diagnosis of pulmonary embolism

Abnormalities in the perfusion scan are checked against a plain chest X-ray; defects on the perfusion scan are not diagnostic if they correspond to radiographic changes. Scans are classified based on the probability of a pulmonary embolism as:

1. Normal – commonly reported as 'low probability'.
2. High probability.
3. Non-diagnostic.

Non-diagnostic scans include those where patients have obstructive diseases such as asthma or COPD which lead to perfusion and ventilation defects; pulmonary embolus cannot be diagnosed if such a pattern is obtained – other investigations (see below) are then indicated.

PULMONARY ANGIOGRAPHY

Pulmonary angiography is the gold standard test for diagnosing pulmonary embolus.

The test is performed by injecting contrast media through a catheter introduced into the main pulmonary artery using the Seldinger technique. Obstructed vessels or filling defects can be seen clearly and emboli show as filling defects. Despite the accuracy of the test, in practice pulmonary angiography is not often performed because it is invasive and time-consuming. A less invasive test involving CT (CTPA) is increasingly preferred.

CT pulmonary angiogram

A special type of CT scan called a CTPA is a non-invasive and accurate method to detect blood clots in the lungs. Unlike *V/Q* scans, it allows visualization of the clot itself, so that the size and number of clots can be assessed accurately. Unlike pulmonary angiography, it is considerably less invasive for the patient.

Computed tomography

CT is the imaging modality of choice for mediastinal and many pulmonary conditions. CT scans provide detailed cross-sectional images of the thorax. The images can be electronically modified to display different tissues (e.g. by using a bone setting compared with a soft-tissue setting).

The patient passes through a rotating gantry which has X-ray tubes on one side and a set of detectors on the other. Information from the detectors is analysed and displayed as a two-dimensional image on visual display units, then recorded.

CT gives a dose of radiation approximately 100 times that of a standard plain film chest radiograph.

Applications of computed tomography

Detection of pulmonary nodules
CT can evaluate the presence of metastases in a patient with known malignancy; however, it cannot distinguish between benign and malignant masses. It can also be a useful imaging modality for biopsy of these lesions.

Mediastinal masses
CT is a useful technique in searching for lymphadenopathy in a person with primary lung carcinoma.

Carcinoma of the lung
CT can evaluate the size of a lung carcinoma, and detect mediastinal extension and staging, including the detection of metastases in other organs.

Pleural lesions
CT is effective at detecting small pleural effusions and identifying pleural plaques (Fig. 11.12).

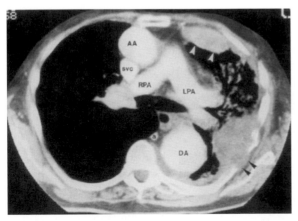

Fig. 11.12 Computed tomography (CT) scan of a pleural mass. Enhanced CT scan at level of bifurcation of main pulmonary artery. The left lung is surrounded by pleural masses (arrowheads), and the posterior mass is invading the chest wall. The vascular anatomy of the mediastinum is well shown. a = azygos vein (left of descending aorta); RPA = right pulmonary artery; LPA = left pulmonary artery; AA = ascending aorta; svc = superior vena cava; DA = descending aorta. (Courtesy of Dr D Sutton and Dr JWR Young.)

Vascular lesions
Contrast studies allow imaging of vascular lesions (e.g. aortic aneurysms).

High-resolution computed tomography

High-resolution CT is useful in imaging diffuse lung disease: thinner sections of 1–2 mm show greater lung detail (Fig. 11.13).

Applications of high-resolution computed tomography

Bronchiectasis
High-resolution CT has replaced bronchography. In dilated bronchi, the technique can show:

* Collapse.
* Scarring.
* Consolidation.

Interstitial lung disease
High-resolution CT is more specific than plain film radiography. Disorders that have specific appearances on high-resolution CT include sarcoidosis, occupational lung disease and interstitial pneumonia.

High-resolution CT can be used for biopsy guidance.

Atypical infections
High-resolution CT provides diagnosis earlier than using plain chest radiography and is useful in monitoring disease and response to treatment. It also provides good delineation of disease activity and destruction.

High-resolution CT is used in imaging of patients with acquired immunodeficiency syndrome (AIDS) (e.g. *Pneumocystis jiroveci* pneumonia).

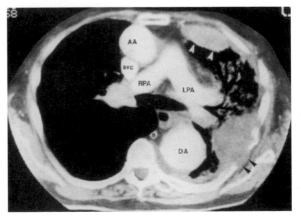

Fig. 11.13 Technical differences between computed tomography (CT) and high-resolution CT (HRCT). For abbreviations, see Figure 11.12.

Diagnosis of lymphangitis carcinomatosa

High-resolution CT can be used in the diagnosis of lymphangitis carcinomatosa.

Chronic obstructive pulmonary disease

High-resolution CT can be used to measure small-airways thickening, gas trapping and emphysema.

ULTRASOUND

Ultrasound uses high-frequency sound waves to image internal structures. In respiratory medicine the technique is primarily used in the investigation of pleural effusions and empyemas. Ultrasound can detect an effusion that is not seen on chest X-ray, or localize an effusion before it is drained by thoracocentesis.

A variation on this technique, Doppler ultrasound, is a non-invasive method for detecting deep vein thrombosis. It is used in investigating patients with suspected pulmonary thromboembolism. The technique examines blood flow and can detect thrombus in the veins above the popliteal fossa.

MAGNETIC RESONANCE IMAGING

MRI uses the magnetic properties of the hydrogen atom to produce images. MRI gives excellent imaging of soft tissues and the heart and its role in respiratory disease is increasing. It was initially not used much because air does not generate a signal on an MRI scan. However, it is being developed as a technique to obtain dynamic images of the lungs, through the inhalation of hyperpolarized inert gases such as xenon. Flowing blood does not provide a signal for MRI, and vascular structures appear as hollow tubes. MRI can be used to differentiate masses around the aorta or in the hilar regions. It has the advantage of not using ionizing radiation.

Useful links

http://www.clinicaltrials.ox.ac.uk/case-studies/imaging-the-invisible-air-we-breathe.

PART 3
RESPIRATORY CONDITIONS

Respiratory emergencies (12)

Objectives

By the end of this chapter you should be able to:
- Describe the presentation of common respiratory emergencies.
- Describe the investigations appropriate for common respiratory emergencies.
- Discuss the management of common respiratory emergencies.

INITIAL ASSESSMENT

When you are called to see a patient, it is important to be able to make a basic assessment of the seriousness of that patient's condition before starting a more thorough examination. It is definitely not good practice to start carefully looking at a patient's hands for clubbing, oblivious to the fact that your patient is extremely short of breath or very hypoxic! The method used by all doctors is very easy to remember, it's as easy as ABC.

A – Airway

Is your patient's airway patent? A simple way of determining this is to ask the patient a question. If the patient can reply, then it is obvious that the airway is patent. Listen for added sounds, such as stridor (a high-pitched wheezing noise) or gurgling, which may indicate obstruction of the upper airways. If this is the case, try simple techniques such as tilting the patient's head and lifting the chin, or thrusting the jaw forward, to open up the upper airways. If this is still not helping, an airway adjunct such as a nasopharyngeal or oropharyngeal airway may be of help. If this is not helping, more complex adjuncts, such as a laryngeal mask airway or even an endotracheal tube, may be necessary. It is important that if you begin to feel out of your depth, you must call a senior for help. Furthermore, only those trained to do so (such as anaesthetists) should intubate a patient.

B – Breathing

Once you have established a patent airway, the next thing to assess is breathing. All patients who have a respiratory emergency will need supplemental oxygen. There are a number of ways in which oxygen can be delivered. These include nasal cannulae, controlled O_2 via a Venturi mask (which ensures only a specific percentage of O_2 is delivered) and a non-rebreather mask.

In an emergency setting, you usually want as much oxygen as possible; therefore, a non-rebreather mask is the most effective, as it delivers 100% O_2.

Next you must assess the breathing itself. What is the patient's respiratory rate? Normal is between 12 and 16 breaths per minute. If the patient is talking to you, can the patient talk in full sentences or is he or she so breathless that he or she has to stop after every couple of words? You can use a finger probe to measure oxygen saturations. In a healthy person at rest, it should be 98–100%. However, in someone with chronic airways disease (such as chronic obstructive pulmonary disease (COPD)), normal for that individual might be anywhere from 88% upwards.

Next, it is time to examine the chest. In this crucial initial assessment, you can omit certain parts of the respiratory examination, such as examining the hands, as this can be done later and any signs will not be immediately helpful in saving the life of your patient.

C – Circulation

Once you are happy with the patient's breathing, you can assess the circulation. What is the patient's pulse and blood pressure? If the patient is tachycardic or hypotensive, now is the time to establish intravenous (IV) access. You should attempt to insert one cannula in each arm, as large a size as possible. Here, IV fluids may be appropriate.

It is important to remember that the ABC approach involves constant reassessment and is a continuous loop. Also, you must never move on to the next step before you are completely satisfied with the current one. There is no point administering oxygen to a patient who does not have a patent airway!

As stated previously, as a junior doctor, you must never be afraid to get senior help in these kinds of situation. If you are worried about a patient and feel you need more support, it is the responsible thing to do.

ACUTE RESPIRATORY DISTRESS SYNDROME (ARDS)

Definition

ARDS is non-cardiogenic pulmonary oedema defined as diffuse pulmonary infiltrates, refractory hypoxaemia, stiff lungs and respiratory distress (see Fig. 12.2, below). ARDS forms part of a systemic inflammatory reaction.

Prevalence

Between 15 and 18% of ventilated patients are affected, with 30–45% mortality.

Aetiology

See Figure 12.1.

Pathogenesis (Fig. 12.2)

The key feature of ARDS is non-cardiogenic pulmonary oedema. Pulmonary venous and capillary engorgement occurs, leading to interstitial oedema. Pulmonary epithelium damage also occurs.

Pulmonary hypertension is common; hypoxic vasoconstriction redirects blood to areas of greater oxygenation.

A protein-rich intra-alveolar haemorrhagic exudate promotes the formation of hyaline membranes that line alveolar ducts and alveoli.

In long-standing cases, pulmonary fibrosis ensues and the alveolar walls become lined by metaplastic cuboidal epithelium.

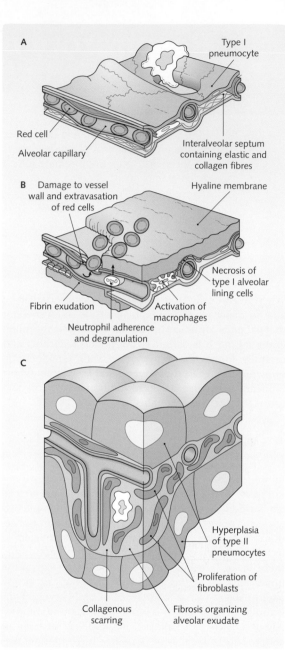

Fig. 12.2 Cell types in adult respiratory distress syndrome (ARDS). (A) Normal alveolar wall; (B) acute phase of ARDS; (C) organization phase of ARDS.

Fig. 12.1 Causes of acute respiratory distress syndrome, divided into pulmonary and extrapulmonary

Pulmonary	Extrapulmonary
Trauma or shock	Gram-negative septicaemia
Infection (e.g. pneumonia)	Pancreatitis
Gas inhalation (e.g. smoke)	Burns
Gastric contents aspiration	Cardiopulmonary bypass
Near drowning	Perforated viscus
Mechanical ventilation	Disseminated intravascular coagulation
	Oxygen toxicity
	Drug overdose (e.g. opiate)

Resolution

Resolution occurs as follows:
- Resorption of oedema.
- Ingestion of red cells and hyaline membranes by alveolar macrophages.
- Regeneration of type II pneumocytes.

Clinical features

Patients with ARDS present with:

- Tachypnoea, often unexplained.
- Dyspnoea.
- Cyanosis.
- Peripheral vasodilation.
- Bilateral fine inspiratory crackles on auscultation.

Investigations

- Blood tests: full blood count, urea and electrolytes, liver function tests, amylase, clotting screen, blood cultures.
- Arterial blood gas (ABG).
- Chest X-ray, which would demonstrate bilateral diffuse shadowing (Fig. 12.3).
- Pulmonary artery catheter to measure pulmonary capillary wedge pressure and demonstrate arterial hypoxaemia, refractory to oxygen therapy.

Management

The aim is to identify and treat the underlying cause whilst providing supportive measures.

Respiratory support: positive end-expiratory pressure (PEEP).

- PEEP prevents the alveolar walls from collapsing during expiration. However, low tidal volume ventilation is used to prevent overstretching the alveoli, which can worsen the lung injury. Also, ventilation in the prone position with ARDS patients has been

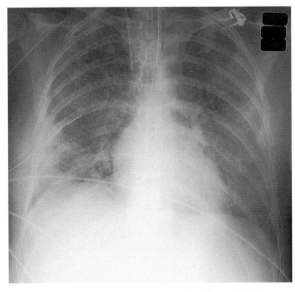

Fig. 12.3 Chest radiograph showing the bilateral diffuse shadowing seen in adult respiratory distress syndrome.

shown to be beneficial as ventilation is more evenly distributed throughout the lung.
- Non-ventilatory management such as the use of inhaled vasodilators (e.g. nitric oxide, prostacyclin) lowers pulmonary pressure and improves the V/Q matching in ARDS patients.
- Steroids have also been shown to be beneficial, especially in the late stages of ARDS, as they can dampen down the inflammation; steroids also have antifibrotic properties.
- The use of surfactant is highly beneficial in infant respiratory distress syndrome but there is no clear evidence of any benefit in ARDS.

Circulatory support

As in pulmonary oedema, the aim to achieve negative fluid balance.

RESPIRATORY FAILURE

Definition

Respiratory failure is defined as a P_aO_2 <8 kPa and can be further subdivided into type 1 or type 2, depending on P_aCO_2 level.

Respiratory failure is not a presentation seen in isolation but a possible outcome of many different respiratory diseases. During the initial stages of lung disease, the body maintains adequate oxygenation by adapting to increased ventilatory demand. However, if the underlying disease progresses, ventilatory workload may become excessive, which results in failure to oxygenate blood adequately as well as possibly failure to remove carbon dioxide by ventilation.

Prevalence

The prevalence of respiratory failure is approximately 78–88 per 100 000 population.

Type 1 respiratory failure

- Acute hypoxaemia: P_aO_2 low (<8 kPa).
- P_aCO_2 is normal or low.

Type 1 respiratory failure is primarily caused by ventilation perfusion (V/Q) mismatch.

Common causes include:

- Severe acute asthma.
- Pneumonia.
- Pulmonary embolism (PE).
- Pulmonary oedema.

Fig. 12.4 Common causes of respiratory failure, divided into categories of aetiology

Pulmonary	Reduced respiratory drive	Neuromuscular
Chronic obstructive pulmonary disease	Trauma	Cervical cord lesions
Asthma	Sedative drugs	Paralysis of diaphragm
Pneumonia	Central nervous system trauma	Myasthenia gravis
Pulmonary fibrosis		Guillain–Barré syndrome
Obstructive sleep apnoea		

Fig. 12.5 Symptoms of hypoxia and hypercapnia

Hypoxia (type 1 and 2 respiratory failure)	Hypercapnia (type 2 respiratory failure only)
Dyspnoea	Headaches
Restlessness and agitation	Drowsiness
Confusion	Confusion
Cyanosis (peripheral and central)	Tachycardia with a bounding pulse
	Tremor in hands
	Peripheral vasodilation
	Papilloedema

Type 2 respiratory failure

- Low P_aO_2 <8 kPa.
- High P_aCO_2 >6.5 kPa.

Type 2 respiratory failure is also known as ventilatory failure; the rise in P_aCO_2 is no longer matched by an increase in alveolar ventilation. This can be because:

- Ventilatory drive is insufficient.
- The work of breathing is excessive.
- The lungs are unable to pump air in and out efficiently.

Common causes are displayed in Figure 12.4.

The commonest cause is an acute exacerbation of COPD. Patients with COPD are often hypoxaemic and hypercapnic for many years, with morning headache being the only sign that P_aCO_2 is slightly raised. An acute exacerbation (e.g. due to respiratory infection) further increases the work of breathing, leading to 'acute-on-chronic' respiratory failure.

Clinical features

Depending on the type of respiratory failure, patients will demonstrate features of hypoxia ± hypercapnia (Fig. 12.5).

Investigations

Investigations should primarily focus on determining the underlying cause of respiratory failure. Some useful investigations include:

- Blood tests and blood cultures.
- ABG.
- Chest X-ray.
- Sputum culture.
- Use of spirometry in acute respiratory failure.

Management

Ultimately, management is dependent on the underlying cause of respiratory failure. However, the type of respiratory support provided depends on the type of respiratory failure.

Type 1 respiratory failure

- Give high-flow O_2 (35–60%) via facemask.
- Consider assisted ventilation if P_aO_2 remains <8 kPa despite 60% O_2 (usually with continuous positive airway pressure).

Type 2 respiratory failure

- Use O_2 therapy conservatively: start at 24% via facemask.
- Recheck P_aCO_2 after 20 minutes (ABG).
- If P_aCO_2 is stable, oxygen can be increased. If P_aCO_2 has risen, consider alternative support, i.e. non-invasive positive pressure ventilation such as biphasic positive airway pressure.

It is important to be cautious in giving oxygen to patients with type 2 respiratory failure on a background of chronic respiratory failure (such as those with severe COPD). Respiratory drive in these patients has become relatively insensitive to high P_aCO_2 (hypercapnia) and so their drive to breathe is stimulated by low P_aO_2 (hypoxic drive to breathe). Thus, giving high concentrations of oxygen will suppress ventilatory drive and P_aCO_2 may rise rather than fall.

PNEUMOTHORAX

Definition

Pneumothorax is the accumulation of air in the pleural space. It may occur spontaneously or following trauma.

Aetiology

Spontaneous

Pneumothorax results from rupture of a pleural bleb, the pleural bleb being a congenital defect of the alveolar wall connective tissue. Patients are typically tall, thin young males. Male-to-female ratio is 6:1. Spontaneous pneumothoraces are usually apical, affecting both lungs with equal frequency.

Secondary

Spontaneous pneumothoraces occur in patients with underlying disease such as COPD, tuberculosis, pneumonia, bronchial carcinoma, sarcoidosis or cystic fibrosis. They are particular common in those with COPD, where emphysematous bullae can spontaneously burst.

The main aim of treatment is to get the patient back to active life as soon as possible.

Clinical features

Pneumothoraces can be asymptomatic, especially if the patient is young and fit or if the pneumothorax is small. However, common symptoms include:

- Sudden-onset unilateral pleuritic chest pain.
- Increasing breathlessness.
- Sudden deterioration in existing lung condition (e.g. COPD).

Examination may reveal:

- Reduced chest expansion on the side of the pneumothorax.
- Hyperresonance to percussion (over the pneumothorax).
- Reduced, absent breath sounds on auscultation.

Investigations

Chest X-ray will demonstrate an area of increased radiolucency without lung markings (Fig. 12.6). The edge of the lung field may be visible away from the chest wall.

Management

Small pneumothoraces often require no treatment but are reviewed 7–10 days following presentation. Patients with moderately sized pneumothoraces are admitted for simple aspiration.

TENSION PNEUMOTHORAX

Tension pneumothorax is a medical emergency. The most common causes include:

- Positive pressure ventilation.
- Stab wound or rib fracture.

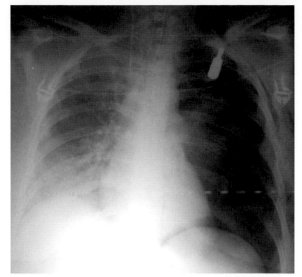

Fig. 12.6 Chest radiograph demonstrating a left-sided pneumothorax.

Air escapes into pleural space and the rise above atmospheric pressure causes the lung to collapse. At each inspiration intrapleural pressure increases as the pleural tear acts as a ball valve that permits air to enter but not leave the pleural space (unlike a simple pneumothorax, where air can flow in and out). Venous return to the heart is impaired as pressure rises and patients experience dyspnoea and chest pain. They may also be cyanotic. In extreme cases, a tension pneumothorax can lead to cardiac arrest.

Clinically:

- Mediastinum is pushed over into the contralateral hemithorax, causing tracheal deviation.
- There is hyperresonance and absence of breath sounds.
- Intercostal spaces are widened on the ipsilateral side.

Investigations

If a tension pneumothorax is suspected, it should be treated immediately before ordering investigations. Where the diagnosis is unclear, the following investigations are useful:

- Chest X-ray (Fig. 12.7):
  - Mediastinal shift and tracheal deviation.
  - Large area of hyperlucency with absent lung markings.
- Electrocardiograph (ECG):
  - Rightward shift in mean frontal QRS complex.
  - Diminution in QRS amplitude.
  - Inversion of precordial T waves.

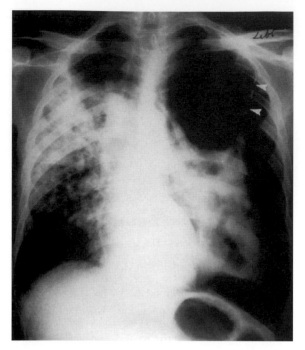

Fig. 12.7 Radiograph of a tension pneumothorax displacing mediastinum and depressing the left hemidiaphragm. Extensive consolidation and cavitation in both lungs are due to tuberculosis. A pleural adhesion (arrowheads) is visible. (Courtesy of Dr D Sutton and Dr JWR Young.)

Management

Immediate management should be a large-bore cannula (the biggest you can find) inserted into the second intercostal space in the mid-clavicular line, on the side of the pneumothorax. Once the immediate pressure has been relieved and the patient stabilized, a chest drain with underwater seal should be inserted.

FOREIGN-BODY ASPIRATION

Aspiration of a foreign body can be life-threatening. It is most commonly seen in children but can occur at any age. The most serious cases are those where the foreign body lodges in the larynx or trachea, as this causes complete airway obstruction. If the object tracks down to below the carina (more commonly to the right main bronchus as it has a more vertical position), it can often go unnoticed for some time, with only mild symptoms.

Prevalence

The prevalence of foreign-body aspiration is variable depending on age group. It is most common in the very young and very old.

Aetiology

Foreign bodies encompass a wide variety of objects. In young children, these tend to be toys and small household objects, which are put in the mouth out of curiosity. However, in the older population, aspiration may occur in those who have a poor swallow (such as following a stroke).

Clinical features

In upper airways:

- Stridor.
- Respiratory distress.
- Cyanosis.
- Respiratory arrest.

Beyond the carina:

- Recurrent cough.
- Pneumonia.
- Shortness of breath.
- Haemoptysis.

Investigations

- Blood tests – may demonstrate an inflammatory response.
- Chest X-ray – will show up any radiopaque objects, and may also demonstrate pneumonia.
- Bronchoscopy – direct visualization of the object.

Management

- If the object is in the proximal airways, try simple techniques such as the Heimlich manoeuvre.
- Airway suction.
- If the object is further down the airways, remove it at bronchoscopy.
- Antibiotics to prevent/treat pneumonia. If secondary to aspiration of gastric contents, antibiotics need to cover gut bacteria.

PULMONARY EMBOLISM

A pulmonary embolus (PE) arises when an embolus (abnormal mass of material) derived from a venous thrombus is transported in the bloodstream and impacts in the pulmonary arterial tree (i.e. the lumen of a pulmonary vessel, which is too small to allow the passage of an embolus). Most thrombi originate in the deep veins of the calf or pelvis.

Prevalence

This is a common condition: the incidence of PE at autopsy has been reported to be 12%.

Aetiology

There are several predisposing factors for PE, including:

- Immobilization (e.g. prolonged bedrest, long-haul flight).
- Oral contraceptive pill (minor risk factor, increased by cigarette smoking).
- Malignancy, especially of pancreas, uterus, breast and stomach.
- Cardiac failure.
- Chronic pulmonary disease.
- Surgery.
- Fractures of the pelvis or lower limb.
- Hypercoagulable states (e.g. pregnancy).

Clinical features

The clinical features of PE depend greatly on the size, distribution and number of PE. A small one may be asymptomatic, whereas a large PE is often fatal.

Symptoms

- Sudden-onset severe chest pain.
- Dyspnoea.
- Haemoptysis.
- Syncope.
- Swollen or tender calf (indicating a deep vein thrombosis and thus the source of the PE).

On examination, features of shock are commonly present, i.e. tachycardia and hypotension. Other features that can be detected include:

- Gallop rhythm.
- Right ventricular heave.
- Prominent a-wave in the jugular venous pulse.
- Hypoxia, especially on exertion.

Investigations

The index of suspicion for a PE can be determined clinically using the Wells score (Fig. 12.8).

- Chest X-ray: usually unremarkable, but valuable in excluding other causes.
- ECG may show signs of right ventricular strain (deep S waves in lead I, Q waves in lead III, and inverted T waves in lead III).
- ABG shows arterial hypoxaemia and hypocapnia (low P_aO_2 and low P_aCO_2).
- A D-dimer test should only performed where there is a low probability of a PE (according to Wells score). It is not diagnostic for a PE, as D-dimer can also be elevated in infection, malignancy and post surgery. However a negative test result makes the presence of an acute PE very unlikely and thus can be used

to exclude PE in patients with a low probability of PE according to Wells score.
- Radioisotope V/Q scans demonstrate ventilated areas of lung and filling defects on the corresponding perfusion scans.
- A computed tomography pulmonary angiogram is now the most commonly used imaging, eclipsing the V/Q scan, as it allows direct imaging of the clot, and thus accurate assessment of clot size, number and location.

Fig. 12.8 The Wells score aids stratification of the likelihood a patient has a pulmonary embolism (PE)	
Clinical signs and symptoms of DVT?	Yes +3
PE is No. 1 diagnosis, or equally likely	Yes +3
Heart rate > 100 bpm?	Yes +1.5
Immobilization at least 3 days, or surgery in the previous 4 weeks?	Yes +1.5
Previous, objectively diagnosed PE or DVT?	Yes +1.5
Haemoptysis?	Yes +1
Malignancy with treatment within 6 months, or palliative?	Yes +1

Patient has none of these: score 0=low probability, 1–2=moderate probability, >3=high probability. DVT=deep vein thrombosis.

Management

Treatment is based on providing supportive management (oxygen and analgesia), anticoagulation and thrombolysis if necessary.

Patients are anticoagulated with low-molecular-weight heparin (e.g. dalteparin), which is given subcutaneously. Oral anticoagulants, i.e. warfarin, should also be started; when the patient's international normalized ratio >2, heparin can be stopped and the patient should remain on warfarin for 6 months. If the patient has more than one PE or deep vein thrombosis, lifelong warfarin should be initiated.

INR

Thrombolysis is indicated in patients who are haemodynamically unstable (e.g. hypotensive). It is possible to break down thrombi by:

- Intravenous streptokinase 250 000 IU infusion over 30 minutes.
- Intravenous streptokinase 100 000 IU hourly for up to 24 hours.

Surgery is performed only on massive PE in patients who fail to respond to thrombolysis.

Prevention

This is achieved by avoidance of deep vein thromboses:

- Early mobilization of patients after operation.
- Use of tight elastic stockings.
- Leg exercises.
- Prophylactic anticoagulation.

ACUTE ASTHMA

Definition

Acute asthma is asthma that is acutely worsening over a period of hours to days and which is not responsive to the patient's normal asthma medications. It requires either an increase in the patient's normal treatments or new, more complex treatment.

Prevalence

There are 77 000 hospital admissions for asthma each year.

Clinical features

See Figure 12.9.

Management

- High-flow oxygen (100%).
- 4–6 puffs, each inhaled separately, of a β_2 agonist (salbutamol or terbutaline) from a metered dose inhaler via a spacer. Repeat every 10–20 minutes. Give via a nebulizer if the asthma is life-threatening.
- Prednisolone 40–60 mg orally or, if the patient cannot swallow tablets, parenteral hydrocortisone 400 mg.
- If there is a poor response to the above, consider the anticholinergic bronchodilator ipratropium bromide (0.5 mg 4–6-hourly via nebulizer) in addition

to a β_2 agonist, or a single dose of magnesium sulphate (1.2–2 mg IV infusion over 20 minutes).
- If the response is still poor, consider the bronchodilator aminophylline IV (5 mg/kg loading dose over 20 minutes, then infusion of 0.5–0.7 mg/kg/hour). If the patient already takes regular aminophylline, the loading dose is not required.

PULMONARY OEDEMA

Definition

Pulmonary oedema is defined as an abnormal increase in the amount of interstitial fluid in the lung. The two main causes are:

1. Increased venous hydrostatic pressures.
2. Injury to alveolar capillary walls or vessels, leading to increased permeability.

Less common causes are blockage of lymphatic drainage and lowered plasma oncotic pressure.

Pathogenesis

High-pressure pulmonary oedema

High-pressure or haemodynamic pulmonary oedema is cardiogenic; it may occur acutely as a result of a myocardial infarction or chronically in aortic and mitral valve disease.

Fluid movement between intravascular and extravascular compartments is governed by Starling forces (Fig. 12.10). Net fluid flow through a capillary wall (out of the blood) is governed by:

- Hydrostatic pressure (arterial blood pressure) at the arteriole end of the capillary bed.
- Capillary permeability.
- Opposing oncotic pressure exerted by serum proteins (mainly albumin); interstitial oncotic pressure may also contribute to the outflow.

Fig. 12.9 Main symptoms and signs of acute asthma, according to severity

Features	Mild/moderate	Severe	Life-threatening
Talking	Complete sentences	Unable to complete sentences	Can't talk at all
Distress	Minimal	Marked	Very severe
Accessory muscles	No	Yes	Yes
Peak flow	>50% predicted	33–50% predicted	<33% predicted
Other		Tachycardic Tachypnoeic	Silent chest Poor respiratory effort Fatigue Coma

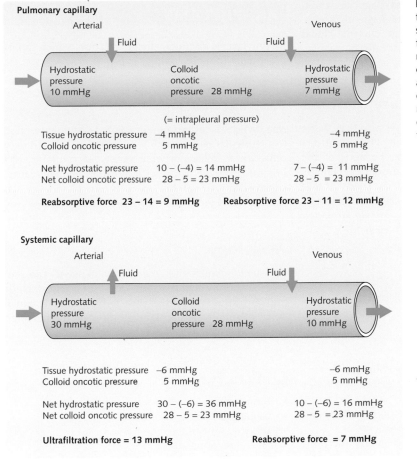

Fig. 12.10 Comparison of Starling's forces between pulmonary and systemic capillary beds. The resorptive force is positive and hence fluid is reabsorbed into the pulmonary capillary. Without surfactant in the alveoli, the tissue hydrostatic pressure could be −23 mmHg and the resorptive force would be −10 mmHg, causing transudation of fluid into the alveolus.

Reabsorption of interstitial fluid is governed by:

- Plasma oncotic pressure (pulling pressure).
- Hydrostatic pressure in the interstitial space (tissue pressure).
- Fall in hydrostatic pressure at the venous end of the capillary.

Imbalances in Starling forces and a reduced plasma oncotic pressure will cause expansion of the interstitial spaces.

No pathological conditions cause a local reduction of plasma protein concentration within the lung capillaries. However, many conditions (e.g. left ventricular failure) cause an elevation of hydrostatic pressure. If left atrial pressure rises, so do pulmonary venous and capillary pressures, thereby raising hydrostatic pressure and causing oedema formation. Pulmonary oedema occurs only after the lymphatic drainage capacity has been exceeded. Lymphatic drainage can increase 10-fold without oedema formation. However, if lymphatic drainage is blocked (e.g. in cancer), oedema occurs more readily.

Oedema due to haemodynamic causes has a low protein content.

Oedema caused by microvascular injury

This is the non-cardiogenic form of pulmonary oedema.

Capillary blood is separated from alveolar air by three anatomical layers:

1. Capillary endothelium.
2. Narrow interstitial layer.
3. Alveolar epithelium.

Damage to capillary endothelium

Normal alveolar capillary endothelial cells are joined by tight junctions containing narrow constrictions. Many conditions can damage the pulmonary capillary endothelium, resulting in movement of fluid and a transcapillary leak of proteins. Interstitial oncotic pressure rises; thus, a natural defence against oedema formation is disabled.

After damage, fibrinogen enters and coagulates within the interstitium. Interstitial fibrosis subsequently occurs, leading to impaired lymphatic drainage. Oedema caused by microvascular damage characteristically has a high protein content.

Progression of pulmonary oedema

Fluid first accumulates in loose connective tissue around the bronchi and large vessels. Fluid then distends the thick, collagen-containing portions of the alveolar wall. The final stage of pulmonary oedema is accumulation of fluid within the alveolar spaces. If pulmonary oedema is chronic, recurrent alveolar haemorrhages lead to the accumulation of haemosiderin-laden macrophages along with interstitial fibrosis.

Clinical features

- Acute breathlessness.
- Wheezing.
- Anxiety.
- Tachypnoea.
- Profuse perspiration.
- Production of pink sputum while coughing.
- Peripheral circulatory shutdown.
- Tachycardia.
- Basal crackles and wheezes heard on auscultation.
- Respiratory impairment with hypoxaemia.
- Overloaded lungs predispose to secondary infection.

Investigations

- Blood tests – brain natriuretic peptide can be elevated in congestive cardiac failure, but it is not specific.
- Chest X-ray – bilateral patchy shadowing, Kerley B lines, increased vascular shadowing (characteristic 'batwing' appearance), upper-lobe diversion and pleural effusions. If it is cardiogenic, the heart size may be enlarged.
- Echocardiogram – can be useful in an outpatient setting once the patient is stable, to establish left ventricular function.

Management

The patient should be placed in a sitting position and 60% O_2 administered. IV diuretics give an immediate and delayed response. Morphine sedates the patient and causes systemic vasodilatation: if systemic arterial pressure falls below 90 mmHg, do not use morphine. Aminophylline can be infused over 10 minutes, but should be used only when bronchospasm is present. A glyceryl trinitrate infusion can also help.

ANAPHYLAXIS

Anaphylaxis is a serious allergic reaction, which can be potentially life-threatening.

Pathogenesis

Anaphylaxis is an immune-mediated systemic reaction to a particular pathogen. It is mediated by IgE and mast cells, which release a wide variety of cytokines and inflammatory mediators such as histamine. This causes constriction of bronchial smooth muscle and vascular leakage throughout the body.

Aetiology

Various foodstuffs and environmental agents can provoke an anaphylactic reaction. Common agents include nuts, bee stings and drugs such as penicillin. The incidence of anaphylaxis is higher in those with other allergic diseases such as asthma or hayfever.

Clinical features

- Rash.
- Generalized itchiness.
- Wheeze and stridor.
- Shortness of breath.
- Tachycardia.
- Hypotension.
- Gastrointestinal symptoms such as nausea and diarrhoea.

Investigations

- The diagnosis of anaphylaxis is clinical.
- However, after the event, skin patch testing can be used to establish the likely cause of the reaction.

Management[1]

- Resuscitation with IV fluids and oxygen.
- Intramuscular (IM) adrenaline 0.5 mL of 1:1000.
- Chlorphenamine (an antihistamine) 10 mg IM or slow IV infusion.
- Hydrocortisone 200 mg IM or slow IV infusion.

Note that all of the above doses are for adults and children over the age of 12. Specific doses should be sought for children under the age of 12.

---

[1]http://www.resus.org.uk/pages/reaction.pdf

CARBON MONOXIDE POISONING

Carbon monoxide poisoning can be difficult to detect and diagnose. However, it is important to include this in a differential diagnosis if the patient is likely to have been exposed to it.

Pathogenesis

Carbon monoxide is an odourless gas which binds to haemoglobin to form carboxyhaemoglobin. This binds irreversibly, meaning that oxygen cannot bind to the haemoglobin, causing hypoxia.

Aetiology

Carbon monoxide poisoning can be caused by old gas heaters and boilers, which have poor oxygen supply and lead to incomplete combustion.

Clinical features

- Confusion.
- Headaches.
- Lightheadedness.
- Cardiac arrest.

Investigations

- Measurement of carbon monoxide levels in the blood.

Management

- 100% oxygen.
- If necessary, hyperbaric oxygen.

VENTILATION

Non-invasive

This is discussed further in Chapter 15.

Invasive

This occurs when a patient has had an endotracheal tube in place. The ventilator can be adjusted to provide different inspiratory and expiratory pressures depending on the patient's needs.

Broadly, mechanical ventilation is used for patients who are unable to maintain their own airway or for those in respiratory failure which is unresponsive to less invasive measures. More objective criteria are based on blood gases, such as a pH of <7.3, a P_aO_2 of <8 kPa or P_aCO_2 of >6 kPa, but these need to be used in combination with clinical features such as apnoea or respiratory distress with altered mental state.

All ventilated patients are managed on intensive therapy units (ITUs), as they almost always need further invasive monitoring and treatment.

It is important that discussions are had with the family of the patient and, if possible, the patient him- or herself, to discuss whether ITU and invasive ventilation are what the patient wants. A clinical judgement needs to be made as to the suitability of the patient for ITU, as a patient with a poor premorbid state may not be fit enough to be weaned off a ventilator and would therefore not survive a stay on ITU.

Useful links

http://www.ncbi.nlm.nih.gov/pmc/articles/PMC270706/.
http://www.patient.co.uk/doctor/Acute-Severe-Asthma-and-Status-Asthmaticus.htm.
http://www.resus.org.uk/pages/reaction.pdf.

Pulmonary hypertension (13)

Objectives

By the end of this chapter you should be able to:
- Define pulmonary hypertension and understand the basic pathophysiology.
- Be aware of the differences between classes of disease.
- Discuss appropriate investigations in the condition.
- Show awareness of pharmacological management options.

DEFINITION AND BACKGROUND

Pulmonary hypertension is a pathophysiological condition characterized by the presence of a sustained mean pulmonary artery pressure of >25 mmHg at rest, as assessed by right heart catheterization. Primary hypertension can be due to numerous medical conditions. Pulmonary arterial hypertension (PAH) is a clinical condition characterized by precapillary primary hypertension in the absence of other causes of precapillary primary hypertension, e.g. pulmonary disease. PAH is thus a far more specific diagnosis (Fig. 13.1). Note that previous definitions of an artery pressure of >30 mmHg during exertion are not supported by published data.

It may be helpful to refer to Chapter 3 for detail on the pulmonary circulation when working through this chapter.

PATHOPHYSIOLOGY

Pulmonary hypertension results from damage to the pulmonary endothelium. This damage can be secondary to numerous factors which cause either precapillary or postcapillary insult. The disorder can be classified by group, as per the 2009 European Society of Cardiology guidelines (Fig. 13.2).

Endothelial damage causes release of vasoconstrictive agents as well as procoagulant factors, leading to an increased constriction of the pulmonary vasculature as well as thrombus formation. The vasculature often attempts to remodel itself in response to the endothelial damage, and this process can lead to irreversible fibrosis of the pulmonary system.

EPIDEMIOLOGY

The incidence of true PAH is between 1 and 3 annual cases per million population, with the incidence of primary hypertension being higher. In particular, patients with connective tissue disease have a significantly increased risk of the condition.

Around 6–12% of cases are likely to be genetic in origin, with an autosomal dominant inheritance pattern. Numerous gene mutations have been implicated, including those involved in tumour growth factor-β.

PRESENTATION

Patients usually have non-specific insidious symptoms with few clinical signs, and as such the condition is often diagnosed late. The commonest signs and symptoms are detailed in Figure 13.3. These are usually due to heart failure secondary to raised pulmonary pressures, so-called cor pulmonale.

INVESTIGATION

Investigations are aimed at looking for both evidence of pulmonary hypertension as well as an underlying condition as cause for the disease. Only once all investigations have been normal, can a diagnosis of true PAH be made.

Common investigations involve an electrocardiograph looking for signs of right ventricular hypertrophy, a chest X-ray to look for evidence of cardiac failure and any underlying respiratory pathology, with progression to a computed tomography scan of the chest if there is suspicion of a fibrosis or emphysema, for example. Likelihood of diagnosis can be assessed with an echocardiogram analysing tricuspid regurgitation velocity. Other underlying causative conditions should be investigated, depending on the level of suspicion raised by the history, such as an autoantibody screen if connective tissue disease is likely. Diagnosis can only be confirmed using right heart catheterization.

Fig. 13.1 Defining pulmonary hypertension (PH)

Definition	Characteristics	Clinical group(s)
Pulmonary hypertension (PH)	Mean PAP ≥25 mmHg	All
Precapillary PH	Mean PAP ≥25 mmHg PWP ≤15 mmHg CO normal or reduced	1. Pulmonary arterial hypertension 3. PH due to lung diseases 4. Chronic thromboembolic PH 5. PH with unclear and/or multifactorial mechanisms
Postcapillary PH	Mean PAP ≥25 mmHg PWP ≥15 mmHg CO normal or reduced	2. PH due to left heart disease
Passive	TPG ≤12 mmHg	
Reactive (out of proportion)	TPG >12 mmHg	

PAP = pulmonary artery pressure; PWP = pulmonary wedge pressure; CO = cardiac output; TPG = transpulmonary artery gradient.

Fig. 13.2 Classification of aetiology of pulmonary artery hypertension (PAH)

PAH type	Main aetiologies
1	Idiopathic, inherited, secondary to connective tissue disease, HIV, portal HTN or congenital cardiac disease
2	Left cardiac disease
3	Pulmonary disease, e.g. COPD, interstitial lung disease
4	Chronic thromboembolic pulmonary hypertension
5	PH with unclear mechanism

HIV = human immunodeficiency virus; HTN = hypertension; COPD = chronic obstructive pulmonary disease; PH = pulmonary hypertension.

Fig. 13.3 Signs and symptoms consistent with a presentation of pulmonary hypertension

Symptoms	Signs (generally of right heart failure)
Shortness of breath	Right ventricular heave
Syncope or presyncope	Increased jugular venous pressure
Malaise and fatigue	Right ventricular third or fourth heart sound Right heart valve regurgitation murmurs Pedal oedema Orthopnoea

MANAGEMENT

Treatment is specific to diagnostic group, as per the guidelines. General principles include initial therapy with warfarin anticoagulation to minimize the risk of thrombosis, as well as calcium channel blockers to reduce the pressure in the pulmonary vasculature. Around 10–15% of patients respond to this therapy regime, at least initially. However, depending on the response from the patient, more advanced treatments can be trialled. These include endothelin receptor antagonists such as bosentan and prostanoid analogues such as nebulized iloprost or oral beraprost. Phosphodiesterase inhibitors such as sildenafil have also shown benefit. Lung transplant may be considered in severe end-stage disease.

Cardiac failure should be aggressively treated with diuretics, digoxin and antihypertensives.

PROGNOSIS

This is poor, as disease is often detected late and can be rapidly progressive and response to treatment is variable. Mean survival is 2–3 years from diagnosis. Death is usually secondary to right heart failure.

Further reading

European Society of Cardiology Clinical Practical Guidelines, 2009. Pulmonary Hypertension (Guidelines on Diagnosis and Treatment of). Available online at: http://www.escardio.org/guidelines-surveys/esc-guidelines/Pages/pulmonary-arterial-hypertension.aspx.

By the end of this chapter you should be able to:
- List the main viruses responsible for the common cold.
- Understand the aetiology and management of allergic rhinitis.
- Understand the key differences in the clinical presentation of croup and acute epiglottitis.
- List the main neoplasms affecting the upper respiratory tract.

DISORDERS OF THE NOSE

Inflammatory conditions

Infectious rhinitis (acute coryza or common cold)

Rhinitis is inflammation of the mucosal membrane lining the nose. Inflammation seen in the common cold is caused by a number of viral infections:

- Rhinovirus (commonest cause).
- Coronavirus.
- Adenovirus.
- Parainfluenza virus.
- Respiratory syncytial virus.

The common cold is a highly contagious, self-limiting condition, with the highest incidence in children. Symptoms are nasal obstruction, rhinorrhoea (runny nose) and sneezing. Complications include sinusitis, otitis media and lower respiratory tract infections.

Pathology
There is acute inflammation with oedema, glandular hypersecretion and loss of surface epithelium.

Treatment
Infections with such viruses are self-limiting and no medical treatment is required. Analgesia and nasal decongestants can be used to relieve symptoms.

Chronic rhinitis

Chronic rhinitis may develop following an acute inflammatory episode. Predisposing factors such as inadequate drainage of sinuses, nasal obstruction caused by polyps and enlargement of the adenoids increase the risk of developing chronic rhinitis.

Allergic rhinitis

Definition
Allergic rhinitis is an inflammatory condition of the nasal mucosa caused by an IgE-mediated response to common environmental allergens.

Epidemiology
Allergic rhinitis is a common condition: prevalence has been estimated to be 15–20%. Symptoms of allergic rhinitis most commonly present in childhood and adolescence; it is estimated that 80% of people with the condition develop symptoms before the age of 20.

The prevalence of allergic rhinitis is equal in men and women; however, the age at which men and women develop symptoms differs. Men are more likely to develop allergic rhinitis in childhood, whereas the peak incidence in women occurs during adolescence. There is a geographical variation in the prevalence of allergic rhinitis – it is much more common in developed countries than in developing countries.

Aetiology
The development of allergic rhinitis cannot be attributed to one single genetic or enviromental factor. It is likely to arise as a result of interaction between multiple genes and specific environmental variables (Fig. 14.1).

A family history of atopy is an important risk factor for developing allergic rhinitis. Studies have suggested that the risk of developing atopic disease in the absence of parental family history is only 13%. This risk increases to 47% if both parents are atopic and 72% if both parents have the same atopic manifestation.

Environmental factors also play a large role in the development of allergic rhinitis; many believe the 'hygiene hypothesis' can account for the increasing prevalence of allergic rhinitis in the Western world. The hygiene hypothesis suggests that lack of exposure to bacteria and microorganisms in childhood (i.e. our

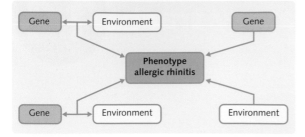

Fig. 14.1 Polygenic inheritance of allergic rhinitis.

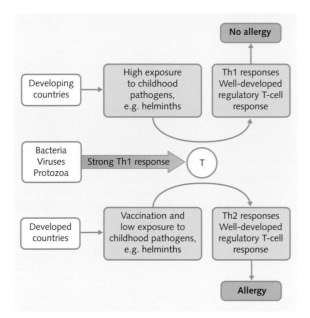

Fig. 14.2 Hygiene hypothesis.

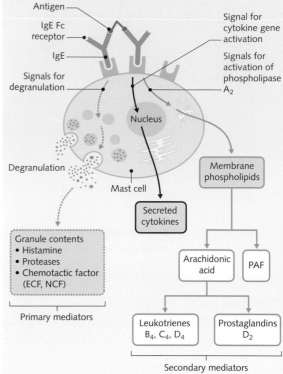

Fig. 14.3 Type I hypersensitivity reactions. ECF = eosinophil chemotactic factor; NCF = neutrophil chemotactic factor; PAF = platelet-activating factor.

Fig. 14.4 Classification of allergic rhinitis

Mild
None of the following items are present:
• Sleep disturbance
• Impairment of daily activities, leisure and/or sport
• Impairment of school or work
• Troublesome symptoms

Moderate/severe
One or more of the following items are present:
• Sleep disturbance
• Impairment of daily activities, leisure and/or sport
• Impairment of school or work
• Troublesome symptoms

environment is too clean) increases the risk of developing allergic rhinitis and other atopic diseases (Fig. 14.2).

Pathology
Symptoms are caused by a type I IgE-mediated hypersensitivity reaction. IgE fixes on to mast cells in nasal mucous membranes. Upon re-exposure to allergen, cross-linking of the IgE receptor occurs on the surface of the mast cells, leading to mast cell degranulation and release of histamine and leukotrienes (Fig. 14.3).

Classification
Allergic rhinitis can be classified into seasonal or perennial rhinitis depending on whether a patient is allergic to pollens (seasonal) or allergens that are present year-round, such as house dust mites, pets and moulds.

However, it is much more useful clinically to classify allergic rhinitis in terms of severity and the impact on a patient's quality of life (Fig. 14.4).

Symptoms
The common symptoms of allergic rhinitis include:
• Nasal congestion.
• Rhinorrhoea.
• Sneezing.
• Itching (eyes/nose/throat).
• Fatigue.

Investigation

Allergic rhinitis is mainly a clinical diagnosis based on taking an accurate history of common symptoms and identifying risk factors and potential allergens.

Skin prick testing can be undertaken to identify specific allergens to which the patient is allergic; however, in clinical practice, a diagnosis is usually made by treating empirically, with trial of antihistamines and nasal corticosteroids producing an improvement in a patient's symptoms.

Management

Management of allergic rhinitis largely depends on the frequency and severity of a patient's symptoms and the extent to which they impact on the patient's life. Figure 14.5 provides broad guidelines for the management of allergic rhinits.

Acute sinusitis

Sinusitis is an inflammatory process involving the lining of paranasal sinuses (Fig. 14.6). The maxillary sinus is most commonly clinically infected. The majority of infections are rhinogenic in origin and are classified as either acute or chronic.

Aetiology

The common causes of acute sinusitis are:

- Secondary bacterial infection (by *Streptococcus pneumoniae* or *Haemophilus influenzae*), often following an upper respiratory tract viral infection.
- Dental extraction or infection.
- Swimming and diving.
- Fractures involving sinuses.

Pathology

Hyperaemia and oedema of the mucosa occur. Blockage of sinus ostia and mucus production increases. The cilia lining the paranasal sinuses stop beating efficiently, leading to stasis of secretions causing secondary infection.

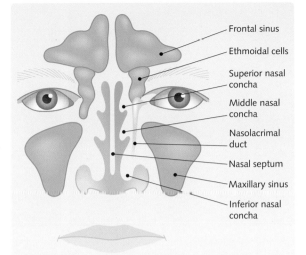

Fig. 14.6   Anatomy of the sinuses.

Frontal sinus
Ethmoidal cells
Superior nasal concha
Middle nasal concha
Nasolacrimal duct
Nasal septum
Maxillary sinus
Inferior nasal concha

Clinical features

Symptoms occur over several days:

- Purulent nasal discharge.
- Malaise.
- Sinus tenderness.
- Disturbed sense of smell.

There may be fullness and pain over the cheeks, maxillary toothache or a frontal headache. Pain is classically worse on leaning forward. Postnasal discharge may lead to cough.

Investigations

Sinusitis is like allergic rhinitis – a clinical diagnosis based on an accurate history. The following investigations may be useful in particularly severe or recurrent cases but are not essential in the majority of cases of sinusitis:

- Bloods – white cell count and inflammatory markers (erythrocyte sedimentation rate/C-reactive protein) may be raised but are often normal.
- Sinus culture.
- Radiology of paranasal sinuses (Fig. 14.7).

Management

Management is mainly symptomatic with:

- Analgesia.
- Nasal decongestants such as carbocisteine.

Where the sinusitis is suspected to be bacterial in origin (a persistent pyrexia and very purulent discharge), patients should be managed with antibiotics. In patients who are immunocompromised, there should be a very low threshold for treating with antibiotics.

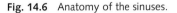

Fig. 14.5 Management of allergic rhinitis	
Mild intermittent symptoms	Allergen avoidance Oral antihistamine
Mild persistent symptoms or moderate-to-severe intermittent symptoms	Allergen avoidance Oral antihistamine Intranasal corticosteroid
Moderate-to-severe persistent symptoms	Allergen avoidance Oral antihistamine Intranasal corticosteroid ± oral corticosteroid

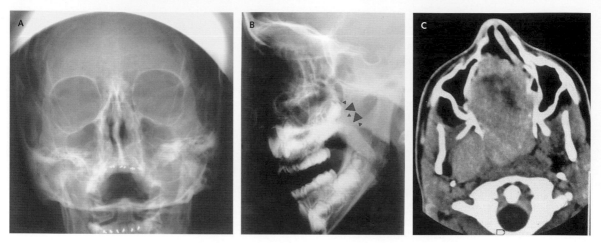

Fig. 14.7 Radiology of the paranasal sinuses. The most commonly used imaging modalities in sinusitis are X-ray (A), which may show an air–fluid level in the affected sinus. Lateral X-rays (B) are useful in children with recurrent sinusitis as they can reveal enlarged adenoids which predispose. Computed tomography scans (C) are useful for assessing the extent of disease and identifying unusual anatomy of the sinuses, which also predisposes to sinusitis.

A referral to an ear, nose and throat (ENT) specialist is warranted in patients with unresolving or recurring symptoms.

Chronic sinusitis

Chronic sinusitis is an inflammation of the sinuses which has been present for more than 4 weeks. It usually occurs after recurrent acute sinusitis and is common in patients who are heavy smokers and work in dusty environments.

Clinical features

Clinical features are similar to those of acute sinusitis but are typically less severe.

Pathology

Prolonged infection leads to irreversible changes in the sinus cavity, including:

- An increase in vascular permeability.
- Oedema and hypertrophy of the mucosa.
- Goblet cell hyperplasia.
- Chronic cellular infiltrate.
- Ulceration of the epithelium, resulting in granulated tissue formation.

Investigations

The investigations are through sinus radiographs, high-definition coronal section computed tomography (CT) and diagnostic endoscopy.

Treatment

This condition is difficult to treat. Treatments are:

- Medical – broad-acting antibiotics and decongestant.
- Surgical – antral lavage, inferior meatal intranasal antrostomy and functional endoscopic sinus surgery.

Rarely, recurrent sinusitis may be caused by Kartagener's syndrome, a congenital mucociliary disorder due to the absence of the ciliary protein dynein. It is characterized by sinusitis, bronchiectasis, otitis media, dextrocardia and infertility.

Neoplasms of the nasopharynx

Nasopharyngeal carcinoma is the most common neoplasm to affect the nasopharynx.

Epidemiology

Nasopharyngeal carcinoma is relatively rare in the UK and, indeed, there are only 80 000 new cases worldwide per year. There is marked geographical variation in incidence; in parts of China the incidence is as high as 25 per 100 000, compared to an incidence of 2 per 100 000 in western Europe. Men are more likely to suffer from the disease than women and peak incidence occurs at 50–70 years.

Aetiology

Risk factors for developing nasopharyngeal carcinoma include:

- Chinese ethnicity.
- Exposure to Epstein–Barr virus.
- Large alcohol intake.

Pathology

Nasopharyngeal carcinomas are predominantly squamous cell carcinomas in origin. They can be classified in terms of histological grade (i.e. high-grade tumours

Fig. 14.8	TNM staging
Tumour (T)	
TX	Primary tumour cannot be assessed
T0	No evidence of primary tumour
Tis	Carcinoma *in situ*
T1	Tumour confined to the nasopharynx, or tumour extends to oropharynx and/or nasal cavity without parapharyngeal extension
T2	Tumour with parapharyngeal extension
T3	Tumour involves bony structures of skull base and/or paranasal sinuses
T4	Tumour with intracranial extension and/or involvement of cranial nerves, hypopharynx, orbit, or with extension to the infratemporal fossa/masticator space
Nodes (N)	
Nx	Regional lymph nodes cannot be assessed
N1	No regional lymph node metastasis
N2	Unilateral metastasis in cervical lymph node(s), ≤6 cm in greatest dimension, above the supraclavicular fossa, and/or unilateral or bilateral, retropharyngeal lymph nodes, ≤6 cm in greatest dimension
N3a	Metastasis in a lymph node(s) >6 cm diameter
N3b	Extension to the supraclavicular fossa
Metastasis	
M0	No distant metastases
M1	Distant metastases

are poorly differentiated, low-grade tumours are well differentiated). They can also be classified in terms of whether they are keratinizing or non-keratinizing. Keratinizing tumours are associated with local invasion of adjacent structures and a poor prognosis.

All tumours are subsequently staged using the TNM system (Fig. 14.8).

Symptoms

Common symptoms include:

- Epistaxis.
- Nasal obstruction.
- Enlarged lymph nodes.
- Tinnitus.
- Recurrent otitis media.
- Cranial nerve palsies.

Investigations

- Endoscopic examination of nasal passages.
- Neurological examination.
- Staging CT/magnetic resonance imaging.

Management

High-dose radiotherapy (external beam radiotherapy) and chemotherapy are first-line management for the majority of nasopharyngeal carcinomas. Surgical resection can be used in those tumours that fail to regress following radiotherapy.

DISORDERS OF THE LARYNX

Inflammatory conditions

Laryngitis

Definition
Laryngitis is an inflammatory condition of the larynx. It is extremely common and usually caused by viral infection.

Epidemiology
The true incidence of laryngitis is hard to quantify as symptoms often go unreported, although the Royal College of General Practitioners in the UK reported a peak average incidence of patients with laryngitis of 23 per 100 000 per week, at all ages, over the period from 1999 to 2005. There is, as expexted, a seasonal variation in laryngitis, with peaks in viral laryngitis in autumn and spring (rhinovirus) and in winter (influenza).

The incidence of bacterial laryngitis has reduced significantly since the introduction of the *Haemophilus influenzae* type B (Hib) vaccine.

Aetiology
Laryngitis is most commonly caused by a viral infection, i.e. rhinovirus. Other infectious causes include:

- Bacterial (diphtheria, *Haemophilus* in unvaccinated children).
- Tuberculosis.
- *Candida* (particularly in immunosuppressed patients).

Symptoms
- Dysphagia.
- Hoarseness.
- Odynophagia.
- Cough.

Investigation and management
Laryngitis is a clinical diagnosis based on accurate history and examination findings. Management is usually supportive with analgesia, and viral infections are self-limiting. Bacterial infections will require treatment with a course of antibiotics. Recurrent laryngitis may warrant referral to an ENT surgeon.

Chronic laryngitis

Chronic laryngitis is inflammation of the larynx and trachea associated with excessive smoking, continued vocal abuse and excessive alcohol.

The mucous glands are swollen and the epithelium hypertrophied. Heavy smoking leads to squamous metaplasia of the larynx. Biopsy is mandatory to rule out malignancy. Management is directed at avoidance of aetiological factors.

Laryngotracheobronchitis (croup) vs acute epiglottitis

Laryngotracheobronchitis (croup) is an extremely common condition in paediatrics, particularly during the winter months, and is caused by a viral infection (Fig. 14.9). In clinical practice it is vitally important to make the distinction between children presenting with croup and those presenting with acute epiglottitis, which is a medical emergency.

The clinical features of these conditions are shown in Figure 14.9. The incidence of epiglottitis has dramatically fallen due to the introduction of the Hib vaccine.

Pathology

In epiglottitis, there is necrosis of epithelium and formation of an extensive fibrous membrane on the trachea and main bronchi. Oedema of the subglottic area occurs, with subsequent danger of laryngeal obstruction.

In croup, there is an acute inflammatory oedema and infiltration by neutrophil polymorphs. No mucosal ulceration occurs.

Treatment

To treat laryngotracheobronchitis, keep the patient calm and hydrated. Nurse in a warm room in an upright position. Drug treatment, if required, includes steroids (oral dexamethasone), oxygen and nebulized adrenaline (epinephrine).

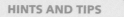

HINTS AND TIPS

Lucy, a 2-year-old girl, came into Accident and Emergency with a cough, difficulty breathing and a sore throat. Her mother said that she had had a cold for the past week. Closer examination revealed that Lucy had a hoarse voice and a cough that sounded like a bark. There was some sternal recession and discomfort when lying down. Lucy was diagnosed as having croup.

She had moderate-to-severe croup and was treated with 100% oxygen, nebulized adrenaline (epinephrine) and budesonide as well as having oral dexamethasone.

Fig. 14.9 Laryngotracheobronchitis (croup) and acute epiglottitis		
	Croup	**Epiglottitis**
Aetiology	Viral	Bacterial
Organism	Parainfluenza, respiratory syncytial virus	Group B *Haemophilus influenzae*
Age range	6 months to 3 years	3–7 years
Onset	Gradual over days	Sudden over hours
Cough	Severe barking	Minimal
Temperature	Pyrexia <38.5 °C	Pyrexia >38.5 °C
Stridor	Harsh	Soft
Drooling	No	Yes
Voice	Hoarse	Reluctant to speak
Able to drink	Yes	No
Active	Yes	No, completely still
Mortality	Low	High

Acute epiglottitis is a medical emergency. Call for the anaesthetist, ENT surgeon and, if appropriate, the paediatric team. Never attempt to visualize the epiglottis. Keep calm and reassure the patient. Never leave the patient alone. As with other serious *Haemophilus influenzae* infections, prophylactic treatment with rifampicin is offered to the close contacts.

Reactive nodules

Reactive nodules are common, small, inflammatory polyps usually measuring less than 10 mm in diameter. They are also known as singer's nodules. They present in patients aged 40–50 years and are more common in men. Reactive nodules are caused by excessive untrained use of vocal cords. Patients present with hoarseness of the voice.

Pathology

Keratosis develops at the junction of the anterior and middle thirds of the vocal cord on each side. Oedematous myxoid connective tissue is covered by squamous epithelium. The reactive nodules may become painful because of ulceration.

Neoplasms

Squamous papilloma

Squamous papilloma is the commonest benign tumour of the larynx; it usually occurs in children aged 0–5 years, but can also affect adults.

Aetiology
The disease is caused by infection of the epithelial cells with human papillomavirus types 6 and 11, and can be acquired at birth from maternal genital warts.

Clinical features
Clinical features include hoarseness of the voice and an abnormal cry (Fig. 14.10).

Fig. 14.10	Features of squamous papilloma	
	Adult	**Child**
Incidence	Rare	Common
Number of lesions	Single mass	Multiple masses
Outcome	Surgical removal	Regress spontaneously at puberty

Pathology
Tumours may be sessile or pedunculated. They can occur anywhere on the vocal cords. Lesions are commoner at points of airway constriction (Fig. 14.11).

Investigations and treatment
Investigations include endoscopy, followed by histological confirmation.

Surgical treatment is by removal with a carbon dioxide laser. Medical treatment is with alpha-interferon.

Squamous cell carcinoma

Squamous cell carcinoma is the commonest malignant tumour of the larynx, affecting men and women in the ratio of 5:1. The disease accounts for 1% of all male malignancies. Incidence increases with age, with peak incidence occurring in those aged 60–70 years. Patients present with hoarseness, although dyspnoea and stridor are late signs.

Predisposing factors include alcohol and tobacco smoking (the condition is very rare in non-smokers).

Pathology
Carcinoma of the vocal cords appears first, and subsequently ulcerates. Carcinoma of the larynx infiltrates and destroys surrounding tissue. Infection may follow ulceration.

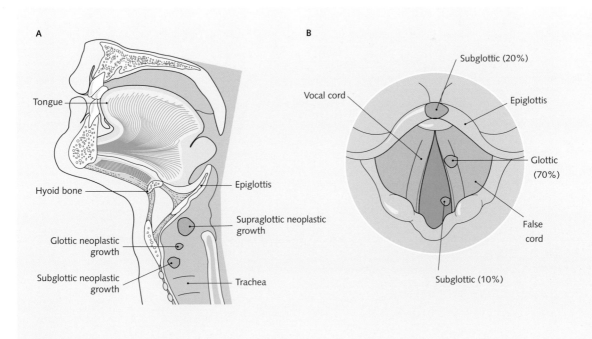

Fig. 14.11   Position of laryngeal carcinoma (A) and as seen on mirror examination (B).

Investigations and treatment

Investigations include chest radiography, full blood count, serum analysis (liver function tests for metastatic disease), direct laryngoscopy under general anaesthesia, and full paraendoscopy and bronchoscopy. Treatment is by radiotherapy and surgery.

Further reading

Birmingham Research Unit of the Royal College of General Practitioners, 2006. Communicable and respiratory disease report for England and Wales. Available online at: http://www.rcgp.org.uk/.

Sleep disorders （15）

Objectives

By the end of this chapter, you should be able to:
- Define and describe the clinical features of sleep apnoea.
- Understand the basic elements of sleep studies.
- Discuss the management and complications of sleep apnoea, including non-invasive ventilation.

SLEEP APNOEA

Definition

Sleep apnoea is the cessation of breathing during sleep. There are two types: obstructive sleep apnoea and central sleep apnoea.

Prevalence

It is estimated that 1 in 10 people over the age of 65 suffer from obstructive sleep apnoea in the USA. It is very common in those who are overweight and obese, affecting up to 70% of these individuals.

Pathogenesis

Obstructive sleep apnoea results from occlusion of the upper airway and is common in overweight, middle-aged men. In inspiration upper-airway pressure becomes negative, but airway patency is maintained by upper-airway muscle (e.g. genioglossus) tone. During sleep these muscles relax, causing narrowing of the upper airways, even in normal subjects. However, if the airway is already narrowed, for example by the weight of adipose tissue in obese patients or a small jaw (micrognathia), the airway collapses and obstructive sleep apnoea results. Other risk factors include:

- Down's syndrome.
- Adenotonsillar hypertrophy.
- Macroglossia – enlarged tongue (seen in hypothyroidism, acromegaly and amyloidosis).
- Nasal obstruction (as in rhinitis).
- Alcohol (which has been shown to reduce muscle tone and reduces the arousal response).

A cycle is generated during sleep in which:

- The upper-airway dilating muscles lose tone (usually accompanied by loud snoring).
- The airway is occluded.
- The patient wakes.
- The airway reopens.

As a consequence of this cycle, sleep is unrefreshing and daytime sleepiness is common, particularly during monotonous situations such as motorway driving. Each arousal also causes a transient rise in blood pressure, which may lead to sustained hypertension, pulmonary hypertension and cor pulmonale, ischaemic heart disease and stroke.

Conversely, in central sleep apnoea, the airway remains patent but there is no efferent output from the respiratory centres in the brain. There is no respiratory effort by the respiratory muscles, causing P_aCO_2 levels to rise. The high P_aCO_2 arouses the patient, who then rebreathes to normalize the P_aCO_2 and then falls asleep again. This cycle can be repeated many times during the night and leads to a disruptive sleep pattern. Central sleep apnoea is rarer than obstructive sleep apnoea but is more common in patients with congestive heart failure and patients with neurological diseases (e.g. strokes). It can also be seen in people with no abnormalities, such as those who live at high altitude.

Clinical features

- Chronic snoring, with pauses in breathing, followed by a choking or gasping sound.
- Daytime somnolence.
- Morning headaches.
- Difficulty concentrating.
- Mood swings.
- Dry throat.

In addition to the above, the patient may appear obese and have a wide neck or small jaw.

Investigations

Patients can have the severity of their suspected sleep apnoea assessed using the Epworth Sleepiness Scale

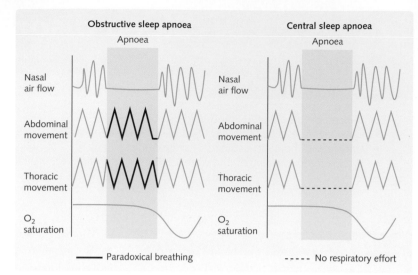

Fig. 15.1 Example results of polysomnographs showing the two types of sleep apnoea. Sleep apnoea can be detected by reduced air flow and a delayed desaturation following the apnoea. Normally the thorax and abdomen move in the same direction; however, in obstructive sleep apnoea the thorax and abdomen move in opposite directions to each other – an abnormal pattern called paradoxical breathing. Conversely, in central sleep apnoea there is neither thoracic nor abdominal movement because the respiratory centre in the brain has stopped instructing the respiratory muscles to move.

(see http://epworthsleepinessscale.com/). A score of 9 or less is normal. Between 10 and 15 indicates likely mild-to-moderate disease, and medical advice should be sought. A score of 16 or over is indicative of severe disease.

Patients are subsequently referred to a sleep or respiratory specialist for overnight sleep study, polysomnography (Fig. 15.1): 15 apnoeas/hypoapnoeas (of 10 seconds or longer) per hour of sleep is diagnostic. The following parameters are measured:

- Brain activity.
- Eye movements.
- Oxygen and carbon dioxide levels.
- Blood pressure and pulse.
- Inspiratory and expiratory flow.

This is the gold standard investigation.

Treatment

Some patients can be managed conservatively and are advised to lose weight and avoid alcohol and sedatives as these relax the upper-airway dilating muscles.

However, for most patients nightly continuous positive airway pressure (CPAP) is recommended. Some success has been obtained with medications which have a stimulator effect on the respiratory system, such as theophylline.

In non-invasive ventilation, respiratory support is given via the patient's upper airway, and intubation is avoided. This method is therefore only suitable if patients can protect their own airway, but has the advantage of reducing the risks of a hospital-acquired infection. The patient breathes spontaneously and the lungs are expanded by a volume of gas delivered, usually at a positive pressure. This decreases the work of the respiratory muscles, particularly the diaphragm.

Two basic types of non-invasive ventilation are available:

- CPAP.
- Bilevel positive airway pressure (BiPAP).

As the name implies, CPAP delivers a continuous positive air pressure throughout the respiratory cycle and is used to keep the upper airway open in obstructive sleep apnoea. BiPAP is an example of intermittent positive-pressure ventilation (IPPV). BiPAP also reduces the work of breathing but differs in that it senses when inspiration is occurring and delivers a higher pressure during the inspiratory part of the cycle.

Some patients find CPAP difficult to use because the mask is uncomfortable, as is the sensation of having air forced in through the mouth and nose. CPAP using just a nasal mask is also available. Patients also often complain that the machine is noisy and cumbersome, thus affecting their relationship with their partner. However, this has to be balanced against the increased health risks associated with sleep apnoea, as well as the noise from snoring!

Complications

Sleep apnoea can have many serious consequences on various aspects of a patient's life. On a personal level, the constant snoring can put a big strain on the relationship between a patient and his or her partner. Furthermore, it can have more widespread consequences for patients who drive, as daytime somnolence significantly increases the risk of falling asleep at the wheel, a dangerous consequence for both the patient and anyone else on the road. It is important to tell patients that they must inform the Driver and Vehicle Licensing Agency of their diagnosis.

Sleep apnoea is also dangerous for the physical health of the patient. As most patients are overweight or obese, they are already at increased risk of heart disease, diabetes and associated complications. However, even taking that into account, these patients are at increased risk for developing hypertension, heart disease and stroke. This is because the constant surges of adrenaline and increases of blood pressure as the body tries to wake the patient and stimulate breathing cause a proinflammatory response. This in turn increases blood pressure, leading to the associated complications.

Associated conditions

Obesity hypoventilation is a disorder of breathing commonly associated with obstructive sleep apnoea, characterized by chronic hypoxia and hypercapnia, in the absence of lung disease. The exact underlying mechanisms are not known, but it is thought to be a combination of a lack of stimulation from the brainstem combined with a large volume of excess weight compressing the chest and upper airways.

The condition presents in a similar way to sleep apnoea, with daytime somnolence, depression and headaches (from hypercapnia). In fact, as patients often have the two conditions, it can be very difficult to distinguish them.

Diagnosis is through a combination of clinical findings (obese patient, cyanosis) and arterial blood gas results, which reveal the characteristic hypoxia and hypercapnia pattern.

Treatment, as with obstructive sleep apnoea, initially involves conservative measures such as weight loss. BiPAP (in order to blow off excess CO_2) is used if this is not effective.

NARCOLEPSY

This is a neurological disorder causing daytime sleep 'attacks' and somnolence. Further information can be found in a neurology textbook.

Useful links

http://sleepmed.com.au/bariatric1.pdf.
http://www.nhlbi.nih.gov/health/health-topics/topics/
 sleepapnea/atrisk.html.

Objectives

By the end of this chapter you should be able to:
- Define asthma.
- Describe the different mechanisms involved in the pathogenesis of asthma.
- Discuss how to investigate a patient with asthma.
- Understand the British Thoracic Soceity stepwise approach to asthma management.

DEFINITION AND BACKGROUND

Asthma is a chronic inflammatory disorder of the lung airways characterized by air-flow obstruction, which is usually reversible (either spontaneously or with treatment), airway hyperresponsiveness and inflamed bronchi.

PREVALENCE

Of the adult population, 5% are receiving therapy for asthma at any one time. Prevalence of asthma in the Western world is rising, particularly in children; up to 20% have symptoms at some time in their childhood. The British Lung Foundation estimates that 5 million people are currently suffering from asthma in the UK. Extrinsic asthma is more common in boys than girls, whilst women tend to more affected by intrinsic disease.

CLASSIFICATION

Bronchial asthma may be categorized as extrinsic (atopic childhood asthma) or intrinsic (adult onset, non-atopic) (Fig. 16.1). Occupational asthma can be considered as a separate group. Precipitating factors in asthma exacerbations are listed below.

Extrinsic asthma

This is classical asthma with onset in childhood, commonly with a previous history of atopy such as food allergy or eczema. It often remits by teenage years.

Intrinsic asthma

This subtype tends to be of adult onset, is more progressive and is less responsive to therapy. It is less likely to be atopy-related.

Occupational asthma is increasing; currently over 200 materials encountered at the workplace are implicated (Fig. 16.2). Occupational asthma may be classified as:
- Allergic (immunologically mediated with a latent period between exposure and symptoms).
- Non-allergic (immediate response after exposure, e.g. to toxic gases).

PRECIPITATING FACTORS

1. Allergen:
   - House dust mite.
   - Flour.
   - Animal danders.

2. Occupational factors:
   - Solder (colophony) fumes.
   - Flour.
   - Isocyanates.

3. Viral infections:
   - Parainfluenza.
   - Respiratory syncytial virus.
   - Rhinovirus.

4. Drugs:
   - Beta-blockers.
   - Non-steroidal anti-inflammatory drugs.

5. Other factors:
   - Cold air.
   - Exercise.
   - Emotion.

PATHOGENESIS

The pathogenesis of asthma is very complex; however, three main processess are responsible for the majority of symptoms. These are bronchospasm, smooth-muscle

	Extrinsic asthma	Intrinsic asthma
...derlying abnormality	Immune reaction (atopic)	Abnormal autonomic regulation of airways
Onset	Childhood	Adulthood
Distribution	60%	40%
Allergens	Recognized	None identified
Family history	Present	Absent
Predisposition to form IgE antibodies	Present	Absent
Association with chronic obstructive pulmonary disease	None	Chronic bronchitis
Natural progression	Improves	Worsens
Eosinophilia	Sputum and blood	Sputum
Drug hypersensitivity	Absent	Present

Fig. 16.2 Factors implicated in occupational asthma

Agents	Workers at risk include:
High-molecular-weight agents	
Cereals	Bakers, millers
Animal-derived allergens	Animal handlers
Enzymes	Detergent users, pharmaceutical workers, bakers
Gums	Carpet makers, pharmaceutical workers
Latex	Health professionals
Seafoods	Seafood processors
Low-molecular-weight agents	
Isocyanates	Spray painters, insulation installers, etc.
Wood dusts	Forest workers, carpenters
Anhydrides	Users of plastics, epoxy resins
Fluxes	Electronic workers
Chloramine	Janitors, cleaners
Acrylate	Adhesive handlers
Drugs	Pharmaceutical workers, health professionals
Metals	Solderers, refiners

hypertrophy and mucus plugging (Fig. 16.3). Allergen-induced airway inflammation results in:

- Smooth-muscle constriction.
- Thickening of the airway wall (smooth-muscle hypertrophy and oedema).
- Basement membrane thickening.
- Mucus and exudate in the airway lumen.

Microscopically, the viscid mucus contains:

- Desquamated epithelial cells.
- Whorls of shed epithelium (Curschmann's whorls).
- Charcot–Leyden crystal (eosinophil cell membranes).
- Infiltration of inflammatory cells, particularly CD4$^+$ T lymphocytes.

INFLAMMATORY MEDIATORS

Inflammatory mediators play a vital role in the pathogenesis of asthma. Inflammatory stimuli activate mast cells, epithelial cells, alveolar macrophages and dendritic cells resident within the airways, causing the release of mediators that are chemotactic for cells derived from the circulation – secondary effector cells (eosinophils, neutrophils and platelets). Mediators that are thought to be involved in asthma include:

- Preformed mediators – present in cytoplasmic granules ready for release. They are associated with human lung mast cells and include histamine, neutral proteases and chemotactic factors for eosinophils. These are responsible for the early response (below).
- Newly generated mediators – manufactured secondary to the initial triggering stimulus after release of preformed mediators. Some of these mediators are derived from the membrane phospholipids and are associated with the metabolism of arachidonic acid (e.g. prostaglandins and leukotrienes). The production of inflammatory cytokines and chemokines is important in the activation and recruitment of inflammatory cells, ultimately leading to a so-called late response (see below).

EARLY AND LATE RESPONSES

Two patterns of response can be considered; in practice most asthmatics show evidence of both responses, although either may be absent.

Immediate (early) reaction

The release of preformed mediators (predominantly from mast cells) causes vascular leakage and smooth-muscle contraction within 10–15 minutes of challenge, with a return to baseline within 1–2 hours. The mast

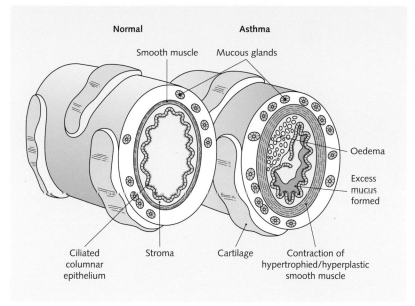

Fig. 16.3 Mechanisms of airway narrowing in asthma.

Normal — Asthma
Smooth muscle — Mucous glands
Oedema
Excess mucus formed
Ciliated columnar epithelium — Stroma — Cartilage — Contraction of hypertrophied/hyperplastic smooth muscle

cells are activated by allergens that cross-link with the IgE molecules that are bound to high-affinity receptors on the mast cell membrane.

Late reaction

The influx of inflammatory cells (predominantly eosinophils) and the release of their inflammatory mediators cause airway narrowing after 3–4 hours, which is maximal after 6–12 hours. This is much more difficult to reverse than the immediate reaction and there is an increase in the level of airway hyperreactivity.

The biphasic nature of asthma attacks is the basis behind patients being admitted for observation for approximately 24 hours after a moderate or severe attack.

The asthmatic process is overviewed in Figure 16.4: part A shows the cellular and mediator response to allergen, whereas part B shows the pathophysiological effects of this process.

AIRWAY REMODELLING

This is a term used to describe the specific structural changes that occur in long-standing asthma with severe airway inflammation. The characteristic features include:

- Increased vascular permeability.
- Loss of surface epithelial cells and hypertrophy of goblet cells.
- Hypertrophy of smooth muscle.
- Myofibroblast accumulation and increased collagen deposition, hence causing basement membrane thickening.

Airway remodelling may cause a fixed airway obstruction which may not be reversible with anti-inflammatory agents or bronchodilators.

CLINICAL FEATURES

Symptoms (breathlessness, chest tightness, cough, wheeze) classically show a diurnal variation, often being worse at night. For example, nocturnal coughing is a common presenting symptom, especially in children.

It is important to try and discern the exact timing of symptoms, as this can be crucial not only in diagnosing the asthma but also in identifying the underlying trigger. Worsening of symptoms at work (with reduction when on holiday or at home) can be very useful in those with occupational asthma.

Other features to look out for in the history include a personal or family history of atopy. Children have often been previously diagnosed with milk allergy and/or eczema as a toddler and then will present with symptoms of asthma once they start school. They can then go on to develop hayfever or allergic rhinitis as teenagers.

Clinical features vary according to the severity of asthma (classified from mild to severe and either intermittent or persistent).

Acute severe asthma in adults is diagnosed if:

- Patient cannot complete sentences in one breath.
- Respiration rate ≥ 25 breaths/min.
- Pulse ≥ 110 bpm.
- Peak expiratory flow rate $\geq 50\%$ of predicted or best.

Life-threatening asthma is characterized by the following:

- Peak expiratory flow rate $< 33\%$ of predicted or best.

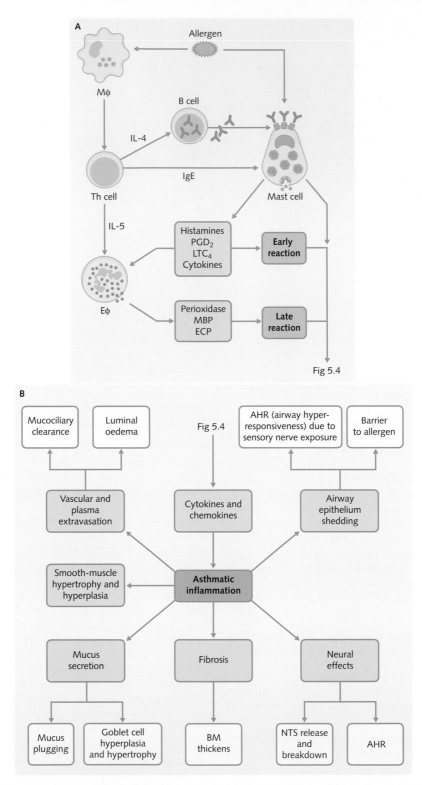

Fig. 16.4 (A) Pathogenesis of asthma. IL-4 = interleukin 4; IL-5 = interleukin 5; MBP = major basic protein; ECP = eosinophil cationic protein; PGD$_2$ = prostaglandin D$_2$; LTC$_4$ = leukotriene C$_4$; IgE = immunoglobulin E. (B) The pathophysiological effects of cellular processess in asthma. BM = basement membrane; AHR = airway hyperresponsiveness; NTS = neurotransmitter substance.

Fig. 16.5 Comparison table: asthma versus chronic obstructive pulmonary disease (COPD)

	Asthma	COPD
Genetic components	Polygenetic	Fewer genes involved, e.g. α_1-antitrypsin
Age of onset	Can occur at any age but more common during childhood	Mainly affects the adult population
Inflammatory cells involved	Eosinophils and mast cells are the main culprits	Mainly neutrophils
Symptoms	Variable – wheeze, cough	Persistent – shortness of breath on exertion, cough
Investigations	Diurnal variation in FEV_1	Progressive decline in FEV_1 over time
Reversibility	Marked	Sometimes
Most effective bronchodilator	β_2-adrenoceptor agonist, e.g. salbutamol	Anticholinergics, e.g. ipratropium bromide
Steroid treatment	Beneficial	Not very beneficial but useful in acute exacerbations

$FEV_1 = $ forced expiratory volume in 1 second.

- Silent chest and cyanosis.
- Bradycardia or hypotension.
- Exhaustion, confusion or coma.
- P_aO_2 <8 kPa.

The management of severe and life-threatening asthma is covered in Chapter 12.

INVESTIGATIONS

- Lung function tests – forced expiratory volume in 1 second (FEV_1)/forced vital capacity is reduced in line with an obstructive flow picture. Residual volume may also be increased secondary to gas trapping; tests demonstrate an improvement in FEV_1 of more than 15% after bronchodilator administration. If there is no improvement with bronchodilators (and the patient has a smoking history), consider a diagnosis of chronic obstructive pulmonary disease (COPD). The main differences between asthma and COPD are described in Figure 16.5.
- Peak expiratory flow rate – morning and evening measurements. Useful in the long-term assessment of asthma; a characteristic morning dipping pattern is seen in poorly controlled asthma (Fig. 16.6). Similarly, in occupational asthma, a reduction in peak flow can be seen during working hours, with return to normal when the patient is off work.
- If peak expiratory flow rate < 50%, arterial blood gases should be tested.
- Exercise laboratory tests.

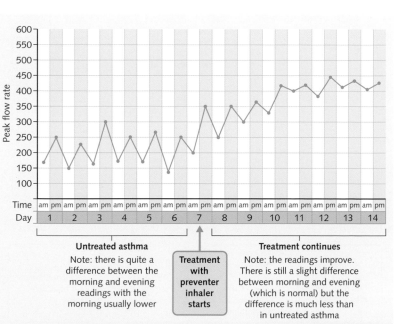

Time: am pm am pm am pm am pm am pm am pm am pm am pm am pm am pm am pm am pm am pm am pm
Day: 1 2 3 4 5 6 7 8 9 10 11 12 13 14

Untreated asthma
Note: there is quite a difference between the morning and evening readings with the morning usually lower

Treatment with preventer inhaler starts

Treatment continues
Note: the readings improve. There is still a slight difference between morning and evening (which is normal) but the difference is much less than in untreated asthma

Fig. 16.6 Characteristic diurnal variation of peak flow in asthma and then improvement with treatment.

- Bronchial provocation tests – performed rarely in normal clinical practice, using histamine or methacholine to demonstrate bronchial hyperreactivity.
- Chest radiography – no diagnostic features of asthma on chest radiograph; used to rule out a diagnosis of allergic bronchopulmonary aspergillosis and pneumothorax in the emergency setting.
- Skin prick tests – allergen injections into the epidermis of the forearm, which are used to identify extrinsic causes. Look for wheal development in sensitive patients.
- Exhaled nitric oxide – an increased level of exhaled nitric oxide is indicative of airway inflammation. It is less commonly used than other, simpler tests.

TREATMENT

It is important to identify and avoid extrinsic factors. However, this may be easier said than done. For example, if the patient is suffering from occupational asthma, this may involve giving up the job. Similarly, it is difficult to avoid house dust mites as they are present on most soft furnishings in a house. However, many items are now available such as protective pillow cases and mattress covers which reduce contact between house dust mites and the patient. Furthermore, it should be emphasized to patients (if they are teenagers and older) and their families that tobacco smoke can trigger asthma and worsen their condition considerably.

The British Thoracic Society has produced guidelines as to how to treat a patient initially presenting with possible asthma (Fig. 16.7).

Follow the British Thoracic Society guidelines with a stepwise approach to drug treatment, as illustrated by Figure 16.8. Each step up the treatment ladder is carried out if the patient's symptoms are not sufficiently controlled. Patients on step 3 of the ladder can be considered for SMART (single maintenance and reliever therapy), which comprises a long-acting β agonist and inhaled steroid in a combination inhaler

Fig. 16.7 A useful approach to asthma diagnosis.

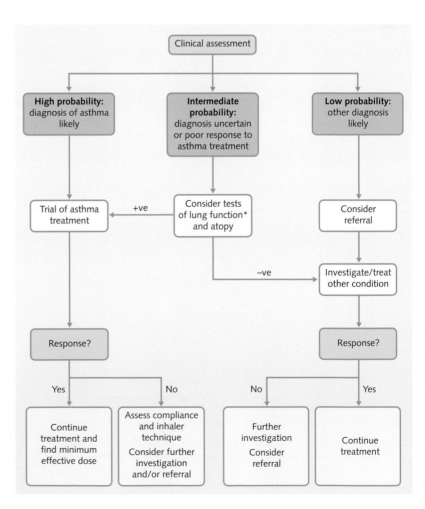

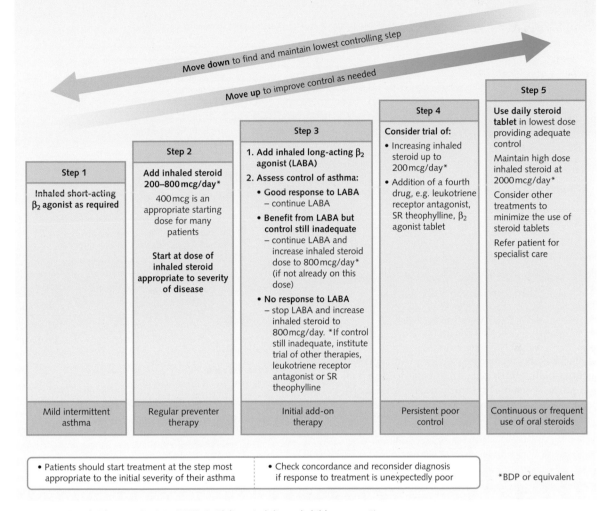

Fig. 16.8 British Thoracic Society (BTS) Guidelines (adults and children over 5).

(Symbicort only and not Seretide). Asthmatics tend to use their steroid inhaler too late in an exacerbation and this regime ensures exacerbations are prevented from worsening. The key point to remember about the stepwise management of asthma is to step down the treatment once the patient has good symptom control.

The pharmacology of the drugs used in treating asthma is discussed in Chapter 7.

ACUTE ASTHMA

Acute asthma should be managed by following the British Thoracic Society guidelines (Fig. 16.9). Continuous monitoring with a pulse oximeter, electrocardiograph and blood pressure is necessary. If possible, serial peak flow measurements can be used to judge response to treatment. Arterial blood gases can also be very useful. If the patient is unresponsive to these treatments, referral to the intensive therapy unit is necessary, with consideration of possible non-invasive or invasive ventilation. This is further discussed in Chapter 12.

EDUCATION

Education with inhaler technique and drug compliance can also contribute to the management of asthma. For younger children, or those who find inhalers difficult to use, a wide variety of spacers are available, which are much simpler to use and allow good delivery of inhaled therapies.

Fig. 16.9 Management of acute
asthma, following British
Thoracic Society guidelines.

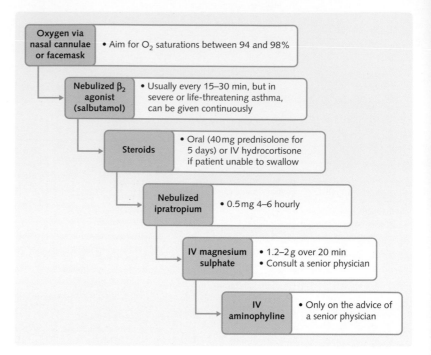

Patients should also be provided with a personalized
asthma plan, which tells them what to do when their
symptoms worsen. This improves outcomes for patients,
reducing hospital admissions and frequency of exacerbations.

Useful links

http://www.asthma.org.uk/how-we-help/publications/
    publications-for-the-public/ucProduct?product=362.
http://www.blf.org.uk/Conditions/Detail/Asthma.

Chronic obstructive pulmonary disease (COPD) 17

● **Objectives**

By the end of this chapter you should be able to:
- Describe the epidemiology and aetiology of COPD.
- Understand the pathophysiology of COPD.
- Describe the common clinical features and explain the diagnostic criteria for COPD.
- Explain the management of stable and acute exacerbations of COPD.

INTRODUCTION

COPD is a progressive lung disease, which is characterized by air flow obstruction with little or no reversibility. The Global Initiative for Obstructive Lung Disease (GOLD) defines COPD as:

> a common preventable and treatable disease, is characterized by persistent air flow limitation that is usually progressive and associated with an enhanced chronic inflammatory response in the airways and the lung to noxious particles or gases.

Patients with smoking-related lung disease were previously thought of as developing either chronic bronchitis or emphysema. However, we now realize that most patients actually develop varying combinations of these two processes (Fig. 17.1). Thus the term COPD represents a spectrum of disease in which several pathological processes occur.

EPIDEMIOLOGY

COPD is a common lung condition and its prevalence is estimated to be 5–15% in industrialized countries. COPD is a major cause of mortality and morbidity. The Global Burden of Disease study predicted that by the year 2020 COPD will be the third most common cause of death and fifth most common cause of disability.

Currently COPD is more common in men and tends to present in those over the age of 50. However, the prevalence is increasing in women and by the next decade it is estimated that COPD will affect both men and women equally.

AETIOLOGY

Worldwide, the most commonly encountered risk factor for developing COPD is tobacco smoke (this includes cigarettes, pipes, cigars, other types of tobacco and environmental exposure, i.e. passive smoking). The relationship between smoking and COPD is well proven; it is estimated that 80% of patients with COPD have a significant smoking history.

Other environmental risk factors:

- Indoor air pollution, i.e. biomass fuels used for indoor cooking and heating – a significant risk factor for women in developing countries.
- Occupational dusts and chemicals.
- Outdoor air pollution (minimal effect in COPD).

A person's risk of developing COPD is related to the total burden of inhaled particles he or she encounters over a lifetime.

GENETIC RISK FACTORS

Despite a strong relationship between smoking and COPD, not all smokers go on to develop COPD. In fact studies have demonstrated that only 15–20% of smokers develop COPD. This implies there must be a genetic susceptibility that predisposes some individuals to developing COPD when exposed to environmental risk factors such as tobacco smoke.

The best-described genetic risk factor is α_1-antitrypsin deficiency, which affects 2% of COPD patients. α_1-Antitrypsin is a serum acute-phase protein produced in the liver; it acts as an antiprotease in the lung and inhibits neutrophil elastase. Deficiency creates a protease–antiprotease imbalance, resulting in

Fig. 17.1	Definitions of chronic bronchitis/emphysema
	Definition
Chronic bronchitis	Clinically defined: Presence of cough and sputum production for most days for 3 months of 2 consecutive years
Emphysema	Histologically defined: Dilatation of the air spaces distal to the terminal bronchioles with destruction of the alveoli

unopposed neutrophil elastase action and, consequently, alveolar destruction and early-onset emphysema. α_1-Antitrypsin deficiency should be suspected in individuals who develop COPD under 40 years of age. Genetic inheritance of this deficiency is autosomal dominant with equal distribution between sexes.

PATHOPHYSIOLOGY

Cigarette smoke and exposure to other environmental noxious particles trigger the pathological processes that occur within the lungs of COPD patients. Tobacco smoke has been shown to damage the lungs via three main mechanisms (Fig. 17.2):

* Inflammatory cell activation: cigarette smoke stimulates epithelial cells, macrophages and neutrophils to release inflammatory mediators and proteases (neutrophil elastase).

* Oxidative stress: oxidants in cigarette smoke act directly on epithelial and goblet cells, causing inflammation.
* Impaired mucociliary clearance, thus leading to retained mucus secretions.

The two main pathological processes in COPD are alveolar destruction (emphysema) and mucus hypersecretion (chronic bronchitis). As previously discussed, there are many different phenotypes of COPD. Whereas some patients may have a more emphysematous or bronchitic phenotype, the majority of patients develop a combination of these two pathological processes and have a mixed phenotype.

ALVEOLAR DESTRUCTION (EMPHYSEMA)

Cigarette smoke and other inhaled noxious particles cause inflammatory cell activation within the lung, inducing cells to release inflammatory mediators and proteases. Importantly, in COPD, cigarette smoke induces the release of neutrophil elastase from neutrophils. In healthy lung tissue, antiproteases neutralise these proteases; however, in COPD the volume of proteases produced overwhelms antiproteases (protease–antiprotease imbalance). Consequently, there is unopposed action of neutrophil elastase within the lung which destroys alveolar attachments. As the distal airways are held open by the alveolar septa, destruction of alveoli causes the airways to collapse, resulting in airway obstruction (Fig. 17.3).

Fig. 17.2 Overall pathogenesis of chronic obstructive pulmonary disease (COPD).

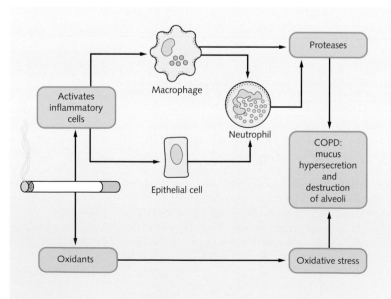

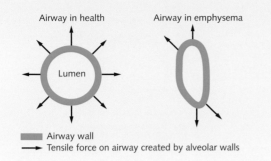

Fig. 17.3 The mechanism of underlying airway obstruction in emphysema.

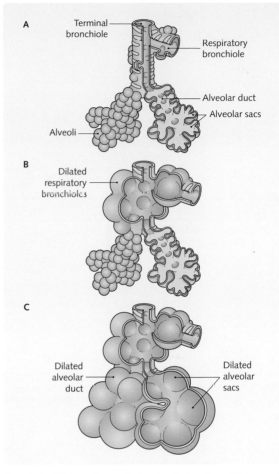

Fig. 17.4 Main patterns of alveolar destruction. (A) Normal distal lung acinus; (B) centriacinar emphysema; (C) panacinar emphysema.

Destruction of the parenchyma increases compliance of the lung and causes a mismatch in ventilation:perfusion. Increased compliance, i.e. reduced elastic recoil of the lungs, means the lungs do not deflate as easily, contributing to air trapping. As more alveolar walls are destroyed, compliance of the lungs increases and bullae (dilated air space >10 mm) form, which may rupture, causing pneumothoraces.

Classification of emphysema is based on anatomical distribution (Fig. 17.4). The two main types are centriacinar and panacinar.

Centriacinar (centrilobular) emphysema

Septal destruction and dilatation are limited to the centre of the acinus, around the terminal bronchiole and predominantly affect upper lobes (Fig. 17.4B). This pattern of emphysema is associated with smoking.

Panacinar (panlobular) emphysema

The whole of the acinus is involved distal to the terminal bronchioles, and lower lobes are predominantly affected. This is characteristic of α_1-antitrypsin deficiency (Fig. 17.4C).

Mucus hypersecretion

Cigarette smoke causes hyperplasia and hypertrophy of mucus-secreting glands found in the submucosa of the large cartilaginous airways. Mucous gland hypertrophy is expressed as gland:wall ratio or by the Reid index (normally <0.4). Hyperplasia of the intraepithelial goblet cells occurs at the expense of ciliated cells in the lining epithelium. Regions of epithelium may undergo squamous metaplasia.

Small airways become obstructed by intraluminal mucus plugs, mucosal oedema, smooth-muscle hypertrophy and peribronchial fibrosis. Secondary bacterial colonization of retained products occurs (Fig. 17.5).

The effect of these changes is to cause obstruction, increasing resistance to air flow. A mismatch in ventilation:perfusion occurs, impairing gas exchange.

CLINICAL FEATURES

The clinical presentation of COPD is variable but patients predominantly complain of:

- Progressive shortness of breath.
- Reduced exercise tolerance.
- Persistent cough.
- Chronic sputum production.
- Weight loss and peripheral muscle weakness or wasting may also occur.

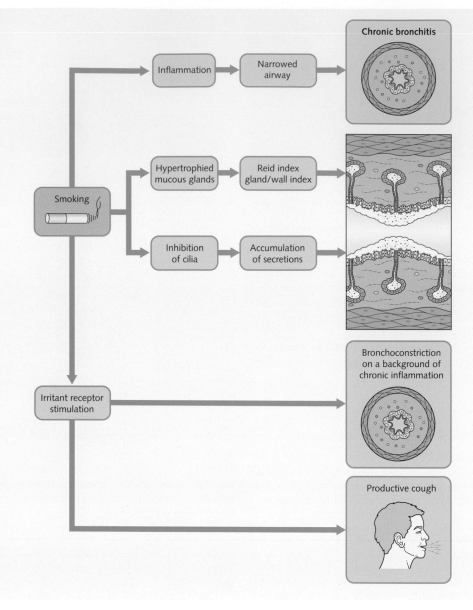

Fig. 17.5 Pathogenesis of mucus hypersecretion.

Breathlessness is one of the primary symptoms of COPD and it is useful to assess this objectively using the Medical Research Council (MRC) dyspnoea scale (Fig. 17.6).

Typical signs found on examination are shown in Figure 17.7.

COMPLICATIONS

Exacerbations

An acute worsening of the patient's condition is usually due to infection, which can be viral (e.g. influenza) or bacterial (commonly *Haemophilus influenzae*). A mild exacerbation may only require an increase in medication at home. If the exacerbation is severe, the patient may deteriorate rapidly and require hospitalization.

Case study

Bob, a 71-year-old man, presented to his GP with a 12-month history of shortness of breath and reduced exercise tolerance. He was noted to have smoked 30 cigarettes a day for the last 25 years. Examination revealed him to be cachectic and breathing through pursed lips. A diagnosis of chronic obstructive pulmonary disease was made on spirometry.

Fig. 17.6 Medical Research Council dyspnoea scale: a useful tool for objectively assessing breathlessness

Grade	Degree of breathlessness related to activities
1	Not troubled by breathlessness except on strenuous exercise
2	Short of breath when hurrying or walking up a slight hill
3	Walks slower than contemporaries on level ground because of breathlessness, or has to stop for breath when walking at own pace
4	Stops for breath after walking about 100 metres or after a few minutes on level ground
5	Too breathless to leave the house, or breathless when dressing or undressing

Fig. 17.7 Signs of chronic obstructive pulmonary disease

On inspection	Central cyanosis
	Barrel chest
	Use of accessory muscles
	Intercostal indrawing
	Pursed-lip breathing
	Flapping tremor
	Tachypnoea
On palpation	Tachycardia
	Tracheal tug
	Reduced expansion
On percussion	Hyperresonant lung fields
On auscultation	Wheeze
	Prolongation of expiration

Respiratory failure

In severe exacerbations the patient may be unable to maintain normal blood gases. This state is known as respiratory failure and is discussed in more detail elsewhere. Respiratory failure is the leading cause of death in patients with COPD and is often hypercapnic (type 2).

Cor pulmonale

Mortality increases in those patients with COPD who develop cor pulmonale, or right ventricular enlargement secondary to disorders affecting the lungs. In COPD it is pulmonary hypertension that causes the right ventricle to hypertrophy and eventually fail.

INVESTIGATION

The gold standard for diagnosis of COPD is spirometry. The presence of a postbronchodilator forced expiratory volume in 1 second (FEV_1)/forced vital capacity (FVC) ratio of <0.70 confirms the presence of persistent airflow limitation and thus of COPD.

The severity of COPD can also be classified in terms of effect on lung function (Fig. 17.8).

Other tests include:

- Pulse oximetry.
- Chest X-ray (classically, hyperinflated lung fields with flattened hemidiaphragms; however, may be normal).
- Full blood count.
- Sputum culture (identify persistent organisms).
- α_1-Antitrypsin level (consider in young patients with COPD).
- Electrocardiograph/echo may be useful in end-stage COPD with features of cor pulmonale.

These tests are helpful but not essential in making a diagnosis of COPD.

MANAGEMENT

Management of COPD is holistic and incorporates both pharmalogical and conservative treatments. There is no cure for COPD and no treatment available that can reverse the damage caused to the lungs by exposure to tobacco smoke or other noxious particles. The aim of treatment in COPD is to control symptoms and reduce exacerbations of disease.

Conservative measures

The single most important intervention in COPD is smoking cessation. Numerous studies have demonstrated that this has the single greatest impact on the natural history of COPD.

Other important conservative measures include:

- Physical activity.
- Improved nutrition.

Fig. 17.8 Classification of chronic obstructive pulmonary disease

Mild	FEV_1 >80+
Moderate	FEV_1 50–80%
Severe	FEV_1 30–39%
Very severe	FEV_1 <30%

FEV_1=forced expiratory volume in 1 second.

- Regular vaccination, i.e. yearly influenza, 5-yearly pneumococcus.
- Counselling and education.

Pulmonary rehabilitation

Pulmonary rehabilitation programmes are increasingly essential in the management of COPD. It is one of the few interventions in COPD (along with smoking cessation) proven to reduce symptoms and improve survival.

Pulmonary rehabilitation normally occurs in an outpatient setting with a multidisciplinary team. Courses usually last 6–12 weeks and aim to improve patients' exercise tolerance and provide management strategies, enabling patients to cope with symptoms of breathlessness.

Pharmacological treatments

Inhaled bronchodilators

The mainstay of treatment in patients with COPD is inhaled bronchodilator therapy used to control symptoms of breathlessness. Initally patients start with a short-acting β_2 agonist (i.e. salbutamol) and/or short-acting anticholinergic (i.e. ipratropium) inhaler, using only when symptomatic.

As the disease progresses, a long-acting inhaler (either β_2 agonist, i.e. salmeterol, or anticholinergic, i.e. tiotropium) is added.

In patients with an FEV_1 <50% or patients still suffering frequent exacerbations, a long-acting β_2 agonist combined with corticosteroid inhaler (i.e. Seretide) can be considered.

In reality, the majority of COPD patients are managed with triple inhaler therapy:

1. Salbutamol PRN (short-acting β_2 agonist).
2. Tiotropium (long-acting anticholinergic).
3. Seretide (long-acting β_2 agonist and corticosteroid).

Two important points to remember when prescribing inhaled bronchodilators for COPD patients are:

1. If introducing a long-acting anticholinergic (tiotropium), then short-acting cholinergic inhalers (ipratropium) need to be stopped.
2. Inhaled corticosteroids are only used in combination with a long-acting β_2 agonist and never alone. They have been shown to reduce the frequency of exacerbations as well as the risk of pneumonia.

Oral medications that can be used include:

- Theophylline.
- Carbocisteine (mucolytic, particularly in patients with chronic productive cough).
- Rescue pack antibiotics (enable patients to treat exacerbations pre-emptively).

Long-term oxygen therapy

Management with home oxygen is an indicator of severe end-stage COPD. National Institute for Health and Clinical Excellence guidance (Fig. 17.9) indicates that patients with the following features should be considered to receive oxygen:

- Non-smokers.
- Patients who have a P_aO_2 less than 7.3 kPa when stable.
- P_aO_2 between 7.3 and 8 kPa, with evidence of one of the following:
  - Polycythaemia.
  - Nocturnal hypoxaemia (S_aO_2 <90%).
  - Peripheral oedema.
  - Pulmonary hypertension.

In order to receive the benefits of long-term oxygen therapy, patients should breathe supplemental oxygen for at least 15 hours per day. If patients are able to adhere to this, an MRC study has demonstrated that long-term oxygen therapy is associated with a 50% reduction in mortality at 3 years.

In patients who become hypercapnic or acidotic on long-term oxygen therapy, regular non-invasive ventilation must be considered – this requires referral to a specialist centre.

Management of acute exacerbations of COPD

An exacerbation is a sustained worsening of the patient's symptoms from his or her usual stable state which is beyond normal day-to-day variations, and is acute in onset. Commonly reported symptoms are worsening breathlessness, cough, increased sputum production and change in sputum colour.

The severity of an exacerbation is assessed using the following tests:

- Blood: evidence of a raised white cell count and C-reactive protein indicates the presence of infection.
- Sputum culture: enables targeted antibiotic use.
- Arterial blood gases: indicators of severity, i.e. hypoxia, hypercapnia and acidosis.
- Chest X-ray.

Management includes:

- Controlled oxygen to maintain oxygen saturations between 88 and 92%; this is normally achieved with a Venturi mask.
- Nebulized short-acting bronchodilators (salbutamol and ipratropium).
- A short course of oral steroids (usually 30 mg prednisolone). If patients have received multiple courses of steroids they will require a reducing-dose regimen to avoid rebound exacerbations when the steroids are stopped.

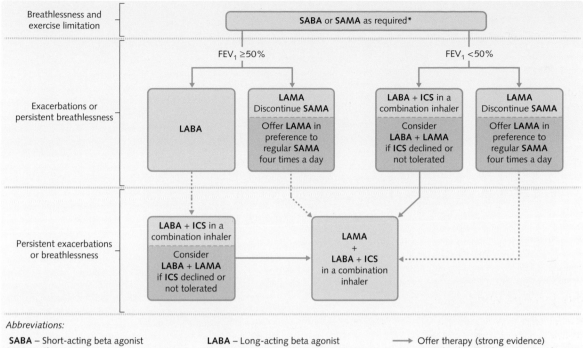

Abbreviations:

SABA – Short-acting beta agonist
SAMA – Short-acting muscarinic antagonist
***SABA** (as required) may continue at all stages

LABA – Long-acting beta agonist
LAMA – Long-acting muscarinic antagonist
ICS – Inhaled corticosteroid

——▶ Offer therapy (strong evidence)
╌╌╌▶ Consider therapy (less strong evidence)

Fig. 17.9   National Institute for Health and Clinical Excellence guidelines for management of chronic obstructive pulmonary disease.

- Antibiotics, e.g. doxycycline if exacerbation is thought to be infective.
- Non-invasive ventilation (i.e. bilevel positive airway pressure) may be required if patients develop respiratory failure and become acidotic – pH <7.3.

Further reading

BMJ learning module: COPD: Diagnosis and management of exacerbations. Available at www.learning.bmj.com.
BTS guidelines for COPD. Available at www.brit-thoracic.org.uk.

GOLD guideline for COPD. Available at www.goldcopd.org.
Lopez, A.D., Murray, C.C., 1998. The global burden of disease, 1990–2020. Nat. Med 4, 1241–1243.
Medical Research Council Working Party, 1981. Long-term domiciliary oxygen therapy in chronic hypoxic cor pulmonale complicating chronic bronchitis and emphysema. Lancet 1, 681–686.
NICE guideline for COPD. Available at www.nice.org.uk.

Disorders of the interstitium (18)

By the end of this chapter you should be able to:
- Describe the different types of interstitial lung disease (ILD).
- Discuss the legal implications of work-related ILD, such as asbestosis and coal worker's pneumoconiosis.
- Discuss the investigation and management of idiopathic pulmonary fibrosis.

INTRODUCTION

The ILDs are a diverse group of over 200 different lung diseases. They all affect the lung interstitium, i.e. the space between the alveolar epithelium and capillary endothelium (see Fig. 2.16) and their pathology can be broadly classed as either granulomatous (e.g. sarcoid) or fibrosis (e.g. idiopathic fibrosing lung disease).

Aetiology is variable but they all present in a similar fashion, typically with shortness of breath and chest-X-ray shadows. Though separately each disease is rare, collectively they affect 1/2000 of the population. Outcome varies between patients and disease, but pulmonary fibrosis represents the common, irreversible end stage of ILD.

Confusion may arise over terminology. To clarify, the term 'diffuse parenchymal lung disease' may be used interchangeably with ILD but not with fibrosing or granulomatous lung disease. This is because fibrosis and granulomas can occur in conditions other than ILD. Additional synonyms are mentioned under each condition.

Some of the most important of the ILDs are discussed below.

PULMONARY FIBROSIS – OVERVIEW

Definition

Pulmonary fibrosis is the end result of many respiratory diseases (Fig. 18.1) and is characterized by scar tissue in the lungs which decreases lung compliance, i.e. the lungs become stiffer.

Pathogenesis

The pathogenesis of pulmonary fibrosis is complex, involving many factors (Fig. 18.2). The main features are:
- A lesion affecting the alveolar-capillary basement membrane.

- Cellular infiltration and thickening by collagen of the interstitium of the alveolar wall.
- Fibroblasts proliferate, leading to further collagen deposition.

The end stage is characterized by a honeycomb lung, a non-specific condition in which cystic spaces develop in fibrotic lungs with compensatory dilatation of unaffected neighbouring bronchioles.

Note from Figure 18.2 that the initial injury to the alveolar-capillary basement membrane may be caused by several different mechanisms. Some (e.g. dusts) are considered below.

Clinical features

Patients become progressively breathless and develop a dry, non-productive cough. On examination, lung expansion is reduced and fine end-inspiratory crackles are heard.

Investigations

Chest X-ray may show fine reticular, nodular or reticulonodular infiltration in the basal areas. High-resolution computed tomography (HRCT) is the gold standard imaging, revealing the characteristic honeycomb and/or ground-glass appearance of pulmonary fibrosis. However, this needs to be interpreted, ideally by a radiologist with a specialist interest in HRCT and/or chest medicine.

Biopsy may be used to aid diagnosis; however, this can be difficult in older patients, who may not be suitable for surgery. Furthermore, there can be considerable differences in the interpretation of histological specimens.

Lung function tests demonstrate a restrictive pattern along with a decreased transfer factor and can help monitor the progression of the disease. Measuring oxygen desaturation on exercise testing (such as the 6-minute

157

Fig. 18.1 Causes of pulmonary fibrosis

Dusts		Inhalants	Infection	Iatrogenic causes	Other causes
Mineral	**Biological**				
Coal	Avian protein	Oxygen	Postpneumonic infection	Cytotoxic drugs	Sarcoidosis
Silica	*Actinomyces*	Sulphur dioxide	Tuberculosis	Non-cytotoxics	Connective tissue disease
Asbestos	*Aspergillus*	Nitrogen dioxide	–	Radiation	Chronic pulmonary oedema

Fig. 18.2 Pathogenesis of pulmonary fibrosis. Macrophages can be activated by several factors (e.g. soluble immune complexes and sensitized T lymphocytes), resulting in the release of various cytokines and leading to fibrosis.

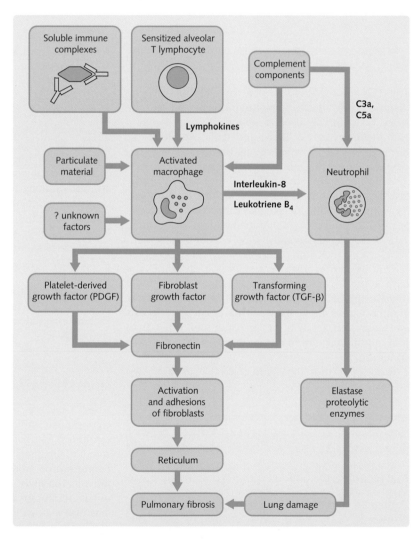

walk test) can be useful for functional assessment. The British Thoracic Society (BTS) recommends integrating the results of both imaging and lung function tests and adopting a multidisciplinary approach, in order to assess the severity and extent of disease best.

Treatment

Treatment for pulmonary fibrosis is variable, depending on the underlying cause. Any underlying triggers or stimuli should be avoided as much as possible, although this may not be practical. The changes seen in pulmonary fibrosis are largely irreversible and there are no definitive treatments.

Medical treatments have variable efficacy. Oral steroids can be used to dampen the inflammatory response. However, there are numerous side-effects to long-term oral steroid treatment, such as osteoporosis and development of cushingoid features. Therefore, steroid-sparing agents such as cyclophosphamide can be used instead. However, the BTS recommends that steroids should not be used in combination with agents such as azathioprine, as a large trial showed that these patients had worse outcomes. *N*-acetylcysteine has been shown in some trials to improve outcomes; however, the evidence is not conclusive. There is very little evidence that inhaled therapies such as salbutamol have any benefit.

When patients develop severe pulmonary fibrosis which is unresponsive to medical therapy, home oxygen therapy may be necessary, progressing to long-term oxygen therapy.

A multidisciplinary approach is recommended by the BTS and subjective and objective benefits may be achieved through pulmonary rehabilitation and other such non-pharmacological interventions.

Complications

Patients can sometimes present in respiratory failure. These patients should be managed in the same way as all other patients in acute respiratory failure (see Ch. 12) and, once stable, an underlying cause can be investigated. It could also be progression of known disease or a superimposed infection. Worsening or first presentation of severe pulmonary fibrosis can be treated initially with intravenous corticosteroids, with cyclophosphamide as second-line therapy. Assessment by an intensive care physician should also be made and decisions about ceiling of care discussed with the patient.

Pulmonary hypertension should be considered in all patients with ILD. The BTS recommends transthoracic echocardiography as the best method to detect pulmonary hypertension in these patients.

One must also consider other diagnoses associated with the underlying cause of the pulmonary fibrosis. This is particularly important in those with asbestosis, as they are at risk of mesothelioma.

THE PNEUMOCONIOSES

Definition

The pneumoconioses are a group of disorders caused by inhalation of mineral or biological dusts. The incidence is decreasing as working conditions continue to improve.

Pathogenesis

Four types of reaction occur:

1. Inert (e.g. simple coal-worker's pneumoconiosis).
2. Fibrous (e.g. asbestosis).
3. Allergic (e.g. extrinsic allergic alveolitis).
4. Neoplastic (e.g. mesothelioma).

Distribution of lung disease depends on the dust involved: particles measuring less than 2–3 μm in diameter reach the distal alveoli.

Coal worker's pneumoconiosis

The incidence of coal worker's pneumoconiosis is related to total dust exposure: it is highest in men who work at the coal face. Two syndromes exist: simple pneumoconiosis and an advanced form, progressive massive fibrosis.

In recent years, thousands of patients have lodged claims for compensation for work-related exposure to coal dust, which in turn has led to the development of coal worker's pneumoconiosis. The Coal Workers Pneumoconiosis Scheme has been set up specifically for this purpose. Although not all claims are successful, many patients are able to get some compensation for the disease that they have subsequently developed. It is also important to note that, when writing a death certificate, one must declare if the cause of death is related to the patient's employment history, as relatives may be eligible for compensation.

Further information in regard to litigation can be found in Chapter 19.

Simple pneumoconiosis

Simple pneumoconiosis is the commonest type of pneumoconiosis, reflecting coal dust deposition within the lung. It is asymptomatic and diagnosis is made on the basis of small round opacities in the upper zone on chest X-rays. Those with severe disease may go on to develop progressive massive fibrosis.

Progressive massive fibrosis

In progressive massive fibrosis, large, round fibrotic nodules measuring more than 10 mm in diameter are seen, usually in the upper lobes. Scarring is present. Nodules may show central liquefaction and become infected by tuberculosis. The associated emphysema is always severe.

Symptoms include dyspnoea, cough and sputum production (which may be black as cavitating lesions rupture). Lung function tests show a mixed restrictive and obstructive pattern.

The disease may progress once exposure has ceased (unlike simple coal worker's pneumoconiosis) and there is no specific treatment.

Caplan's syndrome

Caplan's syndrome is the association of coal worker's pneumoconiosis and rheumatoid arthritis.

Rounded lesions, measuring 0.5–5.0 cm in diameter, are seen on X-ray.

Asbestosis

Asbestosis is diffuse pulmonary fibrosis caused by the inhalation of asbestos, a mixture of silicates of iron, nickel, magnesium, aluminium and cadmium mined from the ground. In the UK, exposure is most likely to occur during building renovations as in the past asbestos was used in housing materials such as insulation. Therefore those with occupations such as plumbers, electricians and builders are at high risk of exposure.

Several types of asbestos exist: serpentine fibres, which do not cause pulmonary disease, and amphibole fibres, which do. The most important type of amphibole asbestos is crocidolite (blue asbestos), a straight fibre 50 µm long and 1–2 µm wide that cannot be cleared by the immune system. Fibres remain in the lung indefinitely and become coated in iron (haemosiderin) to form the classic drumstick-shaped asbestos bodies.

Histology shows asbestos bodies and features of pulmonary fibrosis, affecting the lower lobes more commonly.

A considerable time lag, sometimes as long as 20–40 years, exists between exposure and disease development. The first clinical symptoms are dyspnoea and a dry cough; signs include clubbing. Bilateral end-inspiratory crackles indicate significant diffuse pulmonary fibrosis. No treatment is available.

Exposure to asbestos is a risk factor for mesothelioma. Further information on this can be found in Chapter 19.

EXTRINSIC ALLERGIC ALVEOLITIS

Definition

Hypersensitivity pneumonitis is also known as extrinsic allergic alveolitis. The condition is a widespread diffuse inflammatory reaction caused by a type III hypersensitivity reaction and results from the individual being already sensitized to the inhaled antigen.

Pathogenesis

Antigens that can cause allergic lung disease include:

* Mouldy hay (e.g. farmer's lung).
* Bird faeces (e.g. in bird fancier's lung).
* Cotton fibres (e.g. byssinosis).
* Sugar cane fibres (e.g. bagassosis).

Neutrophils infiltrate small airways and alveolar walls after antigen exposure. Lymphocytes and macrophages then infiltrate, leading to the development of non-caseating granulomas, which may resolve or organize, leading to pulmonary fibrosis.

Clinical features

These consist of cough, shortness of breath, fever and malaise that occur acutely several hours after exposure to antigen. Onset is more insidious in long-term exposure to small amounts. Coarse end-inspiratory crackles can be heard on auscultation.

Investigations

There are many different ways to investigate extrinsic allergic alveolitis. These include polymorphonuclear leucocyte count, precipitating antibodies (evidence of exposure, not disease), nodular shadowing on chest X-ray, lung function tests showing a restrictive pattern and bronchoalveolar lavage.

Treatment

Most diseases will regress once the patient is prevented from further exposure to the antigen. Corticosteroids may speed recovery but do not alter the ultimate level of lung function and are thought to be mostly of benefit in severe disease. HRCT scans can detect disease in patients with normal chest X-rays.

IDIOPATHIC PULMONARY FIBROSIS

Definition

Also known as fibrosing alveolitis or cryptogenic fibrosing alveolitis, idiopathic pulmonary fibrosis is a rare, progressive chronic pulmonary fibrosis of unknown aetiology. It has a peak incidence in patients aged 45–65 years.

Pathology

The alveolar walls are thickened because of fibrosis, predominantly in the subpleural regions of the lower lobes. An increased number of chronic inflammatory cells are in the alveoli and interstitium. This pattern is termed 'usual interstitial pneumonitis' and is a progressive condition.

Patterns of disease also include:

* Desquamative interstitial pneumonitis.
* Bronchiolitis obliterans.

Idiopathic pulmonary fibrosis has been reported with a number of other conditions: connective tissue disorders, coeliac disease, ulcerative colitis and renal tubular acidosis.

Clinical features

Clinical features of idiopathic pulmonary fibrosis include progressive breathlessness and a dry cough. Fatigue and considerable weight loss can occur. There is progression to cyanosis, respiratory failure, pulmonary hypertension and cor pulmonale over time.

Clubbing occurs in two-thirds of patients; chest expansion is reduced and bilateral, fine, end-inspiratory crackles are heard on auscultation.

Investigations

Several investigations are made:

- Transbronchial or open-lung biopsy to confirm histological diagnosis.
- CT scan.
- Blood gases may show arterial hypoxaemia.
- Full blood count may show raised erythrocyte sedimentation rate.
- Lung function test shows a restrictive pattern.
- Bronchoalveolar lavage shows increased numbers of neutrophils.
- Autoantibody tests.
- Antinuclear factor is positive in one-third of patients. Rheumatoid factor is positive in one-half of patients.

Treatment

About 50% of patients respond to immunosuppression. Combined therapy is recommended with:

- Prednisolone 0.5 mg/kg daily for 1 month and then tapered.
- Azathioprine (2–3 mg/kg).

Cyclophosphamide may be substituted for azathioprine.

Single-lung transplantation may be attempted where necessary.

Supportive treatment includes oxygen therapy.

Prognosis

Of patients with the condition, 50% die within 4–5 years.

PULMONARY EOSINOPHILIA

Pulmonary eosinophilia is a group of syndromes characterized by abnormally high levels of eosinophils in the blood, or, in the case of acute eosinophilic pneumonia, in lung lavage fluid. The severity of these diseases can range from mild to fatal (Fig. 18.3).

BRONCHIOLITIS OBLITERANS

In bronchiolitis obliterans, characteristic histological appearance shows:

- Polypoid masses of organizing inflammatory exudate.
- Granulation tissue extending from alveoli to bronchioles.

Fig. 18.3 The causes of pulmonary eosinophilia

Disease	Aetiology	Symptoms	Blood eosinophils (%)	Multisystem involvement	Duration	Outcome
Simple	Passage of parasitic larvae through lung	Mild	10	None	<1 month	Good
Prolonged	Unknown	Mild/moderate	<20	None	>1 month	Good
Asthmatic	Often type I hypersensitivity to *Aspergillus*	Moderate/severe	5–20	None	Years	Fair
Tropical	Hypersensitivity reaction to filarial infestation	Moderate/severe	>20	None	Years	Fair
Hypereosinophilic syndrome	Unknown	Severe	>20	Always	Months/years	Poor
Churg–Strauss syndrome	Possibly immune complex vasculitis	Severe	>20	Always	Months/years	Poor/fair

Aetiology is unknown, although an association with a number of clinical conditions exists:

- Viral infections (e.g. respiratory syncytial virus).
- Aspiration.
- Inhalation of toxic fumes.
- Extrinsic allergic alveolitis.
- Pulmonary fibrosis.
- Collagen or vascular disorders.

Bronchiolitis obliterans is sensitive to corticosteroid treatment.

DESQUAMATIVE INTERSTITIAL PNEUMONITIS

Desquamative interstitial pneumonitis is found in patients with fibrosing alveolitis. It is more diffuse than usual interstitial pneumonitis. A proliferation of macrophages in the alveolar air spaces occurs, along with interstitial thickening by mononuclear inflammatory cells. Lymphoid tissue and a small amount of collagen are sometimes present.

Desquamative interstitial pneumonitis has a distinctly uniform histological pattern. The alveolar walls show relatively little fibrosis.

Corticosteroids may be beneficial, and prognosis is good.

ALVEOLAR PROTEINOSIS

Alveolar proteinosis, also known as alveolar lipoproteinosis, is a rare condition of unknown aetiology and pathogenesis.

Clinically, dyspnoea and cough, and rarely haemoptysis and chest pain, result. Alveolar proteinosis is associated with a high incidence of concomitant fungal infections and may complicate other interstitial disease.

The course of the disease is variable, but the majority of patients enjoy spontaneous remission.

Useful links

http://www.brit-thoracic.org.uk/guidelines/interstitial-lung-disease-%28dpld%29-guideline.aspx.

http://www.brit-thoracic.org.uk/Portals/0/Clinical%20Information/DPLD/Guidelines/Thorax%20Sept%2008.pdf.

http://www.decc.gov.uk/en/content/cms/funding/coal_health/coal_health.aspx.

Malignant lung disease (19)

Objectives

By the end of this chapter you should be able to:
* Show awareness of the epidemiology, risk factors and presentation of bronchial carcinoma.
* Understand the different histological types of bronchial carcinoma and implications for treatment.
* Discuss appropriate investigations in the condition.
* Show awareness of management, including a multidisciplinary team approach.

NEOPLASTIC DISEASE OF THE LUNG

Bronchial carcinoma

Bronchial carcinoma accounts for 95% of all primary tumours of the lung and is the commonest malignant tumour in the Western world. Bronchogenic carcinoma affects men more than women (male-to-female ratio, 3.5:1) but incidence is rising in women and it is now the commonest cancer in both sexes. Typically, patients are aged 40–70 years at presentation; only 2–3% occur in younger patients.

Aetiology

Risk factors are summarized in Figure 19.1. Cigarette smoking is the largest contributory factor:

* It is related to the amount smoked, duration and tar content: 20% of smokers will develop lung cancer.
* The rise in incidence of lung cancer correlates closely with the increase in smoking over the past century.
* In non-smokers, the incidence is 3–5 cases per 100 000. In the UK, there are 100 deaths per 100 000 smokers per year.
* The risk in those who give up smoking decreases with time.
* Passive smoking also increases risk.

Environmental and occupational factors include:

* Radon released from granite rock.
* Asbestos.
* Air pollution (e.g. beryllium emissions).

Histological types

There are four main histological types of bronchogenic carcinoma, subdivided into non-small-cell and small-cell carcinomas.

* Non-small-cell carcinomas (70%):
  * Squamous cell carcinoma (52%).
  * Adenocarcinoma (13%).
  * Large-cell carcinoma (5%).
* Small-cell carcinomas (30%).

The different types of tumour are summarized in Figure 19.2. Tumours may occur as discrete or mixed histological patterns; the development from the initial malignant change to presentation is variable:

* Squamous cell carcinoma: 8 years.
* Adenocarcinoma: 15 years.
* Small-cell carcinoma: 3 years.

Squamous cell carcinoma

Squamous cell carcinoma arises from squamous epithelium in the large bronchi. A strong association between cigarette smoking and squamous cell carcinoma exists. Males are affected most commonly, with a mean age at diagnosis of 57 years.

Squamous cell carcinomas are histologically well differentiated and are associated with paraneoplastic syndromes; the cancer commonly produces a substance similar to parathyroid hormone, which leads to hypercalcaemia and bone destruction (Fig. 19.3).

The major mass of the tumour may occur outside the bronchial cartilage and encircle the bronchial lumen, producing obstructive phenomena. The tumours are almost always hilar and are prone to massive necrosis and cavitation, with upper-lobe lesions more likely to cavitate. Of squamous cell carcinomas, 13% show cavitation on chest radiographs. Peripheral lesions tend to be larger than those seen in adenocarcinomas.

If squamous carcinoma occurs in the apical portion of the lung, it may produce Pancoast's syndrome (see below).

Squamous cell carcinoma is the least likely type to metastasize and, untreated, it has the longest patient survival of any of the bronchogenic carcinomas.

Fig. 19.1 Risk factors in lung cancer

Factor	Relative risk
Non-smoker	1
Smoker, 1–2 packs/day	42
Ex-smoker	2–10
Passive smoke exposure	1.5–2
Asbestos exposure	5
Asbestos plus tobacco	90

Adenocarcinoma

Adenocarcinomas are most common in:

- Non-smoking elderly women.
- The Far East.

Adenocarcinomas are associated with diffuse pulmonary fibrosis and honeycomb lung. Bronchogenic tumours associated with occupational factors are mainly adenocarcinomas. In all, 90% of adenocarcinomas occur between 40 and 69 years of age, with the mean age for diagnosis being 53 years. Two-thirds

Fig. 19.2 Summary of tumour types

	Non-small-cell tumours			Small-cell tumours
	Squamous cell	Adenocarcinoma	Large-cell	
Incidence (%)	52	13	5	30
Male/female incidence	M>F	F>M	M>F	M>F
Location	Hilar	Peripheral	Peripheral/central	Hilar
Histological stain	Keratin	Mucin	–	–
Relationship to smoking	High	Low	High	High
Growth rate	Slow	Medium	Rapid	Very rapid
Metastasis	Late	Intermediate	Early	Very early
Treatment	Surgery			Chemotherapy
Prognosis	2-year survival=50%			3 months if untreated; 1 year if treated

Fig. 19.3 Paraneoplastic disorders associated with lung cancer

	Mechanism	Clinical features	Lung cancer association
SIADH	Excess secretion of ADH	Headache, nausea, muscle weakness, drowsiness, confusion, eventually coma	Small-cell
Ectopic ACTH	Adrenal hyperplasia and secretion of large amounts of cortisol	Cushing's: polyuria, oedema, hypokalaemia, hypertension, increased pigmentation	Small-cell or carcinoid
Hypercalcaemia	Ectopic PTH secretion	Lethargy, nausea, polyuria, eventually coma	Squamous cell (but may be due to bone metastases)
Hypertrophic pulmonary osteoarthropathy	Unknown	Digital clubbing and periosteal inflammation	Adenocarcinoma, squamous cell
Gonadotrophins	Ectopic secretion	Gynaecomastia, testicular atrophy	Large-cell

SIADH=syndrome of inappropriate antidiuretic hormone; ADH=antidiuretic hormone (vasopressin); ACTH=adrenocorticotrophic hormone; PTH=parathyroid hormone.

of adenocarcinomas are found peripherally. Usually, tumours measure more than 4 cm in diameter.

Adenocarcinoma arises from glandular cells such as mucus goblet cells, type II pneumocytes and Clara cells. Histologically, they are differentiated from other bronchogenic tumours by their glandular configuration and mucin production.

As the tumour is commonly in the periphery, obstructive symptoms are rare, so the tumour tends to be clinically silent. Symptoms include coughing, haemoptysis, chest pain and weight loss. A wide range of paraneoplastic syndromes are seen (see below). Malignant cells are detected in the sputum in 50% of patients, and the commonest radiological presentation is a solitary peripheral pulmonary nodule, close to the pleural surface.

Resection is possible in a small proportion of cases; 5-year survival rate is less than 10%. Invasion of the pleura and mediastinal lymph nodes is common, as too is metastasis to the brain and bones.

Metastasis to the gastrointestinal tract, pancreas or ovaries must be excluded after having made a diagnosis.

Large-cell anaplastic tumour

Large-cell anaplastic tumours are diagnosed by a process of elimination. No clear-cut pattern of clinical or radiological presentation distinguishes them from other malignant lung tumours. These tumours are variable in location, but are usually centrally located. The point of origin of the carcinoma influences the symptomatic presentation of the disease: central lesions present earlier than peripheral lesions as they cause obstruction.

The tumour causes coughing, sputum production and haemoptysis. When a tumour occurs in a major airway, obstructive pneumonia can occur. Sputum cytology and bronchoscopy with bronchial biopsy make the diagnosis.

On electron microscopy, these tumours turn out to be poorly differentiated variants of squamous cell carcinoma and adenocarcinoma; they are extremely aggressive and destructive lesions. Early invasion of blood vessels and lymphatics occurs, and treatment is by surgical resection whenever possible.

Small-cell carcinoma

Small-cell carcinomas arise from endocrine cells and their incidence is directly related to cigarette consumption. Cancer of this form is considered to be a systemic disease. Small-cell carcinomas are the most aggressive malignancy of all the bronchogenic tumours.

Most small-cell anaplastic tumours originate in the large bronchi, and obstructive pneumonitis is frequently seen.

These tumours have hyperdense nuclei. Occasionally almost no cytoplasm is present and the cells are compressed into an ovoid form; the neoplasm is then termed an oat-cell carcinoma. On radiography, the oat-cell carcinoma does not cavitate.

There is a high occurrence of paraneoplastic syndromes associated with this type of tumour, so presentation may be varied. The most frequent presenting complaint is coughing. Spread is rapid, and metastatic lesions may be the presenting sign. Small-cell carcinomas metastasize through the lymphatic route.

Prognosis is very poor, with a mean survival time for untreated patients with small-cell carcinoma of 7 weeks after diagnosis. Death is generally caused by metastatic disease. Interestingly, small-cell carcinoma is the only bronchial carcinoma that responds to chemotherapy.

Clinical features

Features specific to the histological types have already been introduced above. There are no specific signs of bronchogenic carcinoma. Diagnosis always needs to be excluded in cigarette smokers who present with recurrent respiratory symptoms:

- Persistent cough – commonest presentation; may be productive if obstruction leads to infection.
- Haemoptysis – occurs at some stage in disease in 50%.
- Dyspnoea – rarely at presentation but occurs as disease progresses.
- Chest pain – often pleuritic, caused by obstructive changes.
- Wheezing – monophonic, due to obstruction.
- Unexplained weight loss.
- Finger clubbing – in 10–30% of patients finger clubbing is present on examination.

Complications

Local complications
Symptoms may be caused by:

- Ulceration of bronchus: occurs in up to 50% of patients and produces haemoptysis in varying degrees.
- Bronchial obstruction: the lumen of the bronchus becomes occluded; distal collapse and retention of secretions subsequently occur. This clinically causes dyspnoea, secondary infection and lung abscesses.
- Central necrosis: carcinomas can outgrow their blood supply, leading to central necrosis. The main complication is then the development of a lung abscess.

Pancoast's syndrome

Pancoast's syndrome can be caused by all types of bronchogenic carcinoma, although two-thirds originate from squamous cells. As the tumour grows outward from the pulmonary parenchymal apex, it encroaches on anatomical structures, including:

- Chest wall.
- Subpleural lymphatics.
- Sympathetic chain.

Pancoast's tumours can affect the sympathetic chain, resulting in loss of sympathetic tone and an ipsilateral Horner's syndrome (mild ptosis, pupil constricted with no reaction to shading, and reduced sweating on ipsilateral side of the head and neck). Intractable shoulder pain occurs when the upper rib is involved. The subclavian artery and vein may become compressed. Destruction of the inferior trunk of the brachial plexus leads to pain in ulnar nerve distribution and may lead to small-muscle wasting of the hand. Pancoast's tumour is diagnosed by percutaneous needle aspiration of the tumour.

Metastatic complications

Metastases to lymph nodes, bone, liver and adrenal glands occur. Metastases to the brain present as:

- Change in personality.
- Epilepsy.
- Focal neurological lesion.

Paraneoplastic syndromes

Paraneoplastic syndromes (Fig. 19.3) cannot be explained by direct invasion of the tumour. They are caused by production by tumour cells of polypeptides that mimic various hormones. Paraneoplastic syndromes are commonly associated with small-cell lung cancer. The commonest of these is syndrome of inappropriate antidiuretic hormone secretion (SIADH), resulting in increased water resorption in the collecting ducts of the kidney, leading to low total body sodium (dilutional hyponatraemia), low serum osmolality and a high urine osmolality. Investigation for this involves paired blood and urine samples to assess their respective osmolalities.

Investigations

Investigations are performed to confirm diagnosis and assess tumour histology and spread.

Chest radiography

Good posteroanterior and lateral views are required. Seventy per cent of bronchial carcinomas arise centrally, and chest radiography demonstrates over 90% of carcinomas. The mass needs to be 1–2 cm in size to be recognized reliably. Lobar collapse and pleural effusions may be present.

CT scan

Computed tomography (CT) scanning gives good visualization of the mediastinum and is good at identifying small lesions. These are essential for staging (via the TNM system) and to assess the operability of the mass. Lymph nodes larger than 1.5 cm are pathological.

Further scans should include brain, liver and adrenals to identify distant metastases.

Fibreoptic bronchoscopy

This involves endoscopic examination of the trachea and first several divisions of the bronchi. It confirms central lesions, assesses operability and allows accurate cell type to be determined. It is used to obtain cytological specimens. Mucus secretions plus sputum can be examined for the presence of malignant cells. If carcinoma involves the first 2 cm of either main bronchus, the tumour is inoperable.

Exciting new techniques such as fluorescence bronchoscopy can detect premalignant lesions, but are currently limited to highly specialized centres.

Transthoracic fine-needle aspiration biopsy

In transthoracic fine-needle aspiration biopsy, the needle is guided by X-ray or CT. Direct aspiration of peripheral lung lesions takes place through the chest wall; 25% of patients suffer pneumothorax due to the procedure. Implantation metastases do not occur.

Staging

Staging can be clinical or histological and is of importance as it affects both prognosis and treatment options. Small-cell and non-small-cell cancers are staged differently. Both are staged using the TNM system (Fig. 19.4), as recommended by the International Union Against Cancer. However, small-cell cancers are often additionally staged using the Veterans Administration Lung Cancer Study Group system as either limited or diffuse. Limited-stage disease is confined to an area that can feasibly be treated by one radiation area; it excludes cancers with pleural and pericardial effusions automatically. All other small-cell lung cancers are extensive-stage in this scheme.

Treatment

Surgery

The only treatment of any value in non-small-cell carcinoma is surgery; however, only 15% of cases are operable at diagnosis. Surgery can only be performed after:

- Lung function tests show the patient has sufficient respiratory reserve.
- CT scan shows no evidence of metastases.

Radiation therapy

This is the treatment of choice if the tumour is inoperable. It is good for slowly growing squamous carcinoma. Radiation pneumonitis develops in 10–15% and radiation fibrosis occurs to some degree in all cases.

Fig. 19.4	Staging in non-small-cell lung cancer		
T1	<3 cm – no evidence of invasion proximal to a lobar bronchus		
T2	≥3 cm or any site involving pleura or hilum; within a lobar bronchus or at least 2 cm distal to the carina		
T3	Any size extending into the chest wall, diaphragm, pericardium (not involving great vessels, etc.)		
T4	Inoperable tumour of any size with invasion of the mediastinum or involving heart great vessels, trachea, oesophagus, vertebral body or carina or malignant pleural effusion		
	Regional lymph nodes	**Distant metastases**	
N0	No nodal involvement	M0	No metastases
N1	Peribronchial and/or ipsilateral hilar nodes	M1	Distant metastases
N2	Ipsilateral mediastinal and subcarinal lymph nodes		
N3	Inoperable contralateral node involvement		

Chemotherapy

This is the only effective treatment for small-cell carcinoma, but it is not undertaken with intent to cure. Platinum compounds can achieve good results.

Terminal care

Endoscopic therapy and transbronchial stenting are used to provide symptomatic relief in patients with terminal disease. Daily prednisolone (maximum dose 15 mg) may improve appetite. Opioid analgesia is given to control pain and laxatives should be prescribed to counteract the opioid side-effects. Candidiasis is a common, treatable problem. Both patients and relatives require counselling. Involvement of Macmillan nurses, palliative care and community teams is paramount for effective management of end-stage disease.

Prognosis

Overall, prognosis is poor; only 6–8% survive 5 years and mean survival is less than 6 months.

NEOPLASMS OF THE PLEURA

Malignant mesothelioma

Malignant mesothelioma is a tumour of mesothelial cells most commonly affecting the visceral or parietal pleura. The incidence of mesothelioma is rising rapidly and has been since the 1960s. Currently, there are approximately 1300 cases per year in the UK. In 90% of cases it is associated with occupational exposure to asbestos, especially fibres which are <0.25 μm in diameter, e.g. crocidolite and amosite. The latent period between exposure and death is long – up to 40 years.

Two histological varieties exist, although 50% of mesotheliomas have elements of both:

1. Epithelial: tubular structure.
2. Fibrous: solid structure with spindle-shaped cells.

The tumour begins as nodules in the pleura and goes on to obliterate the pleural cavity.

Clinical features

Initial symptoms are very vague, with pain being the main complaint, often affecting sleep and resulting from infiltration of the tumour into the chest wall with involvement of intercostal nerves and ribs. Other features include:

- Dyspnoea.
- Weight loss.
- Finger clubbing.

Investigations

Features of the chest radiograph are:

- Pleural effusions.
- Unilateral pleural thickening.
- Nodular appearance.

Mesothelioma should be considered in any patient with pleural thickening or pleural effusion, especially if pain is present. Open-lung biopsy may be needed to confirm diagnosis.

Prognosis

No treatment is available and the condition is universally fatal. Pain responds poorly to therapy. Metastases are common to hilar and abdominal lymph nodes with secondary deposits arising in lung, liver, thyroid, adrenals, bone, skeletal muscle and brain. The patient's symptoms become worse until death occurs, usually within 8–14 months of diagnosis; the cause of death is usually infection, vascular compromise or pulmonary embolus.

Compensation and mesothelioma

This is a booming area of industrial law with increasing awareness of the ability to claim coupled with a more empowered litigious society. Benefits are available from the government in the form of Industrial Injuries Disablement Benefit, paid on a weekly basis to those with mesothelioma who can prove past asbestos exposure.

Additionally, one can sue an employer or former employer, or the insurers of that former employer if no longer in business. For a claim to be successful it must be initiated within 3 years of diagnosis and proven that:

- It is likely that the patient's mesothelioma is due to occupational exposure to asbestos.
- The patient's employer was negligent in not keeping up the standards required by common law.

Lump sum payments are also available under the Pneumoconiosis Workers' Compensation Act of 1979 and from the Diffuse Mesothelioma Scheme 2008 for cases related to self-employment exposure and passive exposure, for example, the relative or spouse of a person exposed occupationally. Relatives who have lost a family member to mesothelioma may also be entitled to compensation.

HINTS AND TIPS

Advice on benefits and living with cancer is available from Macmillan Cancer Support.

Metastatic malignancy to the lung

Metastases to the lung are a common clinical and radiological finding. Metastases are more likely to be multiple

Fig. 19.5 Metastatic malignancy of lung and the resulting radiological appearance

Multinodular		Solitary nodule
Cannonball	Snowstorm	
Salivary gland	Breast	Breast
Kidney	Kidney	Kidney
Bowel	Bladder	Bowel
Uterus/ovarian	Thyroid	
Testis	Prostate	

than solitary. Most haematogenous metastases are sharply circumscribed with smooth edges, and the appearance of multiple smoothly circumscribed nodules is highly suggestive of metastatic disease. Cavitation is unusual in metastatic lesions.

Solitary pulmonary metastases do occur as sarcomas of soft tissue or bone, carcinoma of the breast, colon and kidney. Multinodular lung metastases may be of varying sizes (Fig. 19.5):

- Very large dimensions – cannonball pattern.
- Many small nodules – snowstorm pattern.

Further reading

International Union Against Cancer (UICC), 2012. TNM. Available online at: http://www.uicc.org/resources/tnm.

Macmillan, 2010. Financial help and compensation for mesothelioma. Available online at: http://www.macmillan.org.uk/Cancerinformation/Cancertypes/Mesothelioma/Livingwithmesothelioma/Financialhelpcompensation.aspx.

Micke, P., Faldum, A., Metz, T., et al., 2002. Staging small cell lung cancer: Veterans Administration Lung Study Group versus International Association for the Study of Lung Cancer – what limits limited disease? Lung Cancer 37, 271–276.

Infectious lung disease (20)

INTRODUCTION

In this chapter we will examine the main infectious diseases affecting the lung, focusing on:

- Pneumonia.
- Influenza.
- TB.
- HIV-related lung disease.

PNEUMONIA

Definition and epidemiology

Pneumonia is an acute infection of the lung parenchyma. It is a condition associated with high morbidity and mortality. In the UK alone, pneumonia is responsible for approximately 83 000 hospital admissions per year and is the fifth leading cause of death.

Aetiology

Risk factors for pneumonia are related to processes that impair the lung's natural immune defences. Common risk factors include:

- Smoking.
- Chronic lung disease (i.e. asthma, chronic obstructive pulmonary disease).
- Chronic heart disease.
- Alcohol excess.
- Immunosuppression.

Patients with swallowing impairment, i.e. following a stroke, myasthenia, bulbar palsy, are at increased risk of developing aspiration pneumonia.

Classification and pathology

In clinical practice pneumonia is often classified under four broad terms:

1. Community Acquired Pneumonia (CAP).
2. Hospital Acquired Pneumonia (HAP) after >48 hours in hospital.
3. Aspiration pneumonia, i.e. following inhalation of gastric contents.
4. Pneumonia in immunocompromised patients.

Figure 20.1 highlights the main patient groups affected by these categories and the common organisms which are responsible. This chapter will mainly focus on the presentation, investigation and management of CAP, as this will be most useful in your clinical practice.

Figure 20.2 shows the key pathogens in CAP. *Streptococcus pneumoniae* is the causative organism in 55–75% of cases. Note, however, that in around a third of cases no cause is found.

Clinical features

Patients with pneumonia commonly present with:

- Shortness of breath.
- Cough.
- Sputum production.
- Pleuritic chest pain.
- Fever.
- Confusion (particularly in the elderly).

Patients with an atypical CAP may present with a different constellation of symptoms (Fig. 20.2).

On examination, the patient is typically pyrexial, tachycardic and tachypnoeic. Lung expansion is reduced and signs of consolidation are found (see Ch. 9). Coarse crackles may be heard as the infection resolves.

Fig. 20.1 Classification of pneumonia and common organisms

Pneumonia	Patients at risk	Common organisms
Community-acquired pneumonia (CAP)	Primary (healthy adults) Secondary (underlying lung disease), e.g. • Chronic obstructive pulmonary disease • Interstitial lung disease • Bronchial cancer	• *Streptococcus pneumoniae* • *Haemophilus influenzae* • *Mycoplasma pneumoniae*
Hospital-acquired pneumonia (HAP)	• Elderly • Immobile • Pain (causes basal atelectasis) • Immunosuppression • Immunocompromise	• *Staphylococcus aureus* • Gram-negative enterobacteria • *Pseudomonas* • *Klebsiella*
Aspiration	• Alcohol excess • Impaired consciousness • Swallowing problems, i.e. stroke	• Anaerobes • Gram-negative enterobacteria • *Staphylococcus aureus*
Immunocompromised	• HIV • Transplant patients • Chemotherapy • Leukaemia/lymphoma	• CAP organisms • HAP organisms • Viruses (CMV, VZV) • Fungi (*Aspergillus*) • Mycobacteria

HIV = human immunodeficiency virus; CMV = cytomegalovirus; VZV = varicella-zoster virus.

Fig. 20.2 Organisms causing community-acquired pneumonia (CAP)

Organism	Features of pneumonia	% cases
Streptococcus pneumoniae	Most common cause of CAP Gram-positive alpha-haemolytic cocci Polysaccharide capsule determines virulence and is detectable serologically; responsible for a high mortality unless treated appropriately	55–75
Influenza	Epidemics common Affects patients with underlying lung disease (can be severe): *Staphylococcus aureus, Streptococcus pneumoniae, Haemophilus influenzae* occur secondarily	8
Haemophilus influenzae	Gram-negative rod Causes exacerbations of chronic obstructive pulmonary disease	4–5
Staphylococcus aureus	Gram-positive diplococci Often complication of influenza Severe, often cavitating pneumonia (commonly fatal)	1–5
Atypical bacteria		
Mycoplasma pneumoniae	Epidemics every 3–4 years, usually in young patients Flu-like symptoms (headache, myalgia, arthralgia) followed by dry cough Extrapulmonary features: haemolytic anaemia, erythema multiforme, Guillain–Barré (rare), Stevens–Johnson syndrome (rare) Penicillin ineffective as no bacterial cell wall	5–18
Legionella pneumophila	Gram-negative Found in cooling towers and air conditioning (outbreaks of legionnaires' disease) Flu-like symptoms with dry cough and shortness of breath Extrapulmonary features: diarrhoea and vomiting, hepatitis, hyponatraemia Severe pneumonia with high mortality	2–5
Chlamydia pneumoniae	Biphasic illness with headache, otitis media and pharyngitis followed by pneumonia Usually serological diagnosis	2–5

Fig. 20.3 Investigations in pneumonia

Investigation	Use
Sputum culture	Identify causative organism
Blood	
Full blood count	Raised white cell count and neutrophilia confirm infection
C-reactive protein/erythrocyte sedimentation rate	Raised inflammatory markers confirm infection
Urea and electrolytes	Dehydration common in pneumonia (raised urea and creatinine)
Liver function tests	Can become deranged in atypical pneumonia, i.e. *Legionella*
Cultures	Only if patient is pyrexial; identify organism
Arterial blood gases	Identify respiratory failure
Electrocardiograph	Atrial fibrillation common in pneumonia; rule out cardiac cause of chest pain
Chest X-ray	May be evidence of consolidation or effusion

Investigation

Common investigations are shown in Figure 20.3. In patients with an atypical presentation, a severe pneumonia or pneumonia that is not responding to antibiotics, it is useful to do an atypical pneumonia screen. This includes:

- Urinary *Legionella* antigen.
- Cold agglutinins (present in *Mycoplasma*).
- *Mycoplasma, Chlamydia* serology.
- Pneumococcal antigen.

Management

When managing a patient with pneumonia it is important to assess the severity objectively. This is done using the CURB-65 score (Fig. 20.4). The score correlates with severity and will guide your management:

Fig. 20.4 CURB-65 score

C: confusion	Abbreviated mental test score <8
U: urea	Urea >7 mmol/L
R: respiratory rate	>30 breaths/min
B: blood pressure	Systolic blood pressure <90 mmHg
65: age	>65 years

- CURB-65 0–1: Mild pneumonia: can consider treatment at home with oral antibiotics.
- CURB-65 2: Moderate pneumonia will require treatment in hospital.
- CURB-65 3+: Severe pneumonia: consider high-dependency unit – high mortality.

In general, the management of pneumonia involves:

- Oxygen (maintain O_2 saturations >94%).
- Intravenous (IV) fluids to correct dehydration (be cautious in patients with heart failure).
- Antibiotics (oral or IV depending on severity).

Figure 20.5 provides overall guidance for antibiotic use; however, you should always follow local antibiotic guidelines when selecting an antibiotic as they consider local antibiotic resistance patterns. In simple terms, a penicillin will treat most 'typical' organisms whilst a macrolide antibiotic will treat any 'atypical' organisms.

Complications

The key complications are:

- Respiratory failure.
- Parapneumonic effusions.
- Empyema.
- Lung abscess.
- Atrial fibrillation

TUBERCULOSIS

Definition and epidemiology

TB arises as a result of infection with *Mycobacterium tuberculosis*. TB is the world's leading cause of death from an infectious disease. In the UK, 6000 new cases occur per year, with the highest incidence among immigrants, who are 40 times more likely to develop the disease than the native Caucasian population. The prevalence of TB is increasing in the UK, most notably in urban areas.

Fig. 20.5 Antibiotics in pneumonia

Mild community-acquired pneumonia	Oral penicillin and macrolide, e.g. amoxicillin + clarithromycin
Severe community-acquired pneumonia	Intravenous broad-spectrum penicillin and oral macrolide, e.g. co-amoxiclav + clarithromycin
Hospital-acquired pneumonia	Intravenous antipseudomonal penicillin and aminoglycoside, e.g. Tazocin + gentamicin
Aspiration pneumonia	Broad-spectrum + antianaerobic, e.g. co-amoxiclav + metronidazole

Risk factors for developing TB include:

- Close contact (relative) with TB.
- Immunocompromise, e.g. HIV.
- Homelessness.
- Drug or alcohol abuse.

Pathology

Transmission and dissemination

Initial infection usually occurs in childhood and transmission of TB is via droplet infection or direct contact. A cough, sneeze or exhalation from an infected person discharges droplets of viable mycobacteria. The droplet nuclei are then inhaled by an uninfected person and can lodge anywhere in the lungs or airways.

Primary tuberculosis

The initial lesion is usually solitary, 1–2 cm in diameter, and subpleural in the middle or upper zones of the lung. The focus of primary infection is termed the Ghon complex.

The primary infection has two components:

1. Initial inflammatory reaction.
2. Secondary inflammation in surrounding lymph nodes.

Within 3–8 weeks of infection the initial lesion becomes a tubercle (granulomatous inflammation). The tubercle undergoes necrosis in a process called caseation and is surrounded by multinucleated giant cells and epithelioid cells (both derived from macrophages). The caseous tissue may liquefy, empty into an airway and be transmitted to other parts of the lung. Lymphatic spread of mycobacteria occurs. The combination of tuberculous lymphadenitis and the Ghon complex is termed the primary complex.

In most cases, the primary foci will organize and form a fibrocalcific nodule in the lung with no clinical sequelae.

Secondary tuberculosis

Secondary TB results from reactivation of a primary infection or reinfection. Any form of immunocompromise may allow reactivation. The common sites are posterior or apical segments of the upper lobe or the superior segment of the lower lobe. Tubercle follicles develop and lesions enlarge by formation of new tubercles. Infection spreads by lymphatics and a delayed hypersensitivity reaction occurs.

In secondary TB, the lesions are often bilateral and usually cavitating.

Progressive tuberculosis

Progressive TB may arise from a primary lesion or may be caused by reactivation of an incompletely healed primary lesion or reinfection. TB progresses to widespread cavitation, pneumonitis and lung fibrosis (Fig. 20.6).

Miliary tuberculosis

In miliary TB, an acute diffuse dissemination of tubercle bacilli occurs through the bloodstream. Numerous small granulomas form in many organs, with the highest numbers found in the lungs. These form a characteristic pattern on chest X-ray (see Fig. 20.8, below).

Miliary TB may be a consequence of either primary or secondary TB and is fatal without treatment.

Clinical features

Primary TB is usually asymptomatic; however it may be associated with a mild febrile illness and erythema nodosum (Fig. 20.7).

Patients with secondary or progressive TB classically present with:

- Cough.
- Sputum production (mucopurulent).
- Haemoptysis.
- Fevers.
- Night sweats.
- Fatigue.
- Weight loss.

Extrapulmonary TB

TB can affect most organs, including gut, skin, kidney, genital tract and bone. The most common extrapulmonary manifestations involve:

- Skin – erythema nodosum (Fig. 20.7A).
- Spine – tuberculoma causing vertebral collapse (Pott's disease) (Fig. 20.7B and C).
- Brain – TB can cause chronic meningitis or a space-occupying lesion (Fig. 20.7B).

TB of the adrenal glands is now rare in the UK. It is a historically important cause of Addison's disease.

Investigation

If you suspect from clinical history or examination that a patient may have TB, the National Institute for Health and Clinical Excellence recommends a chest X-ray is performed. Features of TB on chest X-ray include (Fig. 20.8):

- Hilar lymphadenopathy.

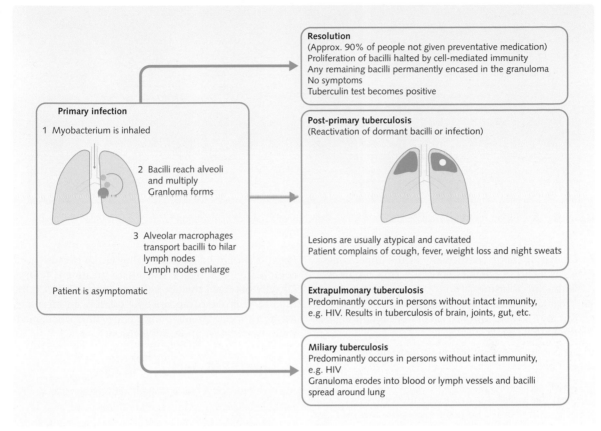

Fig. 20.6 The pathogenesis of tuberculosis with different outcomes following primary infection. HIV = human immunodeficiency virus.

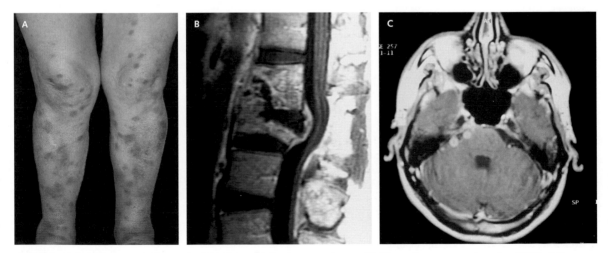

Fig. 20.7 Extrapulmonary features of tuberculosis. (A) Erythema nodosum. (B) Magnetic resonance imaging (MRI) of the spine demonstrating Pott's disease. (C) MRI/computed tomography of the brain showing a tuberculoma.

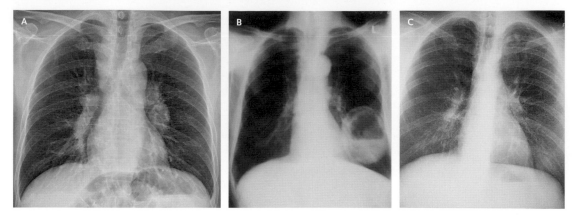

Fig. 20.8 (A–C) Features of tuberculosis on chest X-ray. Selection of X-rays demonstrating features described in the text.

- Cavitating lesion (particularly in the upper zones).
- Consolidation/pleural effusion (in conjunction with clinical history).
- Irregular nodule (upper zones).
- Miliary TB (disseminated small nodules throughout the lung field).

In the presence of X-ray features consistent with TB you should obtain:

- Three sputum samples (including one early-morning sample) for culture and microscopy.
- If sputum cannot be produced spontaneously, use induced sputum or bronchoalveolar lavage.

The samples should be taken before starting treatment if possible. Sputum is initially stained (Ziehl–Neelsen) and then examined under microscopy to look for acid-fast bacilli (the bacilli appear red on a blue background) and then sent for culture.

Sputum culture is the gold standard for TB diagnosis, however, this takes several weeks, therefore if the patient has clinical symptoms treatment is normally started whilst awaiting the culture results. Similarly, if the patient is smear-positive (i.e. staining reveals acid-fast bacilli), then treatment is also started.

Other useful investigations in TB include:

- TB ELISPOT.
- Biopsy of any organs thought to be affected.

Management

Treatment is typically with four drugs: isoniazid, rifampicin, ethambutol and pyrazinamide. Patients are treated for 6 months:

- Initial phase, lasting 2 months (rifampicin, isoniazid, pyrazinamide plus streptomycin or ethambutol).
- Continuation phase, lasting 4 months (isoniazid and rifampicin).

Patients should be regularly followed up because non-compliance is a major reason for treatment failure. Directly observed therapy short course (DOTS) can be used to improve compliance by offering an incentive, e.g. a free meal, for attending a daily clinic where medications are taken under supervision.

> **HINTS AND TIPS**
>
> When in hospital, patients with active tuberculosis should be managed in a side room (preferably negative-pressure). You should wear a facemask and gloves. If the patient leaves the side room, ask him or her to wear a facemask.

Contact tracing

TB is a notifiable disease and any close contacts of the patient will be traced in order to assess their risk of having contracted TB.

- If contacts are <35 years old, test for latent TB; consider bacille Calmette-Guérin (BCG) or treatment for latent TB infection once active TB has been ruled out.
- If older than 35, do a chest X-ray and further investigation for active TB if needed.

Prevention

The BCG vaccine is made from non-virulent tubercle bacilli. It is offered to newborns in high-risk areas, i.e. inner-city London. Other groups that receive the BCG are:

- Health workers.
- New immigrants from countries with high levels of TB.
- Close contacts of patients infected with respiratory TB.

BCG is given to individuals who are tuberculin-negative. A positive tuberculin test indicates prior infection and those testing positive are screened with a chest X-ray. A 0.1 mL intradermal dose of the vaccine (chosen dilution is usually 1:1000) is given to children and adults either as a subcutaneous injection (Mantoux test) or using a multipuncture device (Heaf test). Immunization decreases the risk of developing TB by up to 70%. Once an individual has been vaccinated, subsequent tuberculin tests are positive.

INFLUENZA

Definition and epidemiology

Influenza is an acute viral infection that usually affects the nose, throat and bronchi and occasionally the lungs. Influenza occurs in yearly seasonal epidemics (autumn/winter). Worldwide, these annual epidemics result in 3–5 million cases of severe illness and 250 000–500 000 deaths.

Pandemic influenza occurs when a new subtype of influenza arises, which is capable of spreading worldwide. Unlike seasonal influenza, pandemic influenza can occur at any time and can be associated with huge mortality.

HINTS AND TIPS

In 1918–1919 a new H1N1 influenza emerged – 'Spanish flu'. In 2 years over 40 million people died in the Spanish flu pandemic.

In 2009 a new H1N1 emerged in Mexico – 'swine flu'. It caused mild or asymptomatic disease in the majority of cases but severe illness and death in a small proportion.

HINTS AND TIPS

Definitions

Epidemic

An epidemic is the occurrence of more cases of a disease than would be expected in a community or region during a given time period

Pandemic

A pandemic is a worldwide epidemic that, according to the World Health Organization (WHO), has to meet three conditions:
1. The microbe infects and causes serious illness in humans.
2. Humans do not have immunity against the virus.
3. The virus spreads easily from person to person and survives within humans.

Pathology

There are three types of influenza virus:
1. Influenza A.
2. Influenza B.
3. Influenza C.

Type A influenza viruses are further subtyped according to different kinds and combinations of virus surface proteins (Fig. 20.9). Currently, influenza A (H1N1) and A (H3N2) subtypes are circulating in the human population.

As with many other organisms, there is a large animal reservoir of influenza virus (mainly in domestic animals such as birds, cattle and pigs). Different strains of influenza affect animals and humans. If an animal strain of virus combines with a human strain in a process called reassortment, then a new hybrid strain of influenza is formed. If this new strain is able to replicate well and can be easily transmitted from person to person, then a pandemic is born (Fig. 20.10).

Influenza is spread by droplet infection and patients become infective one day before the onset of symptoms (making the control of spread very difficult).

Clinical features

Symptoms of influenza include:
* High fever.
* Dry cough.
* Coryza.
* Myalgia.
* Arthralgia.
* Headache.

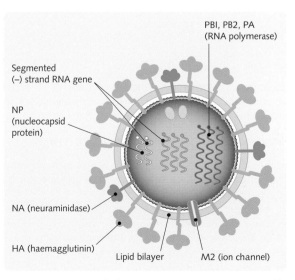

Fig. 20.9 Structure of influenza A virus. It is the highly variable haemagluttinin surface proteins that we develop immunity to.

Fig. 20.10   Stages of a pandemic.

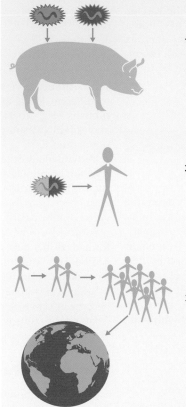

1. **Reassortment**
   - Pig infected with both human and swine virus
   - Reassortment occurs
   - New strain of influenza virus

2. **Transmission of virus to human population**
   - Human population has no immunity to new strain of influenza

3. **Spread**
   - Virus spreads by droplet infection days before infection symptoms occur. Thus spread is difficult to control

In the majority of patients these symptoms will resolve within 1 week; however, certain groups are at risk of developing complications. Patients at risk include:

- Children <2 years.
- Elderly.
- Underlying lung disease.
- Heart disease.
- Diabetes.
- Immunocompromised.

Common complications include secondary bacterial pneumonia (*Staphylococcus aureus*), otitis media, sinusitis and encephalitis.

Investigation and management

Influenza is a clinical diagnosis;, however, in cases of pandemic influenza a nasopharyngeal aspirate can be taken for culture.

Management is usually symptomatic, with paracetamol and bed rest.

In the case of pandemic influenza, antiviral drugs are available. There are two classes of such drugs:

1. Adamantanes (amantadine and rimantadine).
2. Neuraminidase inhibitors (oseltamivir and zanamivir).

Prevention

Vaccination is the most effective way to prevent influenza and severe illness. Among healthy adults, influenza vaccine can prevent 70–90% of influenza-specific illness.

Vaccination is especially important for people at higher risk of serious influenza complications, and for people who live with or care for high-risk individuals.

The World Health Organization recommends annual vaccination for (in order of priority):

- Nursing-home residents (the elderly or disabled).
- Elderly individuals.
- Patients with chronic medical conditions.
- Other groups, i.e. pregnant women, healthcare workers, children aged 6 months to 2 years.

HIV-RELATED LUNG DISEASE

Definition and epidemiology

Human Immunodeficiency Virus (HIV) is one of the leading causes of mortality from an infectious disease. It is estimated that 25 million people have died worldwide as a result of HIV in the past 30 years. It is estimated that over 34 million people worldwide are living with HIV.

Sixty per cent of patients living with HIV are in sub-Saharan Africa; however, HIV is a significant problem in the UK and has a large impact on certain communities, such as:

- Immigrants from sub-Saharan Africa.
- Homosexual men.
- Intravenous drug users.

Pathology

HIV can be transmitted via several methods:

- Sexual intercourse.
- Transfusion of contaminated blood.
- Sharing contaminated needles.
- Mother-to-child (during pregnancy, childbirth or breastfeeding).

HIV targets the immune system, destroying and impairing the function of CD4 cells. Patients become immunodeficient and are susceptible to infections and cancers to which normal healthy individuals are not susceptible.

There are multiple ways in which HIV affects the lung.

TB

TB is an important complication of HIV. It is estimated that 40% of people with acquired immunodeficiency syndrome (AIDS) also have TB. In patients with HIV, TB often presents atypically in a number of ways:

- Atypical symptoms (patients are more likely to have extrapulmonary features).
- Reactivation of latent TB is increased.
- The Mantoux and sputum stains are often negative.
- Chest X-ray features can be atypical.
- Greater risk of developing multidrug-resistant TB.

Pneumonia

Patients with HIV are at greater risk of developing normal CAP and HAP. They are also at risk of pneumonia from atypical organisms such as (Fig. 20.11):

- *Pneumocystis jiroveci* pneumonia.
- Viruses i.e. cytomegalovirus or varicella-zoster.
- Fungi, i.e. *Aspergillus*.

Kaposi's sarcoma

Kaposi's sarcoma is a malignancy of connective tissue cause by human herpesvirus 8. It occurs in epidemics in patients with HIV. Kaposi's sarcoma is characterized by malignant cells and abnormal growth of blood vessels.

Kaposi's sarcoma commonly affects the skin, causing erythematous purple nodules that are occasionally associated with pain and swelling. They can develop in any organ, including the lung, where they cause dyspnoea.

Fig. 20.11 Atypical pneumonia in human immunodeficiency virus (HIV)

Organism	Presentation	Pathology	Diagnosis	Treatment
Pneumocystis jiroveci (fungi)	Dry cough Fever Shortness of breath Rarely, pleural effusions	Interstitial infiltrate of mononuclear cells Alveolar air spaces filled with eosinophilic material	Immunofluorescent stains with monoclonal antibodies Chest X-ray: bilateral alveolar and interstitial shadowing	High dose co-trimoxazole 100% mortality if untreated. 20–50% mortality in treated patients
Cytomegalovirus (CMV) (DNA virus)	90% of AIDS patients are infected Rarely causes pneumonia Disseminated CMV can occur, e.g. encephalitis	Interstitial infiltrate of mononuclear cells, scattered alveolar hyaline membranes, protein-rich fluid in alveoli and intranuclear inclusion bodies in alveolar epithelial cells	Characteristic 'owl's eyes' intranuclear inclusions in tissues on histology Can also be detected by direct immunofluorescence	Ganciclovir
Aspergillus fumigatus (fungi)	Invasive aspergillosis can cause necrotizing pneumonia, abscesses or solitary granulomas		Microabscesses show characteristic fungal filaments	Amphotericin (poor prognosis)

AIDS = acquired immunodeficiency syndrome.

Management of Kaposi's sarcoma in HIV patients is normally with antiretrovirals.

Further reading

NICE guidance on management of pneumonia. Available online at: http://guidance.nice.org.uk/index.jsp?action=byID&o=13666.

NICE guidance on management of tuberculosis. Available online at: http://publications.nice.org.uk/tuberculosis-cg117/other-versions-of-this-guideline#full-guideline.

WHO website (advice on tuberculosis, pandemic influenza and HIV). Available online at: http://www.who.int/topics/en/.

Suppurative lung disease (21)

Objectives

By the end of this chapter you should be able to:
• Describe the clinical features, investigations and management of bronchiectasis.
• Describe the clinical features, investigations and management of cystic fibrosis.
• Discuss lung transplant, including complications.
• Describe the pathogenesis and treatment of lung abscesses.

Suppurative lung diseases are associated with chronic inflammation and dilatation of the bronchi. This may be associated with chronic mucus plugging and recurrent infection. This category includes bronchiectasis, Kartagener's syndrome and cystic fibrosis. Treatment mainly involves control of infection and ultimately lung transplant may be required.

BRONCHIECTASIS

Definition

Bronchiectasis is defined as an abnormal and permanent dilatation of the bronchi and is associated with chronic infection. Most cases arise in childhood.

Aetiology

Bronchiectasis can either be acquired or, less commonly, has a congenital cause. However, about 50–60% of cases are idiopathic.

Acquired bronchiectasis

Bronchiectasis is usually caused by a severe childhood infection (e.g. bronchopneumonia, measles or whooping cough). Inflammation can damage and weaken the bronchial wall, leading to dilatation. It may also be caused by bronchial obstruction (e.g. by a foreign body, tuberculous lymph nodes or tumour) followed by infection in the lung distal to the obstruction.

Other conditions associated with bronchiectasis include allergic bronchopulmonary aspergillosis, inflammatory bowel disease and rheumatoid arthritis. In particular, the British Thoracic Society recommends that allergic bronchopulmonary aspergillosis should be ruled out in all patients with suspected bronchiectasis. This is done by measuring *Aspergillus*-specific IgE and IgG.

Congenital bronchiectasis

Congenital abnormalities that interfere with ciliary function (e.g. primary ciliary dyskinesia, Kartagener's syndrome and Young's syndrome) impair the transport of mucus and cause recurrent infection.

Kartagener's syndrome, which is a rare cause, is also associated with dextrocardia and sinusitis. The viscous mucus and recurrent infections of cystic fibrosis may also lead to bronchiectasis. Recurrent infections are also a feature of immunoglobulin deficiencies (e.g. of IgA and other primary antibody deficiencies); therefore these are also associated with bronchiectasis. This should be considered in all patients with serious, persistent and recurrent infections with subsequent bronchiectasis. These patients should be managed under the joint care of a chest physician and immunologist.

Pathogenesis

Infection leads to obstruction, dilatation of bronchi and often loss of cilia. Destruction of the alveolar walls and fibrosis of lung parenchyma occur and pulmonary haemodynamic changes can take place. The dependent portions of the lungs, usually the lower lobes, are affected most commonly.

Clinical features

Cough is the most common symptom; this is often persistent and accompanied by sputum which may be mucopurulent or copious, purulent and foul-smelling. Systemic features of infection such as fever and malaise also occur.

Haemoptysis may be present and can be massive. Clubbing occurs and coarse inspiratory crackles are heard on auscultation in the infected areas.

Investigations

According to the British Thoracic Society guidelines, bronchiectasis should be investigated in the following patients:

Children

- Chronic cough.
- Symptoms of asthma which are non-responsive to treatment.
- Severe or recurrent pneumonia.
- High risk of aspiration or oesophageal disorder.
- Haemoptysis.

Adults

- Persistent productive cough, especially if onset at a young age or associated with haemoptysis.
- Patients with recurrent exacerbations of chronic obstructive pulmonary disease or who are non-smokers.

Bronchiectasis can be investigated through:

- Radiology – chest radiograph may be normal or show bronchial wall thickening. If disease is advanced, cystic spaces may be seen.
- High-resolution computed tomography – the investigation of choice to detect bronchial wall thickening and dilatation.
- Sputum tests – Gram stain, anaerobic and aerobic culture, and sensitivity testing are vital during an infective exacerbation. Major pathogens include *Staphylococcus aureus*, *Pseudomonas aeruginosa*, *Haemophilus influenzae* and anaerobes. It can also be useful to quantify sputum production by asking the patient to do a 24-hour sputum collection.
- Tests for cystic fibrosis where appropriate (cystic fibrosis sweat test and looking for specific CFTR gene mutations: see below).
- Lung function spirometry (may show an obstructive pattern).
- Immunoglobulin levels – may demonstrate a specific deficiency, especially IgA, IgM and IgG. *Aspergillus*-specific immunoglobulins can also rule out allergic bronchopulmonary aspergillosis. Other more complex immunological investigations should be managed by an immunologist.
- Bronchoscopy does not have a role in the routine investigation of bronchiectasis. However, it can be used to rule out a foreign body in children with single-lobe bronchiectasis. It can also be used for bronchoalveolar lavage and washout for obtaining samples for microbiology.

Treatment

Aims of treatment are twofold:

- Control of infection and maintainence of lung function/stopping progression of disease.
- Removal of secretions.

Infections should be eradicated with antibiotics if progression of the disease is to be halted. Treatment regimens depend on infecting organism (e.g. flucloxacillin 500 mg 6-hourly to treat *Staphylococcus aureus* infection) and, as much as possible, sputum cultures should be taken before antibiotics are commenced.

The British Thoracic Society guidelines suggest amoxicillin as first-line therapy if no underlying organism is identified, with clarithromycin if the patient is allergic to penicillin. If there is no improvement with treatment, the patient is likely to be infected with *Pseudomonas aeruginosa*: treat with ceftazidime or ciprofloxacin parenterally.

In severe cases, intravenous antibiotics may be necessary, either one or in combination, depending on the underlying cause. In all cases, you should refer to local trust guidelines and consult a microbiologist if there is no response to initial therapy.

The BTS recommends long-term antibiotic therapy for those with more than three infections a year or signficant infections requiring hospitalization.

Respiratory secretions are cleared by using a combination of small and deep breaths that move secretions up the bronchial tree. These are called active cycle breathing techniques and are used while the patient is lying in a position that encourages drainage of the lung (each lobe has a different position). Secretions are removed by postural drainage for 10–20 minutes three times a day. Patients are trained in the method by specialist chest physiotherapists.

Bronchodilators are useful if demonstrable air flow limitation exists.

Surgery is of limited value but may be indicated in a young patient with adequate lung function, if disease is localized to one lung or segment.

Complications

Complications of bronchiectasis include:

- Pneumonia.
- Pneumothorax.
- Empyema.
- Meningitis.
- Metastatic abscess (e.g. in brain).
- Amyloid formation (e.g. in kidney).

CYSTIC FIBROSIS

Definition

Cystic fibrosis is a disorder characterized by the production of abnormally viscid secretions by exocrine glands and mucus-secreting glands, such as those in the pancreas and respiratory tract. Impaired mucociliary clearance in the airways leads to recurrent infections and bronchiectasis.

Prevalence

Cystic fibrosis is the commonest genetically transmitted disease in Caucasians. It is an autosomal recessive condition occurring in 1:2000 live births. The gene has been identified on the long arm of chromosome 7. Prevalence of heterozygous carriers is 4%. Approximately 300 people were diagnosed with cystic fibrosis in 2010.

Aetiology

The commonest mutation is a specific gene deletion in the codon for phenylalanine at position 508 in the amino acid sequence (ΔF508). This results in a defect in a transmembrane regulator protein known as the cystic fibrosis transmembrane conductance regulator (CFTR).

Mutation causes a failure of opening of the chloride channels in response to elevated cAMP in epithelial cells, leading to:

- Decreased excretion of chloride into the airway lumen.
- Increased reabsorption of sodium into the epithelial cells.
- Increased viscosity of secretions.

Pathology

The thick secretions produced by the epithelial cells cause:

- Small-airway obstruction, leading to recurrent infection and ultimately bronchiectasis.
- Pancreatic duct obstruction, causing pancreatic fibrosis and ultimately pancreatic insufficiency.

Cystic fibrosis patients are prone to respiratory infections, especially *Pseudomonas aeruginosa*. It is thought that the naturally occurring antibiotic peptides (defensins) become inactive in cystic fibrosis patients, as these peptides are salt-sensitive.

Fig. 21.1 Manifestations of cystic fibrosis	
Respiratory manifestations	**Gastrointestinal manifestations**
Recurrent bronchopulmonary infection Bronchiectasis	Meconium ileus Rectal prolapse Diarrhoea Failure to thrive Malabsorption

Clinical features

Presentation depends on age. Usually, the condition presents in infancy with gastrointestinal manifestations such as meconium ileus or malabsorption (Fig. 21.1).

Stools are bulky, greasy, and offensive in smell. Respiratory signs are normal and symptoms are non-specific:

- Lungs are normal at birth.
- There are frequent infections with cough and wheeze as the child gets older.
- Clubbing and dyspnoea occur.

Almost all men with cystic fibrosis are infertile; females may be subfertile.

Investigations

Family history is sought (e.g. affected siblings). Genetic screening is available for couples with a family history. Prenatal diagnosis is available by chorionic villous sampling or amniocentesis.

A massive advance in the early detection of cystic fibrosis is the National Neonatal Screening Programme, which involves the Guthrie test (see below).

Tests include:

- Guthrie test – heel prick test.
- Immunoreactive trypsin test – positive test shows low levels.
- Sweat test – raised levels of sodium and chloride in sweat (>60 mmol/L). It is thought that because of the CFTR mutation the sweat ducts are unable to reabsorb Cl^- from the ductal lumen into the interstitium, resulting in sweat having an increased salt content.
- Genetic testing – can be useful if the patient has the ΔF508 mutation. However, this only accounts for around 75% of cases and other mutations cannot be detected.
- Chest X-ray – may show accentuated bronchial markings and small ring shadows.

The complications of cystic fibrosis are described in Figure 21.2.

Fig. 21.2 Complications of cystic fibrosis

Respiratory complications	Other complications
Allergic aspergillosus	Abdominal pain
Bronchiectasis	Biliary cirrhosis
Cor pulmonale	Delayed puberty
Haemoptysis	Diabetes mellitus
Lobar collapse	Gallstones
Nasal polyps	Growth failure
Pneumothorax	Male infertility
Sinusitis	Portal hypertension
Wheezing	Rectal prolapse

Treatment

Patients with cystic fibrosis should be managed by a multidisciplinary team. Cystic fibrosis clinics are unique in that the patient remains in the consultation room and the various members of the team come into the patient's room. This prevents cystic fibrosis patients from being in close contact with each other, which would signficantly increase their risk of being colonized with resistant bacteria.

Treatment (Fig. 21.3) is based on:

- Physiotherapy.
- Antibiotics (see below).
- DNase (see below).
- Anti-inflammatory drugs (steroids).
- Nutritional support.

Intravenous antibiotics may be given at home (e.g. through implantable venous access devices) to reduce hospital admissions and improve patient independence. However, these have their own complications and place the patient at risk of sepsis.

DNA fragments from decaying neutrophils can accumulate within the lung lining fluid in cystic fibrosis patients. This makes the sputum more viscous and more difficult to expectorate. Human DNase has been cloned, sequenced and expressed by recombinant techniques. When DNase is given in a nebulized form it is capable of degrading the DNA and has been shown to improve the forced expiratory volume in 1 second. This treatment is expensive but very effective in combination with regular physiotherapy.

Nebulized hypertonic saline has been shown to increase mucociliary clearance, reduce exacerbations and improve quality of life in some studies. It has to be administered with bronchodilators.

Heart–lung and liver transplantations are possible in severely affected patients.

Research into replacing the CFTR gene by using viral vectors and liposomes has been trialled in patients, but gene therapy is extremely far from being an effective treatment for cystic fibrosis.

Prognosis

Prognosis is improving: currently, mean survival is 29 years but patients diagnosed today have a mean life expectancy of 41 years. Death is mainly caused by respiratory complications.

LUNG TRANSPLANTATION

Single lung transplantation is preferred to double transplantation because of donor availability. Bilateral lung transplantation is required in infective conditions to prevent bacterial spill-over from a diseased lung to a single lung transplant.

Patients must have end-stage lung or pulmonary vascular disease with no other treatment options (Fig. 21.4).

Fig. 21.3 Summary of treatment of cystic fibrosis

Respiratory	Gastrointestinal
Drain secretions, postural drainage	Pancreatic enzyme supplements with all meals and snacks
Prevent infection where possible	High-energy, high-protein diet
Exercise encouraged	Do not restrict fat in diet
Regular sputum cultures	Vitamin A, D and E supplements
Immunization against measles and influenza	

Fig. 21.4 Indications and diseases treated by lung transplantation

Indications	Diseases treated by transplantation
Age <60 years	Pulmonary fibrosis
Life expectancy <18 months without transplantation	Primary pulmonary hypertension
No underlying cancer	Bronchiectasis and cystic fibrosis
No serious systemic disease	Emphysema, including α_1-antitrypsin deficiency

Fig. 21.5 Summary of the complications of lung transplantation	
Complication	**Time**
Hyperacute rejection	Seconds/minutes
Pulmonary oedema	12–72 hours
Bacterial lower respiratory tract infection: Donor-acquired Recipient-acquired	Hours/days Days/years
Acute rejection	Day 5/years
Airway complications	Week 1/months
Opportunistic infection	Week 4/years
Chronic rejection (e.g. bronchiolitis obliterans)	Week 6/years

Currently, around 120 lung transplants take place every year in the UK in seven specialist centres.

Complications

The complications of lung transplantation are listed in Figure 21.5.

Strategies for avoiding rejection

Lung transplantation does not require any significant degree of matching based on tissue type. The main criteria are compatibility of blood group and size match between organ and recipient.

Suppression of the immune system

All transplant patients require immunosuppression for life. This begins immediately before transplantation; drugs used include:

- Prednisolone.
- Azathioprine.
- Ciclosporin.

Large doses are given in the initial postoperative period. Lower maintenance doses are achieved after a few months. Rejection episodes are treated with high-dose intravenous corticosteroids.

Prognosis

One-year survival rates are 60–70%, with 5-year survival around 50%.

LUNG ABSCESS

Definition

Lung abscess is a localized area of infected parenchyma, with necrosis and suppuration.

Aetiology

A lung abscess may occur due to:

- Aspiration of infected material (e.g. in alcoholism, unconscious patients).
- Complications of pneumonia.
- Infection of cavities in bronchiectasis or tuberculosis.
- Bronchial obstructions (e.g. tumours or foreign body).
- Pulmonary infarction.

Clinical features

Onset may be acute or insidious, depending on the cause of the abscess. Acute symptoms include malaise, anorexia, fever and a productive cough. Copious foul-smelling sputum is present, caused by the growth of anaerobic organisms.

In large abscesses there may be dullness to percussion. Pallor is common, caused by anaemia. Clubbing is a late sign.

Investigations

- Investigations must exclude necrosis in a malignant tumour or cavitation caused by tuberculosis; bronchoscopy may be indicated to sample cells or exclude an obstruction. Chest radiography shows a walled cavity with fluid level.
- Sputum culture may identify a causative organism.
- Blood culture and full blood count show that the patient is often anaemic with high erythrocyte sedimentation rate. Patients usually have mild-to-moderate leucocytosis.

Treatment

Follow disease carefully with regular chest radiographs and sputum collections. Resolution of disease is prompt after institution of appropriate antibiotics. In the initial stages these should be broad-spectrum, covering aerobic, anaerobic and atypical organisms. Antifungals should also be considered, especially if the host is thought to be immunocompromised.

Postural drainage should be used. Surgery is not usually indicated.

Complications

Abscesses can heal completely, leaving a small fibrous scar. Complications include empyema, bronchopleural fistula, pyopneumothorax, pneumatoceles, haemorrhage caused by erosion of a bronchial or pulmonary artery, meningitis and cerebral abscess.

Useful links

http://www.brit-thoracic.org.uk/guidelines/bronchiectasis-guideline-%28non-cf%29.aspx.
http://www.brit-thoracic.org.uk/Portals/0/Clinical%20Information/Cystic%20Fibrosis/UK%20CF%20Registry%20-%20Annual%20Data%20Report%202010.pdf.
http://www.cfmedicine.com/cfdocs/cftext/hypertonicsaline.htm.
http://www.blf.org.uk/Page/Lung-transplantation.

By the end of this chapter you should be able to:
- Define a pleural effusion and list the main causes.
- Discuss the investigation and management of a pleural effusion with reference to tapping and analysis of these results.

INTRODUCTION

A pleural effusion is the presence of fluid between the visceral and parietal pleura. Effusions can be categorized as transudative or exudative, depending on the protein concentration (Fig. 22.1). Transudative pleural effusions (<25 g/L of protein) occur as a result of an imbalance between hydrostatic and osmotic forces, for example in congestive cardiac failure. Exudative pleural effusions (>35 g/L of protein) occur when local factors influencing pleural fluid formation and reabsorption are altered, specifically through injury or inflammation. Effusions of 25–35 g/L protein must be analysed using Light's criteria (see below). Causes of each type of effusion are shown in Figure 22.1.

GROSS APPEARANCE

On examination, the pleural fluid may be clear and straw-coloured, turbid (signifying infection) or haemorrhagic. If a haemorrhagic effusion exists, neoplastic infiltration, pulmonary infarction and tuberculosis need to be excluded. Leading malignancies that have associated pleural effusions are breast carcinoma, bronchial carcinoma and lymphomas/leukaemia.

CLINICAL FEATURES

Pleural effusions are typically asymptomatic until >500 mL of fluid is present. Pleuritic chest pain may develop in addition to dyspnoea, which is dependent on the size of the effusion. There are often constitutional symptoms related to the underlying cause, e.g. weight loss, night sweats and fevers.

Signs on examination include a stony dull percussion note, reduced or absent breath sounds and reduced vocal resonance over the area of effusion. Bronchial breathing is often present above an effusion.

INVESTIGATIONS

Features on a chest radiograph include blunting of costophrenic angles with 'white-out' and a meniscus demonstrating a fluid level. Ultrasound is used to detect small effusions not seen on chest X-ray and for guiding aspiration, which is performed for microbiological examination (diagnostic tap) or, if the patient is compromised by the effusion, therapeutically. A pleural biopsy with Abrams' needle may be necessary if the aspiration is inconclusive.

Simple blood tests looking for evidence of infection, anaemia or underlying organ disease should be conducted. Computed tomography scanning may be required if either malignancy or empyema is suspected.

LIGHT'S CRITERIA

Pleural fluid with a protein concentration of 25–35 g/L requires analysis against Light's criteria. These state that if:

- Fluid/serum protein of >0.5 or
- Fluid serum lactate dehydrogenase >0.6 or
- Fluid lactate dehydrogenase >2/3 the upper limit of normal serum

then the the fluid is an exudate. That is, if any of Light's criteria are met, then the effusion is exudative.

TREATMENT

Treatment is largely by treating the underlying disease. Figure 22.2 gives details of the British Thoracic Society guidelines for the investigation and treatment of pleural effusion. If the patient is symptomatic, then the effusion should be drained. This can either be done using a conventional chest drain or by aspirating fluid with

Fig. 22.1	Type of pleural effusions by cause and frequency	
Effusion type	**Cause**	**Frequency**
Transudate (protein <25 g/L)	Heart failure (secondary to oncotic pressure)	Common
	Hepatic failure (secondary to low albumin)	Common
	Renal failure (secondary to fluid overload)	Common
	Hypothyroidism	Uncommon
	Pulmonary embolus	Uncommon
	Meigs' syndrome	Rare
Exudate (protein >35 g/L)	Malignancy	Common
	Infection (parapneumonic effusion)	Common
	Rheumatoid disease	Rare
	Tuberculosis	Rare
	Empyema	Rare
	Sarcoidosis	Rare

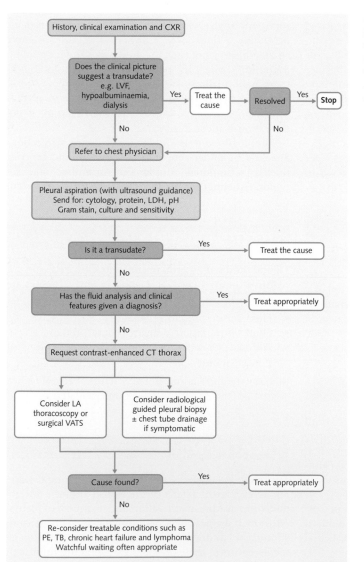

Fig. 22.2 British Thoracic Society algorithm for investigation and treatment of pleural effusion. CXR = chest X-ray; LVF = left ventricular failure; LDH = lactate dehydrogenase; CT = computed tomography; LA = left atrium; VATS = video-assisted thoracic surgery; PE = pulmonary embolism; TB = tuberculosis.

a needle and syringe. Fluid should be drained slowly. Transudative effusions will recur quickly unless the underlying imbalances are corrected and, as such, are usually only tapped symptomatically. Details on chest drain insertion can be found below.

Chemical pleurodesis can provide temporary relief in malignant effusions using bleomycin/tetracycline.

EMPYEMA

Also known as a pyothorax, empyema is a collection of pus within the pleural cavity caused by:

* Complication of thoracic surgery.
* Rupture of lung abscess into the pleural space.
* Perforation of oesophagus.
* Mediastinitis.
* Bacterial spread of pneumonia.

The empyema cavity can become infected by anaerobes. The patients are pyrexial and ill. The pus must be drained and appropriate antibiotic treatment should be initiated immediately.

HAEMOTHORAX

Haemothorax refers to blood in the pleural cavity. It is common in both penetrating and non-penetrating injuries of the chest and may cause hypovolaemic shock and reduce vital capacity through compression. Due to the defibrinating action that occurs with motions of respiration and the presence of an anticoagulant enzyme, the clot may be defibrinated and leave fluid that is radiologically indistinguishable from effusions of another cause.

Blood may originate from lung, internal mammary artery, thoracoacromial artery, lateral thoracic artery, mediastinal great vessels, heart or abdominal structures via the diaphragm.

Haemothoraces can be classified as either massive (estimated blood volume >1.5 L) or small (<1.5 L). Massive haemothoraces usually require thoracotomy, whereas smaller ones can be treated expectantly with chest drains and medical management.

CHYLOTHORAX

A chylothorax is an accumulation of lymph in the pleural space. Commonest causes are rupture or obstruction of the thoracic duct due to surgical trauma or neoplasm,

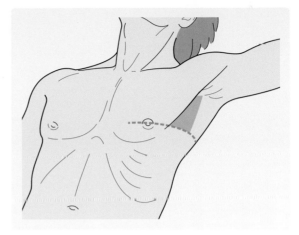

Fig. 22.3 The safe triangle for chest drain insertion. (From Laws et al., 2003).

e.g. lymphoma. A latent period between injury and onset of 2–10 days occurs. The pleural fluid is high in lipid content and is characteristically milky in appearance. Interestingly, octreotide has been found to be effective in the treatment of chylothoraces. Prognosis is generally good.

CHEST DRAIN INSERTION

Chest drains can be used for the drainage of air, pus or liquid (effusion or blood) from the pleural space. They must be inserted into the 'safe triangle' (Fig. 22.3). This is the triangle bordered by the anterior border of the latissimus dorsi, the lateral border of the pectoralis major muscle, a line superior to the horizontal level of the nipple, and an apex below the axilla. Full details of insertion are beyond the scope of this text; however, indications, procedural details and risks are available in the BTS guidelines.

Further reading

Laws, D., Neville, E., Duffy, J., et al., 2003. BTS guidelines for the insertion of a chest drain. Thorax 58, ii53–ii59.

Respiratory manifestations of systemic disease

23

INTRODUCTION

This chapter will examine the main respiratory manifestations of systemic diseases, focusing on:

- Sarcoidosis.
- Vasculitis.
- Rheumatoid arthritis.

SARCOIDOSIS

Definition and epidemiology

Sarcoidosis is a multisystem granulomatous disorder of unknown aetiology. Pulmonary involvement is common and non-caseating granulomas form within the lung.

Sarcoidosis is a relatively rare condition and prevalence in the UK is estimated to be 19 per 100 000. It is more common in women and the peak age of incidence is 20–40 years. Women of black African origin are more likely to suffer with severe disease.

Pathology

Sarcoidosis is characterized by the formation of non-caseating granulomas. These granulomas are infiltrated by Th1 lymphocytes and macrophages, which fuse to form multinucleated epithelioid cells.

Often these granulomas resolve, leading to spontaneous remission; however, in 10–20% the persistent inflammation results in interstitial fibrosis.

Clinical features

The clinical presentation of sarcoidosis is dependent on the organ involved; however, the majority of patients (>90%) have pulmonary involvement causing:

- Dyspnoea.

- Chest pain.
- Dry cough.

Other non-specific features include:

- Lymphadenopathy.
- Fever.
- Fatigue.
- Weight loss.

Common extrapulmonary features include:

- Skin (erythema nodosum/lupus pernio) (Fig. 23.1).
- Arthralgia.
- Uveitis.
- Cranial nerve palsies (in neurosarcoid).
- Cardiomyopathies (rare).

Investigation

Figure 23.2 demonstrates useful investigations in a patient with suspected sarcoidosis. The Global Initiative for Obstructive Lung Disease (GOLD) standard diagnosis for sarcoidosis remains biopsy, showing epithelioid non-caseating granulomas on histology.

Chest X-rays can be useful in staging disease and determining prognosis (Fig. 23.3). It is important to remember that staging disease in sarcoidosis does not reflect disease progression, i.e. stage III disease can develop with a patient never having developed stage I.

Management

Treatment

If the patient has hilar lymphadenopathy and no lung involvement, then no treatment is required.

If infiltration has occurred for more than 6 weeks, treat with corticosteroids (20–40 mg/day for 4–6 weeks, then reduced dose for up to 1 year).

Prognosis is dependent on disease stage. Mortality is less than 5% in UK Caucasians and approximately 10% in Afro-Americans. If shadowing is present on chest

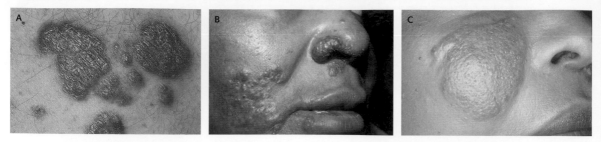

Fig. 23.1 Skin manifestations of sarcoidosis. (A) Erythema nodosum. (B) Lupus pernio. (C) Sarcoid nodules.

Fig. 23.2 Useful investigations in sarcoidosis	
Test	**Use**
Full blood count	May show a normochromic normocytic anaemia
Erythrocyte sedimentation rate	Often raised; can be used to monitor disease activity
Serum calcium	Granulomas secrete vitamin D, causing hypercalcaemia
Serum angiotensin-converting enzyme (ACE)	Granulomas secrete ACE. Can be twice normal levels. Used to monitor disease activity
Chest X-ray	Typical features. Useful in staging disease
High-resolution computed tomography	Disease staging, identifying pulmonary fibrosis
Biopsy	GOLD standard for diagnosis

radiographs for more than 2 years, the risk of fibrosis increases.

VASCULITIS

Vasculitis is a broad term incorporating a heterogeneous group of disorders that share a common underlying feature – inflammation of blood vessels.

They tend to be multiorgan diseases primarily affecting the kidney, lungs, joints and skin. This chapter will consider three vasculitides with well-described pulmonary manifestations:

- Goodpasture's syndrome.
- Wegener's granulomatosis.
- Churg–Strauss disease.

Goodpasture's syndrome

Goodpasture's syndrome is characterized by glomerulonephritis and respiratory symptoms. The syndrome is driven by a type II hypersensitivity reaction whereby

Fig. 23.3 The staging of sarcoidosis by chest radiographs					
Stage	**0**	**I**	**II**	**III**	**IV**
Chest radiograph					
Chest X-ray changes	Normal chest X-ray	Bilateral hilar lymphadenopathy	Bilateral hilar lymphadenopathy and pulmonary infiltration	Pulmonary infiltration without bilateral hilar lymphadenopathy	Pulmonary fibrosis
% of patients entering spontaneous remission		55–90%	40–70%	10–20%	0%

IgG autoantibodies to the glomerular basement membrane (anti-GBM) attach to the glomerulus, causing glomerulonephritis. In the lung, anti-GBM antibodies cross-react with the alveolar basement membrane, causing pulmonary haemorrhage.

Patients present with haemoptysis, haematuria and anaemia. Treatment is by corticosteroids or plasmapheresis to remove antibodies. The course of the disease is variable: some patients resolve completely, whereas others proceed to renal failure.

Wegener's granulomatosis

Wegener's granulomatosis is a rare, necrotizing vasculitis of unknown aetiology affecting small blood vessels. It classically involves midline structures, including the nose (Fig. 23.4), lungs and kidneys, where it causes glomerulonephritis.

In the lung, mucosal thickening and ulceration occur, producing the clinical features of rhinorrhoea, cough, haemoptysis and dyspnoea. Wegener's granulomatosis can be diagnosed with an autoantibody screen by the presence of cytoplasmic antineutrophil cytoplasmic antibodies; however, the GOLD standard of diagnosis remains biopsy (renal).

If untreated, mortality after 2 years is 93%, but the disease responds well to high-dose prednisolone and cyclophosphamide.

Churg–Strauss disease

Churg–Strauss disease is a small-vessel vasculitis. It classically presents with a triad of:

- Late-onset asthma.
- Eosinophilia.
- Small-vessel vasculitis.

Vasospasm is also a common feature and patients are at risk of developing myocardial infarction, pulmonary embolism or deep vein thrombosis. Treatment is usually with high-dose corticosteroids or interferon.

RESPIRATORY MANIFESTATIONS OF SYSTEMIC RHEUMATOLOGICAL DISEASES

Respiratory involvement is often a cause of high morbidity and a sign of poor prognosis in patients with autoimmune diseases, such as:

- Rheumatoid arthritis.
- Systemic lupus erythematosus (SLE).
- Systemic sclerosis.
- Ankylosing spondylitis.

Rheumatoid arthritis

Rheumatoid arthritis is a chronic inflammatory condition characterized by a symmetrical deforming polyarthropathy. It has many extra-articular features, including manifestations in the lung.

In all, 10–15% of patients with rheumatoid arthritis have lung involvement and usually these patients have severe disease. Patients can develop:

- Diffuse pulmonary fibrosis.
- Bronchiolitis obliterans.
- Follicular bronchiolitis.
- Pleural fibrosis.
- Pleural effusions.
- Rheumatoid nodules within the lung (rare).

Systemic lupus erythematosus

SLE is a multisystem autoimmune disease in which multiple autoantibodies form immune complexes, which deposit in a variety of organs, including the skin, joints, kidneys and lung.

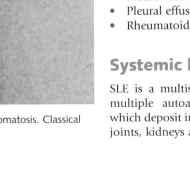

Fig. 23.4 Features of Wegener's granulomatosis. Classical saddle-shaped nose deformity.

Respiratory involvement is usually in the form of pleurisy, with or without an effusion, and pulmonary fibrosis is rare.

Systemic sclerosis

Systemic sclerosis is a severe autoimmune connective tissue disorder. Pulmonary involvement is a sign of severe disease and is associated with a poor prognosis. Patients typically develop pulmonary fibrosis and rapidly progressive pulmonary hypertension, which leads to cor pulmonale.

Ankylosing spondylitis

Ankylosing spondylitis is a chronic inflammatory condition of the spine and sacroiliac joints, which predominantly affects men. It has several extra-articular manifestations, including:

- Acute iritis.
- Aortic regurgitation.
- Apical lung fibrosis.

SELF-ASSESSMENT

Single best answer questions (SBAs)

1. Overview of the respiratory system

1. Which of the following is *not* an obstructive lung disorder?
   A. Asthma.
   B. Chronic bronchitis.
   C. Pulmonary fibrosis.
   D. Chronic obstructive pulmonary disease (COPD).
   E. Bronchiectasis.

2. Which of these is *not* a function of the respiratory system?
   A. Hormonal activity.
   B. Metabolism.
   C. Acid–base regulation.
   D. Control of electrolytes.
   E. Body temperature control.

2. Organization of the respiratory tract

1. Which of the following is true of the larynx?
   A. Is a structure discontinuous with the trachea.
   B. Protects the trachea and bronchi during swallowing.
   C. Contains multiple external muscles.
   D. Innervated by the pharyngeal plexus.
   E. Is unimportant in phonation.

2. The hilum of the lung contains:
   A. The vagus nerve.
   B. The pulmonary ligament.
   C. The recurrent laryngeal nerve.
   D. Mucosa-associated lymphoid tissue (MALT).
   E. The bronchial circulation.

3. The nasal cavity:
   A. Contains Clara cells.
   B. Is lined with columnar epithelium in the upper region.
   C. Is important in gas exchange.
   D. Is covered in olfactory epithelium in the lower region.
   E. Is important in defence against infection.

4. The following is true of the lower respiratory tract:
   A. The trachea is encircled by rings of cartilage.
   B. The left main bronchus is more acutely angled than the right.
   C. Both type I and type II pneumocytes exist.
   D. It contains respiratory bronchioles where the majority of gas exchange occurs.
   E. It lacks MALT.

5. Alveolar macrophages:
   A. Are neutrophil-derived blood cells.
   B. Circulate in the blood in macrophage form.
   C. Phagocytose foreign material.
   D. Are a prominent physical defence against infection.
   E. Exist mainly outside the respiratory zone.

6. Which of the following comments regarding the respiratory tree is most accurate?
   A. The main bronchi turn to segmental bronchi at the carina.
   B. Bronchioles contain no cartilage in their walls.
   C. There are approximately 12–14 divisions of the respiratory tree.
   D. Three main airway zones are described.
   E. Approximately 500 mL of the respiratory tree by volume is described as anatomical dead space in a 75-kg man.

7. The following is true regarding physical airway defences:
   A. S-fibres are the main irritant airway receptor stimulated by infective material.
   B. Filtering of air by the nasopharynx removes fine particulate matter from inspired air.
   C. Cough involves a high-velocity expiration against a closed glottis.
   D. Mucociliary clearance removes the majority of large particulate matter.
   E. Cilia beat at around 10 000 strokes per minute.

8. Components of cellular and humoral lung defences include:
   A. A predominance of IgG antibody.
   B. Surfactant produced by type I pneumocytes.
   C. A predominant basophilic response to bacterial infection.
   D. Filtration of air by the nasopharynx.
   E. Antiproteases, including hepatic α_1-antitrypsin.

3. Pulmonary circulation

1. Which of the following best describes the pulmonary circulation?
   A. A high-pressure, high-resistance system.
   B. A high-pressure, low-resistance system.
   C. A low-pressure, high-resistance system.
   D. A low-pressure, low-resistance system.
   E. A negative-pressure, low-resistance system.

2. Which one of the following statements is true?
   A. Blood vessels at the lung bases are subjected to a lower hydrostatic pressure than those at the apices.
   B. Blood flow is greater at the apices of the lungs.
   C. Blood flow is greater at the bases of the lungs.
   D. The pressure in the pulmonary circulation is normally equal to that of the systemic circulation.
   E. The pressure in the pulmonary circulation is normally greater than that of the systemic circulation.

3. An 80-year-old woman with severe pneumonia and extensive consolidation of the right lung desaturates whenever the nurses turn her on to her right side. Why is this?
   A. Increased ventilation of the right lung increasing ventilation:perfusion mismatch.
   B. Reduced ventilation of the right lung reducing ventilation:perfusion mismatch.
   C. Reduced blood flow to the right lung increasing ventilation:perfusion mismatch.
   D. Increased blood flow to the right lung increasing ventilation:perfusion mismatch.
   E. Increased blood flow to the right lung reducing ventilation:perfusion mismatch.

4. Physiology, ventilation and gas exchange

1. The functional residual capacity (FRC) is defined as which of the following?
   A. Volume of air remaining in lungs at the end of a normal expiration.
   B. Volume of air that can be breathed in by a maximum inspiration following a maximum expiration.
   C. Volume of air remaining in lungs at the end of a maximum expiration.
   D. Volume of air that can be expelled by a maximum effort at the end of a normal expiration.
   E. Volume of air breathed in by a maximum inspiration at the end of a normal expiration.

2. A patient with COPD has become increasingly breathless and tachypnoeic over the past 6 months. On examination the patient is hyperexpanded and has a barrel chest. Which of the following answers best accounts for these findings?
   A. Increased functional residual capacity.
   B. Increased inspiratory capacity.
   C. Increased tidal volumes.
   D. Increased residual volume.
   E. Reduced inspiratory capacity.

3. An elderly man attends the outpatient clinic complaining of breathlessness on exertion and weight loss. On examination he has clubbing, is cyanosed and

has fine inspiratory crackles. The patient is sent for spirometry. Which of the following is most likely?
   A. Reduced forced expiratory volume in 1 second (FEV_1) and normal forced vital capacity (FVC).
   B. Reduced FEV_1 and FVC.
   C. Normal FEV_1 and reduced FVC.
   D. Normal FEV_1 and FVC.
   E. Increased FEV_1 and FVC.

5. Perfusion and gas transport

1. Which best describes the ideal ventilation–perfusion relationship?
   A. One where the flow of gas and flow of blood are closely matched.
   B. One where the flow of gas exceeds the flow of blood.
   C. One where the flow of blood exceeds the flow of gas.
   D. One where regional differences in gas flow predominate.
   E. One where regional differences in blood flow predominate.

2. Which of the following best describes gas transport in the blood?
   A. Once oxygen is bound to the haem group of haemoglobin, the ferrous (Fe^{2+}) ion changes to the ferric state (Fe^{3+}).
   B. Myoglobin has a lower affinity for oxygen than haemoglobin A.
   C. Carbon dioxide and oxygen have similar diffusing capacity in the lung.
   D. During exercise an individual will hyperventilate in order to blow off carbon dioxide.
   E. Increase in carbon dioxide and decrease in pH enhance dissociation of oxygen from oxyhaemoglobin.

3. Which of the following is true of the $V:Q$ ratio?
   A. Ventilation increases towards the apex of the lung.
   B. Perfusion decreases towards the base of the lung.
   C. V_A/Q is dependent on lung volume and posture.
   D. V_A/Q is uniform throughout the lung in the healthy patient.
   F. Perfusion is increased to those areas of lung which are underventilated.

4. Which of the following statements regarding acid–base balance is most accurate?
   A. Uncomplicated respiratory acidosis results from an increase in PCO_2.
   B. Renal compensation returns the blood gases and pH to normal in respiratory acidosis.
   C. Metabolic acidosis may cause respiratory compensation, increasing ventilation and therefore increasing PCO_2.

D. The bicarbonate buffer system is important in the acid–base balance because its pK is very close to physiological pH.
E. Normal physiological pH range is 7.25–7.45.

5. Which of the following statements regarding haemoglobinopathies is correct?
   A. The thalassaemias are inherited in an X-linked manner.
   B. Those heterozygous for sickle cell disease are often profoundly anaemic.
   C. Sickling of red blood cells relates to polymerization at low oxygen tensions.
   D. Thalassaemia is caused by defective haemoglobin gamma chain production.
   E. Treatment of a sickle crisis involves fluid restriction.

6. Control of respiratory function

1. Which of these factors do *not* affect ventilatory response to P_aCO_2?
   A. P_aO_2.
   B. Psychiatric state.
   C. Genetics.
   D. Pulmonary disease.
   E. Fitness.

2. Which of these is *not* a way in which the body can combat hypoxia at altitude?
   A. Increasing the amount of haemoglobin in the blood.
   B. Hyperventilation.
   C. Shifting the oxygen dissociation curve.
   D. Increasing myoglobin.
   E. Alteration of blood pH through renal excretion.

7. Basic pharmacology

1. Which of the following regarding salbutamol is correct?
   A. It is used predominantly in the treatment of allergic rhinitis.
   B. It has a prolonged duration of action.
   C. It exerts its action via β_1 receptors.
   D. It is highly receptor-specific.
   E. It commonly causes a tachycardic response.

2. Which of the following statements on formoterol is correct?
   A. It is a partial receptor agonist.
   B. It is a full receptor agonist.
   C. It has near identical pharmacokinetics to salmeterol.
   D. It is unsuitable for use in single maintenance and reliever therapy (SMART).
   E. It is more effective than anticholinergic agents in the treatment of COPD.

3. Which of the following makes theophyllines challenging to use clinically?
   A. They exert effects in a similar manner to β_2 agonists.
   B. Both oral and intravenous formulations exist.
   C. Hepatic enzyme activity varies markedly between patients.
   D. Their complete mechanism of action is not understood.
   E. They are only useful in severe asthma attacks.

4. The British Thoracic Society guidelines on the management of asthma state that:
   A. Step 2 should be reached when reliever medication is used more than once monthly
   B. Step 4 introduces oral glucocorticosteroids.
   C. Leukotriene receptor antagonists are a useful adjunct to step 4.
   D. Patients should not be stepped down the algorithm as their disease will likely worsen.
   E. Patients should all commence treatment at step 1 and work up as needed.

5. All of the following are recognized smoking cessation strategies except:
   A. Nicotine replacement therapy.
   B. Bupropion
   C. GP-led counselling.
   D. Acamprosate.
   E. Stop smoking media campaigns.

8. The respiratory patient – taking a history and exploring symptoms

1. Which of these is *not* an important cause of haemoptysis?
   A. Bronchial carcinoma.
   B. Tuberculosis.
   C. COPD.
   D. Pulmonary embolism.
   E. Acute/chronic bronchitis.

9. Examination of the respiratory system

1. Which of the following is *not* a physical sign of hypercapnia?
   A. Palmar erythema.
   B. Bounding pulse.
   C. Clubbing.
   D. CO_2 retention flap.
   E. Reduced Glasgow Coma Scale.

2. An 18-year-old male basketball player attends Accident and Emergency (A&E) complaining of

shortness of breath and chest pain. On examination there is markedly reduced chest expansion of the left side with hyperresonant percussion and absent breath sounds on that side. What is the most likely diagnosis?
A. Pleural effusion.
B. Lung collapse.
C. Lung fibrosis.
D. Consolidation.
E. Pneumothorax.

3. A 60-year woman with a new diagnosis of breast cancer attends A&E with a 4-day history of increasing shortness of breath. On examination there is markedly reduced chest expansion on the left side with stony dull percussion and absent breath sounds at the left base. Vocal resonance is reduced at the left base. What is the most likely diagnosis?
A. Pleural effusion.
B. Lung collapse.
C. Lung fibrosis.
D. Consolidation.
E. Pneumothorax.

4. A 49-year-old smoker with a 6-month history of weight loss attends A&E with shortness of breath and a dry cough. On examination there is reduced chest expansion on the right side with dull percussion and absent breath sounds at the right base. What is the most likely diagnosis?
A. Pleural effusion.
B. Lung collapse.
C. Lung fibrosis.
D. Consolidation.
E. Pneumothorax.

10 and 11. The respiratory patient: clinical and imaging investigations

1. What is a normal value for peak expiratory flow rate (PEFR) in a healthy adult?
A. 50–150 L/min.
B. 150–250 L/min.
C. 250–350 L/min.
D. 350–450 L/min.
E. 450–600 L/min.

2. Which of these tests assesses breathlessness by having patients walk a 10-metre distance during increasingly short time intervals?
A. 6-minute walk test.
B. Exercise electrocardiograph.
C. Shuttle test.
D. Treadmill test.
E. Spirometry.

3. Which of these investigations is the gold standard for diagnosis of a pulmonary embolism?
A. D-dimer.
B. Computed tomography (CT) pulmonary angiogram.
C. Pulmonary angiography.
D. CT chest.
E. Spirometry.

12. Respiratory emergencies

1. Which of these is *not* a pulmonary cause of adult respiratory distress syndrome?
A. Infection.
B. Cardiopulmonary bypass.
C. Near drowning.
D. Aspiration.
E. Gas inhalation.

2. Which of these is not a common cause of secondary pneumothorax?
A. COPD.
B. Bronchial carcinoma.
C. Tuberculosis.
D. Sarcoidosis.
E. Pulmonary fibrosis.

3. Which of this factors is not taken into account in the Wells scoring system?
A. Previous pulmonary embolism.
B. Oral contraceptive pill.
C. Malignancy.
D. Haemoptysis.
E. Evidence of deep vein thrombosis.

4. Which of these is first-line therapy for the management of acute asthma?
A. Intravenous (IV) hydrocortisone.
B. IV salbutamol.
C. Nebulized ipratropium.
D. Inhaled salbutamol.
E. Oxygen.

13. Pulmonary hypertension

1. Which of the following regarding pulmonary hypertension is true?
A. The condition results from respiratory epithelium damage.
B. The gold standard for diagnosis is echocardiography.
C. It is defined as a mean pulmonary artery pressure of >30 mmHg during exertion.
D. Pulmonary hypertension includes those cases secondary to other factors.
E. Pulmonary arterial hypertension is more common than pulmonary hypertension.

2. Which of the following is not a pathophysiological step in pulmonary hypertension?
A. Endothelial cell damage.
B. Vasculature remodelling.
C. Vasoconstrictive agent release.
D. Procoagulant factor production.
E. Bronchiectatic airway change.

14. The upper respiratory tract

1. An anxious mother brings her 2-year-old son to the GP surgery with a 3-day history of cough and fevers. The child's cough is particularly bad at night and as a result he has not been sleeping. On examination the child is irritable and has a characteristic barking cough. What is the most likely diagnosis?
A. Asthma.
B. Epiglottitis.
C. Croup.
D. Bronchiolitis.
E. Virus-induced wheeze.

15. Sleep disorders

1. Which of these is *not* a symptom of sleep apnoea?
A. Daytime somnolence.
B. Morning headaches.
C. Snoring.
D. Shortness of breath.
E. Mood swings.

2. Which of these features is not measured during somnography?
A. Blood pressure.
B. Eye movements.
C. Brain activity.
D. Peak expiratory flow.
E. Pulse.

16. Asthma

1. Which of these is *not* a symptom of asthma?
A. Wheeze.
B. Chest tightness.
C. Cough.
D. Breathlessness.
E. Weight loss.

2. Which of these is not a symptom of life-threatening acute asthma?
A. PEFR 50% predicted.
B. P_aO_2 <8 kPa.
C. Silent chest.
D. Confusion.
E. Bradycardia.

17. Chronic obstructive pulmonary disease (COPD)

1. Which of the following interventions has been shown to have the greatest impact on slowing the progression of COPD?
A. Pulmonary rehabilitation.
B. Inhaled bronchodilators.
C. Steroids.
D. Influenza vaccination.
E. Smoking cessation.

2. A 75-year-old man with a 100-pack-year smoking history attends the GP surgery complaining of shortness of breath and a productive cough every day for the past 6 months. Which of the following investigations would be most helpful in making a diagnosis of COPD?
A. Chest X-ray.
B. Spirometry.
C. Echo.
D. Full blood count.
E. Sputum culture.

3. A 75-year-old man has been admitted to hospital with an acute exacerbation of COPD. He is managed with 35% oxygen on facemask, nebulized bronchodilators, antibiotics and steroids. The patient develops type 2 respiratory failure and his most recent blood gas demonstrates pH 7.18, PO_2 7.9 kPa, PCO_2 11 KPa. What is the most appropriate management?
A. Give 15 L oxygen through non-rebreather mask.
B. Reduce level of oxygen.
C. Refer to intensive care.
D. Start patient on non-invasive ventilation (bilevel positive airway pressure).
E. Increase the dose of steroids.

18. Disorders of the interstitium

1. Which of these is the gold standard investigation for idiopathic pulmonary fibrosis?
A. High-resolution CT chest.
B. Spirometry.
C. Arterial blood gas.
D. Blood tests, including erythrocyte sedimentation rate.
E. Bronchoalveolar lavage.

2. Which of these is not a commonly recognized cause of extrinsic allergic alveolitis?
A. Bird faeces.
B. Cotton fibres.
C. House dust mite.
D. Sugar cane fibres.
E. Mouldy hay.

19. Malignant lung disease

1. Which one of the following statements regarding bronchial carcinoma is false?
   A. It accounts for 70% of all primary lung tumours.
   B. Men are affected more than women.
   C. Cigarette smoke is the largest contributory factor.
   D. It is the commonest malignant tumour in the Western world.
   E. Risk falls with time in those who have given up smoking.

2. Which of the following is not associated with Pancoast's syndrome?
   A. Anhydrosis.
   B. Ptosis.
   C. Hypertrophic pulmonary osteoarthropathy.
   D. Miosis.
   E. Facial palsy.

3. A 67-year-old retired plumber presents with progressive shortness of breath and right-sided chest pain. His GP refers him for a plain chest radiograph which is reported as 'right pleural thickening'. Which of the below is the most likely diagnosis?
   A. Small-cell carcinoma.
   B. COPD.
   C. Mesothelioma.
   D. Large-cell carcinoma.
   E. Pleuritis.

4. A 63-year-old woman has been diagnosed with mesothelioma 5 years ago, likely due to her previous factory work in her 30s and 40s. The company she worked for is now out of business. She consults her GP regarding compensation for her illness. Which of the following should her GP advise?
   A. She can claim against the company's insurers as the company is no longer in operation.
   B. She needs to seek legal representation to clarify whether her former employer was negligent.
   C. She has no capacity to claim due to her date of diagnosis.
   D. She is eligible for compensation under the Industrial Injuries Disability Benefit scheme.
   E. She has no capacity to claim as the company is no longer trading.

20. Infectious lung disease

1. Which of the following is the most common causative organism in community-acquired pneumonia?
   A. *Staphylococcus aureus.*
   B. *Klebsiella pneumoniae.*
   C. *Streptococcus pneumoniae.*
   D. *Moraxella catarrhalis.*
   E. *Haemophilus influenzae.*

2. A 75-year-old man with COPD is admitted to hospital following 1 week of flu-like symptoms. Over the past 2 days he has developed a productive cough, fevers and progressive dyspnoea. Sequential chest X-rays show a rapidly progressive left-sided consolidation with evidence of cavitation. What is the most likely causative organism?
   A. *Staphylococcus aureus.*
   B. *Klebsiella pneumoniae.*
   C. *Streptococcus pneumoniae.*
   D. *Moraxella catarrhalis.*
   E. *Haemophilus influenzae.*

3. A 55-year-old man with a history of alcoholism is admitted to A&E with a reduced Glasgow Coma Scale. A chest X-ray done on admission shows a right basal consolidation. What would be the most appropriate choice of antibiotics in this case?
   A. Oral amoxicillin.
   B. Oral ciprofloxacin.
   C. IV meropenem.
   D. IV co-amoxiclav and clarithromycin.
   E. IV co-amoxiclav and metronidazole.

4. A 25-year-old male is admitted to A&E with a dry cough and worsening dyspnoea over several weeks. He appears very cachectic and discloses that 6 months ago he was diagnosed with human immunodeficiency virus (HIV) but he has not attended any clinic appointments. What is the most likely causative organism?
   A. *Moraxella catarrhalis.*
   B. *Pneumocystis jiroveci.*
   C. *Aspergillus.*
   D. Cytomegalovirus.
   E. Influenza.

21. Suppurative lung disease

1. Which of these is not an acquired cause of bronchiectasis?
   A. Childhood measles.
   B. Foreign body.
   C. Tumour.
   D. Cystic fibrosis.
   E. Whooping cough.

2. Which of these is not a useful investigation of bronchiectasis?
   A. High-resolution CT scan.
   B. Sweat test.
   C. Sputum test.
   D. Spirometry.
   E. Blood tests, including full blood count and C-reactive protein.

22. Pleural effusions

1. Which of the following is not a recognized cause of pleural effusion?
   A. Hepatic failure.
   B. Chronic kidney disease.
   C. Malnourishment.
   D. Leukaemia.
   E. Hypocalcaemia.

2. A 67-year-old smoker presenting with weight loss and malaise is found to have a unilateral pleural effusion on chest X-ray. A diagnostic tap drains bloody fluid. What is the most likely diagnosis?
   A. Bronchial carcinoma.
   B. Hepatocellular carcinoma.
   C. Bronchiectasis.
   D. Cardiac failure.
   E. Sarcoidosis.

Extended matching questions (EMQs)

1. Overview of the respiratory system

Respiratory muscles

A. Diaphragm.
B. External intercostals.
C. Internal intercostals.
D. Levator scapulae.
E. Quadratus lumborum.
F. Sternocleidomastoids.
G. Thoracis transversus.

Match the respiratory muscle to its description:

1. These muscles are attached to the inferior border of a rib and the superior border of the rib below. They slope downwards and forward.
2. The aorta traverses this muscle at the level of T12.
3. The central part of this domed muscle is tendinous and the outer margin is muscular.
4. These muscles play the greatest role in preventing chest wall recession during quiet inspiration.
5. In addition to the diaphragm and scalene muscles, these muscles raise the ribs anteroposteriorly to produce movement at the manubriosternal joint during forced inspiration.

Ventilation and gas exchange

A. Partial pressure.
B. Diffusion.
C. Perfusion.
D. Restrictive disorder.
E. Obstructive disorder.
F. Ventilation.
G. Expiration.
H. Tidal volume.
I. Respiration.

Match the statement to the best answer as given above.

1. The movement of air in and out of the respiratory system.
2. A passive process, due to the elastic recoil of lung tissue.
3. A disorder because of difficulty expanding the lungs, such as due to stiffening of the lung tissue or weakness of the respiratory muscles.
4. Occurs at the gas-exchange surface, using partial pressures.
5. Can be determined by the gas content of liquids.

2. Organization of the respiratory tract

Cells and tissues of the lower respiratory tract

A. Alveolar ducts.
B. Alveolar macrophages.
C. Alveoli.
D. Bronchiole.
E. Bronchus.
F. Respiratory bronchiole.
G. Mucosa-associated lymphoid tissue (MALT).
H. Trachea.
I. Type I pneumocytes.
J. Type II pneumocytes.

Match the cell or tissue to its description:

1. This structure contains no cartilage and no glands in the submucosa. This part does not have a role in gas exchange.
2. This structure has no contractile element and contains loose submucosa and glands.
3. These cells have flattened nuclei and few mitochondria.
4. These cells have rounded nuclei and are rich in mitochondria. Also, microvilli are present on their exposed surface.
5. These structures have perforations between cells to communicate with adjacent similar structures.

4. Physiology, ventilation and gas exchange

A. Vital capacity.
B. Forced expiratory volume in 1 second (FEV_1).
C. Total lung capacity.
D. Functional residual capacity.
E. Residual volume.
F. Expiratory reserve volume.
G. Tidal volume.
H. Inspiratory capacity.

Match the above terms to their definition below:

1. The volume of air remaining in lungs at end of a maximum expiration.

2. The volume of air remaining in lungs at the end of a normal expiration.
3. The volume of air that can be breathed in by a maximum inspiration following a maximum expiration.
4. The volume of air breathed in and out in a single breath.
5. The volume of air that can be expelled by a maximum effort at the end of a normal expiration.

---

5. Perfusion and gas transport

Acid–base balance

A. Compensated respiratory acidosis.
B. Compensated respiratory alkalosis.
C. Compensated metabolic acidosis.
D. Compensated metabolic alkalosis.
E. Metabolic acidosis.
F. Metabolic alkalosis.
G. Respiratory acidosis.
H. Respiratory alkalosis.

(Normal values: pH 7.35–7.45: $PO_2 = 90$–110 mmHg; $PCO_2 = 34$–45 mmHg; [HCO_3^-] 21–27 mmol/L.)

Match the acid–base imbalance to the following blood gas results:

1. pH 7.4; PO_2 49 mmHg; PCO_2 26 mmHg; [HCO_3^-] 15 mmol/L.
2. pH 7.4; PO_2 94 mmHg; PCO_2 20 mmHg; [HCO_3^-] 14 mmol/L.
3. pH 7.6; PO_2 94 mmHg; PCO_2 40 mmHg; [HCO_3^-] 35 mmol/L.
4. pH 7.2; PO_2 80 mmHg; PCO_2 55 mmHg; [HCO_3^-] 22 mmol/L.
5. pH 7.2; PO_2 100 mmHg; PCO_2 40 mmHg; [HCO_3^-] 16 mmol/L.

---

6. Control of respiratory function

A. Pontine neurons.
B. Botzinger complex.
C. Medullary neurons.
D. Chemoreceptors.
E. Carotid bodies.
F. C-fibres.
G. Rapidly adapting receptors.
H. Slowly adapting receptors.

Match the description below to the best answer from the list above.

1. Form part of the cough reflex.
2. Situated rostral to the nucleus ambiguus.
3. Regulate the dorsal respiratory group.

4. Sensitive to P_aO_2, P_aCO_2, pH, blood flow and temperature.
5. Stimulation of these results in bradycardia and hypotension.

---

7. Basic pharmacology

Asthma drugs

A. Short-acting β_2 agonist.
B. Long-acting β_2 agonist.
C. Theophyllines.
D. Leukotriene antagonist.
E. Inhaled corticosteroid.
F. Oral corticosteroid.

Match the drug to its description in the following clinical scenarios:

1. The drug prescribed to an asthmatic adult who uses a reliever (but no other medications) more than once a day.
2. Phosphodiesterase inhibitor which prevents the breakdown of cAMP to cause bronchodilatation.
3. A long-term asthmatic woman suffering from side-effects of her medication including osteoporosis, diabetes and recurrent infections.
4. A mild asthmatic complaining that his medication causes oral candidiasis and a hoarse voice.
5. The first medication to try in a newly diagnosed asthmatic.

---

8. The respiratory patient – taking a history and exploring symptoms

Cough

A. Asthma.
B. Bronchiectasis.
C. Carcinoma of bronchus.
D. COPD.
E. Cystic fibrosis.
F. Gastro-oesophageal reflux disease (GORD).
G. Iatrogenic.
H. Inhaled foreign body.
I. Pulmonary embolism.
J. Tuberculosis.

Match the most likely diagnosis to the following clinical scenarios:

1. A 3-year-old boy attends hospital having an acute bout of coughing. On auscultation the doctor hears a monophonic inspiratory wheeze.
2. A 12-year-old boy attends hospital after having an acute bout of coughing. On auscultation the doctor hears a polyphonic expiratory wheeze.

3. A 27-year-old man presents with a (at least) 5-month history of purulent sputum. He has never smoked and he tells you he had whooping cough as a child.
4. A 48-year-old woman who is being managed for diabetes and hypertension complains of a constant dry cough.
5. A 60-year-old woman, who smokes 25 cigarettes per day, presents with a 5-week history of cough, malaise and weight loss.

9. Examination of the respiratory system

A. Pleural effusion.
B. Consolidation.
C. Pneumothorax.
D. Atelectasis.
E. Asthma.
F. Pulmonary oedema.
G. Interstitial lung disease.
H. Tension pneumothorax.

For each of the following select the most likely diagnosis:

1. An 80-year-old woman is admitted to hospital with shortness of breath. She is tachypnoeic and desaturates on air. On examination you notice a raised jugular venous pressure and fine inspiratory crackles on auscultation.
2. An 80-year old woman is admitted to hospital with shortness of breath. On examination there is reduced chest expansion on the left side with dull percussion and reduced breath sounds at the left base. Vocal resonance is reduced.
3. An 80-year-old woman is admitted to hospital with shortness of breath. On examination there is reduced chest expansion on the left side with dull percussion and reduced breath sounds with coarse crackles at the left base. Vocal resonance is increased.
4. An 80-year-old woman is admitted to hospital with shortness of breath. On examination there is reduced chest expansion on the left side with hyperresonant percussion and absent breath sounds. The trachea is deviated to the right.
5. An 80-year-old woman is admitted to hospital with shortness of breath. On examination there is reduced chest expansion bilaterally and fine inspiratory crackles are audible at both apices of the lungs.

10 and 11. The respiratory patient: clinical and imaging investigations

A. Shuttle test.
B. Bronchoalveolar lavage.

C. Flexible fibreoptic bronchoscopy.
D. Peak expiratory flow rate.
E. Body plethysmography.
F. 6-minute walk test.

Match the investigation with the following clinical scenarios:

1. A patient whom you suspect to have asthma is asked to keep a diary of peak flow measurements.
2. A camera that is passed through the upper airways to visualize pathology directly and take samples for histology in a lifelong smoker complaining of a new-onset cough with haemoptysis.
3. Saline that is squirted through a bronchoscope and then sucked back up again to collect cells for cytology in a lifelong smoker complaining of new-onset cough with haemoptysis.
4. A sealed box the size of a telephone box, in which the patient whom you suspect of having an interstitial lung disease is asked to sit and perform respiratory manoeuvres. Changes in lung volume are measured.
5. A test of exercise capacity whereby the patient complaining of reduced exercise tolerance is asked to walk up and down between two cones, placed 10 metres apart, in a set period of time. The time in which the patient is allowed to complete the course is progressively reduced.

12. Respiratory emergencies

A. Positive end-expiratory pressure.
B. Nitric oxide.
C. Surfactant.
D. Obstructive sleep apnoea.
E. Paralysis of the diaphragm.
F. Confusion.
G. Headaches.
H. Type 1 respiratory failure.
I. Type 2 respiratory failure.

Select the appropriate response from the options above for the following statements:

1. A pulmonary cause of respiratory failure.
2. Treatment with conservative oxygen therapy.
3. A symptom of hypoxia.
4. Useful in infant respiratory distress syndrome.
5. Prevents alveolar collapse during expiration.

13. Pulmonary hypertension

A. Type 1.
B. Type 2.

C. Type 3.

D. Type 4.

E. Type 5.

F. True PAH.

Match the category of pulmonary hypertension to its description in the following clinical scenarios:

1. A 70-year-old woman has suffered with recurrent deep vein thrombosis and pulmonary emboli secondary to antiphospholipid syndrome.
2. A 65-year-old man with a long history of ankle swelling and worsening left ventricular function on echocardiography.
3. A 42-year-old former intravenous drug user with falling CD4 count is increasingly short of breath.
4. A 67-year-old with a history of heavy smoking complains of shortness of breath on lying flat and general fatigue.
5. A 46-year-old woman with pulmonary hypertension but no evidence of any medical condition despite comprehensive investigation for her shortness of breath.

16. Asthma

Pathogenesis of asthma

A. Preformed mediators.

B. Secondary effector cells.

C. Smooth-muscle constriction.

D. Prostaglandins.

E. Early response.

F. Late response.

G. Hypertrophy of smooth muscle.

Match the statements below with the single best answer from the list:

1. Occurs in long-standing asthma.
2. Includes histamine and neutral proteases.
3. Associated with the metabolism of arachidonic acid.
4. Includes eosinophils and platelets.
5. The process of the influx of inflammatory cells.

17. Chronic obstructive pulmonary disease (COPD)

A. Pulmonary rehabilitation.

B. Inhaled bronchodilators.

C. Antibiotics.

D. Long-term oxygen therapy.

E. Long-term oral steroids.

F. Non-invasive ventilation.

G. Smoking cessation.

H. Carbocisteine.

For each of the following select the most appropriate management:

1. A 45-year-old female smoker attends her GP concerned that she has developed a chronic cough. The cough is productive and is present most days of the year, particularly during the winter months.
2. A 77-year-old man with severe COPD is admitted to hospital with an acute exacerbation of COPD. During the admission an echo is performed which shows a mildly dilated right ventricle and pulmonary artery pressure of 50 mmHg.
3. A 77-year-old man with severe COPD is admitted to hospital with an acute exacerbation of COPD. An arterial blood gas performed on admission demonstrates pH 7.17, PO_2 7.1 and PCO_2 8.9 on 35% oxygen (Venturi mask).
4. A 65-year-old female with COPD is recently discharged from hospital and still complains of breathlessness despite stopping smoking and starting inhalers.
5. A 65-year-old ex-smoker is diagnosed with COPD following spirometry which demonstrates an FEV_1:FVC ratio of 0.65.

18. Disorders of the interstitium

A. Simple pneumoconiosis.

B. Pulmonary fibrosis.

C. Asbestosis.

D. Coal worker's pneumoconiosis.

E. Progressive massive fibrosis.

F. Caplan's syndrome.

G. Extrinsic allergic alveolitis.

H. Bronchiolitis obliterans.

Match the descriptions below to the best answer above.

1. A type III hypersensitivity reaction.
2. Most common type of pathogen is crocidolite.
3. Associated with rheumatoid arthritis.
4. Characterized by large, round fibrotic nodules.
5. Characterized by polypoid masses and granulation tissue.

19. Malignant lung disease

Bronchial carcinoma

A. Squamous cell.

B. Adenocarcinoma.

C. Small-cell carcinoma.

D. Palliative care.

E. Paraneoplastic syndrome.

F. Pancoast's syndrome.

Match the correct letter above to its description in the following clinical scenarios:

1. A 62-year-old woman has suffered with some weight loss and is found to be anaemic. She has never smoked.
2. An 87-year-old woman is found to have a suspected primary small-cell carcinoma with multiple metastases. She has a background of COPD and diabetes. Her main complaints are of breathlessness and pain.
3. A 54-year-old man is concerned by a drooping of his left eyelid. He is a smoker and found to have a microcytic anaemia on blood tests.
4. A 70-year-old man with known lung cancer presents to his GP with his wife who is concerned he is becoming increasingly confused.
5. A 55-year-old woman who is a heavy smoker is found to have cytological findings of hyperdense nuclei with minimal cellular cytoplasm.

Malignancy on chest X-ray

A. Primary renal tumour.

B. Likely soft-tissue sarcoma.

C. Small-cell carcinoma.

D. Mesothelioma.

E. Likely thyroid primary.

F. Squamous cell carcinoma.

Match the correct letter above to its description in the following clinical scenarios:

1. A 56-year-old man with multiple, large well-circumscribed nodules throughout both lung fields.
2. A solitary large hilar mass with evidence of cavitation.
3. The chest X-ray of a 67-year-old man shows a thickened diaphragm with a lumpy appearance.
4. A 34-year-old man who presented with a swollen thigh appears to have a large, well-circumscribed nodule in his left lung.
5. A 70-year-old lifelong smoker is found to have a mass originating from his right main bronchus.

20. Infectious lung disease
Organisms in pneumonia

A. *Staphylococcus aureus.*

B. Influenza.

C. *Streptococcus pneumoniae.*

D. *Pseudomonas aeruginosa.*

E. Tuberculosis.

F. *Mycoplasma pneumoniae.*

G. *Haemophilus influenzae.*

H. *Legionella pneumophila.*

For each of the following, which is the most likely causative organism?

1. A 45-year-old man returns from a business conference with shortness of breath, a dry cough and diarrhoea and vomiting. After 24 hours in hospital he develops type I respiratory failure and is transferred to the intensive care unit (ICU) for ventilation.
2. A 19-year-old develops shortness of breath and a dry cough following a week of flu-like symptoms.
3. An elderly patient who has required ventilation on the ICU for several weeks begins spiking fevers and is noted to have purulent secretions.
4. A 70-year-old smoker is admitted to hospital with shortness of breath and a productive cough following a week of flu-like symptoms. The patient rapidly deteriorates and is transferred to ICU for ventilation.
5. A 70-year-old male is admitted to hospital with confusion, fevers and a productive cough.

Treatment of respiratory infections

A. Isoniazid.

B. Amoxicillin.

C. Clarithromycin.

D. Co-trimoxazole.

E. Metronidazole.

F. Oseltamivir.

G. Meropenem.

H. Trimethoprim.

For each of the following choose the most appropriate treatment:

1. A 48-year-old immigrant from Bangladesh with a 3-month history of fevers, productive cough and weight loss. Tuberculosis ELISPOT is positive.
2. A 75-year-old man recovering from a recent stroke with a right lobar pneumonia.
3. A 75-year-old patient ventilated on ICU. Sputum cultures have grown a Gram-negative rod.
4. A 30-year-old human immunodeficiency virus (HIV)-positive male with a 2-week history of shortness of breath and a dry cough. CD4 count is found to be 50 cells/mm^3.
5. A 19-year-old with shortness of breath and a dry cough following a week of flu-like symptoms.

21. Suppurative lung disease
Cystic fibrosis

A. Guthrie test.

B. Sweat test.

C. Immunoreactive trypsin test.

D. DNase.

E. CFTR.

F. ΔF508.

G. Liposome.

Select the appropriate response from the options above for the following statements:

1. Low levels indicate a positive test.
2. The most common mutation in cystic fibrosis.
3. A vector used in experimental treatment to replace the affected gene.
4. Performed as a screening test on newborn babies.
5. Shown to improve FEV_1 in cystic fibrosis patients.

22. Pleural effusions

Management of pleural effusion

A. Diagnostic tap.

B. Transudative effusion.

C. Exudative effusion.

D. Therapeutic tap.

E. Light's criteria.

F. Empyema.

Match the correct letter above to its description in the following clinical scenarios:

1. A 51-year-old woman presents with a unilateral pleural effusion. She is otherwise well.
2. A 63-year-old man has a chest X-ray suggestive of pleural effusion. However on chest drain insertion only minimal fluid is drained.
3. A 39-year-old man presents acutely unwell with elevated respiratory rate and oxygen saturations of 87% on air. Chest X-ray shows a large left-sided effusion.
4. On diagnostic tap an effusion is found to have an albumin content of 27 g/L.
5. A 57-year-old woman with an ejection fraction of 19% is found to have bilateral pleural effusions.

Diagnosis of effusion fluid

A. Transudate.

B. Exudate.

C. Light's criteria.

D. Conservative management.

E. Therapeutic tap.

F. Investigation for underlying malignancy.

Match the correct letter above to its description in the following clinical scenarios:

1. A man with hepatic failure has small bilateral transudative effusions on diagnostic tap.
2. A diagnostic tap shows effusion fluid with an albumin content of 40 g/L.
3. A diagnostic tap shows effusion fluid with an albumin content of 27 g/L that meets Light's criteria.
4. A diagnostic tap shows effusion fluid with an albumin content of 16 g/L.
5. A large right-sided effusion is compromising a 59-year-old woman's breathing.

23. Respiratory manifestations of systemic disease

Vasculitis

A. Churg–Strauss.

B. Wegener's granulomatosis.

C. Rheumatoid arthritis.

D. Ankylosing spondylitis.

E. Systemic lupus erythematosus.

F. Sarcoid.

G. Scleroderma.

H. Goodpasture's disease.

For each of the following, which is the most likely diagnosis?

1. An elderly man has severe arthritis of the spine. On auscultation he has an early diastolic murmur heard best in the aortic region and fine inspiratory crackles at the apices of both lungs.
2. A young woman of Afro-Caribbean origin attends her GP surgery with a 3-month history of dry cough and increasing shortness of breath. A chest X-ray is organized and shows evidence of hilar lymphadenopathy.
3. A young man attends A&E with haemoptysis and is also found to be in acute renal failure. An autoantibody screen reveals that he is cytoplasmic antineutrophil cytoplasmic antibody (c-ANCA)-positive.
4. An 18-year-old female is admitted to hospital with shortness of breath and pleuritic chest pain. On examination you notice the patient has an erythematous rash on both cheeks that spares her nasolabial folds.
5. A 45-year-old woman with severe arthritis affecting both hands develops shortness of breath. On examination the patient is clubbed, cyanotic and has widespread fine inspiratory crackles on auscultation.

1. Overview of the respiratory system

1. C. Pulmonary fibrosis. This is a restrictive lung disease.
2. D. Control of electrolytes.

2. Organization of the respiratory tract

1. B. The larynx is continuous with the trachea, and moves back during swallowing to cover the trachea and direct food down the oesophagus, preventing aspiration. The larynx has one external muscle, the cricothyroid, and multiple internal muscles. Innervation is from the vagus nerve. It is crucial to phonation (speech).
2. B. The hilum of the lung contains the main bronchi, the pulmonary artery and vein, nerves, lymph nodes and the pulmonary ligament. The bronchial circulation delivers oxygenated blood to the lung parenchyma and does not pass through the hilum.
3. E. The nasal cavity comprises the nose and nasopharynx. The upper third of the nasal cavity is lined with olfactory, and the remainder with columnar epithelium. It plays no role in gas exchange but is important in warming and humidifying air. Ciliated cells in the lower two-thirds trap particulate matter and prevent it reaching the lower airways.
4. C. The trachea is surrounded by C-shaped cartilage rings and is not encircled. The right main bronchus is more acute than the left, and, as such, foreign bodies are more likely to lodge here than in the left bronchus. The majority of gas exchange occurs in the alveoli, although exchange does occur in the respiratory bronchioles. MALT is present in the walls of the lower respiratory tract.
5. C. Alveolar macrophages exist predominantly in the alveoli and are derived from circulating monocytes. They are a key cellular defence mechanism and phagocytose bacteria and foreign material.
6. B. Bronchioles are the first point in the tree to contain non-cartilaginous walls. The carina describes the division of the trachea into left and right main bronchi. There are more than 20 divisions of the respiratory tree, with two main zones (the conducting zone and respiratory zone). The dead space consists of around 150 mL.

7. D. Large material is predominantly removed by mucociliary clearance, whether in the nasopharynx or lower down the respiratory tract. Cilia waft at approximately 1000 strokes per minute. Irritant C-fibres stimulate the cough reflex.
8. E. Antiproteases are a key humoral lung defence. IgA, not IgG, is the most prevalent antibody and neutrophils, not basophils, are the key cellular response to bacterial infection. Filtration of air is a physical defence. Surfactant is a cellular response but from type II pneumocytes.

3. Pulmonary circulation

1. D. The pulmonary circulation is a low-pressure, low resistance system.
2. C. Hydrostatic pressure is larger in blood vessels supplying the lung bases; therefore blood flow is greater at the lung bases compared to the apices.
3. D. Blood flow is gravity-dependent. Therefore when this patient is turned on to her right side blood flow to the right lung is increased, and because this lung is poorly ventilated due to extensive consolidation, ventilation:perfusion mismatch is increased, causing the patient to desaturate.

4. Physiology, ventilation and gas exchange

1. A. The FRC is the volume of air remaining in lungs at the end of a normal expiration.
2. D. Increased residual volume.
3. B. This patient has symptoms and signs in keeping with pulmonary fibrosis. Such patients usually develop a restrictive lung disorder characterized by a reduced FEV_1 and FVC.

5. Perfusion and gas transport

1. A. The flow of gas and blood should be equal for an ideal ventilation–perfusion relationship. In theory this is not exact as the flow of both blood and gas differs throughout the lung.
2. E. This enhanced dissociation at high carbon dioxide levels is termed the Bohr effect. The association between oxygen and haemoglobin is not an oxidation; it is an oxygenation. Myoglobin accepts

the oxygen molecule from oxyhaemoglobin and temporarily stores it for skeletal muscle. Carbon dioxide has a 20-fold greater diffusing capacity than oxygen. In exercise there is increase in depth of breathing (hyperpnoea), not hyperventilation.

3. C. Changes in posture do alter the $V{:}Q$ ratio. Ventilation and blood flow are decreased at the apices compared to the bases, and thus the $V{:}Q$ is not uniform across the lung, even in health. Perfusion is reduced to underventilated areas of lung by hypoxic vasoconstriction.

4. A. CO_2 is an acidic gas: an uncompensated increase causes acidosis. Metabolic compensation returns acid–base disturbances towards normal but cannot completely correct them. Increasing ventilation decreases PCO_2. pK is low relative to pH of the blood. It is 7.35–7.45. For more information see Chapter 10.

5. C. The abnormal HbS polymerizes at low oxygen levels causing deformation or 'sickling' of the red blood cell. Thalassaemias are inherited in an autosomal recessive manner and relate to abnormal alpha or beta Hb chain synthesis. A mild, usually asymptomatic anaemia is present in those with heterozygous sickle disease, so-called sickle cell trait. Sickle cell homozygotes can present in sickle vaso-occlusive crisis with infarction and severe pain. Treatment is with analgesia and fluids.

6. Control of respiratory function

1. D. Pulmonary disease. Although this may affect levels of P_aCO_2, it does not affect the body's response to it.
2. E. Alteration of blood pH through renal excretion.

7. Basic pharmacology

1. E. Salbutamol is a short-acting β_2-receptor agonist used to treat lower-airways disease. It has a degree of non-specific receptor activity and side-effects such as headache, fine tremor and tachycardia result from cross-stimulation of β_1 receptors.
2. B. Formoterol is a full agonist of the β_1 receptor, unlike salmeterol, which is a partial agonist. For this reason formeterol can be used in SMART. Anticholinergics are more useful in COPD due to evidence of increased vagal tone in the airway smooth muscle.
3. C. Wide variations in enzyme activity and thus breakdown across patient populations lead to varying levels of theophyllines in the blood. This is challenging as theophyllines have a narrow therapeutic window and, as such, levels in the blood must be checked regularly.

4. C. Leukotriene receptor antagonists are a component of step 4 of the guidelines. Patients should be initiated at a step that corresponds to the severity of their asthma at that time and stepped down to the lowest step possible that maintains good disease control.

5. D. Acamprosate is licensed for use in alcohol dependence through reducing cravings. It has no use in nicotine addiction.

8. The respiratory patient – taking a history and exploring symptoms

1. C. COPD does not cause haemoptysis. If a patient with COPD presents with haemoptysis, you must rule out another cause, such as lung cancer. These patients will be high-risk due to smoking as a common risk factor in both diseases.

9. Examination of the respiratory system

1. C. Clubbing.
2. E. These are the classical findings in a patient with pneumothorax.
3. A. These are the classical features of a pleural effusion.
4. B. Given the history of smoking and weight loss it is most likely this patient has an obstructing bronchial tumour that has caused collapse of the right lower lobe.

10 and 11. The respiratory patient: clinical and imaging investigations

1. E. 450–600 L/min.
2. C. Shuttle test.
3. B. CT pulmonary angiogram is the gold standard investigation. Although pulmonary angiography is useful, it has considerably more risks associated with it.

12. Respiratory emergencies

1. B. This is an extrapulmonary cause.
2. E. Pulmonary fibrosis.
3. B. Although a risk factor, the oral contraceptive pill is not on the Wells score.
4. E. Oxygen. Although salbutamol is a key part of acute asthma management, oxygen should be the first treatment.

13. Pulmonary hypertension

1. D.   Pulmonary arterial hypertension is a far more specific diagnosis as it relates to primary and not secondary pulmonary hypertension. Damage is to endothelial and not epithelial cells. The gold standard diagnosis is on right heart catheterization. You may find it helpful to review the European Society of Cardiology Guidelines on pulmonary hypertension.
2. E.   All the above are aspects of pulmonary hypertension except bronchiectatic airway change.

14. The upper respiratory tract

1. C.   Croup.

15. Sleep disorders

1. D.   Shortness of breath.
2. D.   Peak expiratory flow.

16. Asthma

1. E.   Weight loss.
2. A.   PEFR in life-threatening asthma is <33% predicted.

17. Chronic obstructive pulmonary disease (COPD)

1. E.   Smoking cessation.
2. B.   Spirometry with an FEV_1/FVC ratio <0.70 is the Global Initiative for Obstructive Lung Disease (GOLD) standard for diagnosis of COPD.
3. D.   This patient has become acidotic and hypercapnic when managed on facemask oxygen and now requires non-invasive ventilation. If, after a trial of non-invasive ventilation, the patient does not respond or cannot tolerate it, then he might need referral to intensive care for invasive ventilation. Giving high-flow oxygen or simply reducing the amount of oxygen (as the patient is already hypoxic) is likely to make the situation worse.

18. Disorders of the interstitium

1. A.   Although all tests are useful in the diagnosis and work-up of a patient with idiopathic pulmonary fibrosis, high-resolution CT chest remains the gold standard.
2. C.   House dust mite is a common cause of asthma.

19. Malignant lung disease

1. A.   Bronchial carcinoma accounts for 95% of primary lung tumours. All the other statements regarding this cancer are true.
2. E.   Facial palsy is not associated with Pancoast's syndrome. Hypertrophic pulmonary osteoarthropathy can result from disruption to the nervous supply to the arm from invasion of the sympathetic plexus.
3. C.   Mesothelioma. This patient has a history of probable occupational exposure to asbestos with clinical features of malignancy. Furthermore, his chest X-ray shows the hallmark of mesothelioma – pleural thickening.
4. C.   Sadly she has no claim as all claims must be initiated within 3 years of diagnosis. Full details are available in the 'neoplasms of the pleura' section in Chapter 19.

20. Infectious lung disease

1. C.   *Streptococcus pneumoniae.*
2. A.   *Staphylococcus aureus* is a common cause of secondary bacterial infection following influenza. *S. aureus* pneumonia is often rapidly progressive and characteristically causes cavitation on X-ray.
3. E.   IV co-amoxiclav and metronidazole. Given the history of alcohol use and reduced Glasgow Coma Scale, and the fact the pneumonia is right-sided, it is likely this patient has developed aspiration pneumonia. In this case the most appropriate choice of antibiotics is E (co-amoxiclav and metronidazole). Co-amoxiclav is broad-spectrum and metronidazole provides good anaerobic cover.
4. B.   *Pneumocystis jiroveci.*

21. Suppurative lung disease

1. D.   Cystic fibrosis. This is a congenital cause of bronchiectasis.
2. E.   Although they may be useful in a superimposed infection, routine blood tests are not of any real diagnostic value for bronchiectasis.

22. Pleural effusions

1. E.   Hypocalcaemia is not a recognized cause of pleural effusion. Organ failure and malignancy (including haematological malignancies) as well as low-albumin states from poor nutrition are all common causes of pleural effusion.
2. A.   A blood-stained effusion is highly suggestive of pulmonary malignancy, whether bronchial carcinoma or a pleural malignancy.

EMQ answers

1. Overview of the respiratory system

Respiratory muscles

1. B. External intercostals.
2. A. Diaphragm.
3. A. Diaphragm.
4. C. Internal intercostals.
5. F. Sternocleidomastoids.

Ventilation and gas exchange

1. F. Ventilation.
2. G. Expiration.
3. D. Restrictive disorder.
4. B. Diffusion.
5. A. Partial pressure.

2. Organization of the respiratory tract

Cells and tissues of the lower respiratory tract

1. D. Bronchiole.
2. H. Trachea.
3. I. Type I pneumocytes.
4. J. Type II pneumocytes.
5. C. Alveoli.

4. Physiology, ventilation and gas exchange

1. E. Residual volume.
2. D. Functional residual capacity.
3. H. Inspiratory capacity.
4. G. Tidal volume.
5. F. Expiratory reserve volume.

5. Perfusion and gas transport

Acid–base balance

1. A. Compensated respiratory alkalosis.
2. C. Compensated metabolic acidosis.
3. F. Metabolic alkalosis.
4. G. Respiratory acidosis.
5. E. Metabolic acidosis.

6. Control of respiratory function

1. G. Rapidly adapting receptors.
2. B. Botzinger complex.
3. A. Pontine neurons.
4. E. Carotid bodies.
5. F. C-fibres.

7. Basic pharmacology

Asthma drugs

1. E. Inhaled corticosteroid.
2. C. Theophyllines.
3. F. Oral corticosteroid.
4. E. Inhaled corticosteroid.
5. A. Short-acting β_2 agonist

8. The respiratory patient – taking a history and exploring symptoms

Cough

1. H. Inhaled foreign body.
2. A. Asthma.
3. B. Bronchiectasis.
4. G. Iatrogenic.
5. C. Carcinoma of bronchus.

9. Examination of the respiratory system

1. F. Pulmonary oedema.
2. B. Consolidation.
3. A. Pleural effusion.
4. H. Tension pneumothorax.
5. G. Interstitial lung disease.

10 and 11. The respiratory patient: clinical and imaging investigations

1. D. Peak expiratory flow rate.
2. C. Flexible fibreoptic bronchoscopy.

3. B. Bronchoalveolar lavage.
4. E. Body plethysmography.
5. A. Shuttle test.

12. Respiratory emergencies

Management of respiratory emergencies

1. D. Obstructive sleep apnoea.
2. I. Type 2 respiratory failure.
3. G. Headaches.
4. C. Surfactant.
5. A. Positive end-expiratory pressure.

13. Pulmonary hypertension

1. D. Type 4.
2. B. Type 2.
3. A. Type 1.
4. C. Type 3.
5. E. Type 5.

16. Asthma

Pathogenesis of asthma

1. G. Hypertrophy of smooth muscle.
2. A. Preformed mediators.
3. D. Prostaglandins.
4. B. Secondary effector cells.
5. F. Late response.

17. Chronic obstructive pulmonary disease (COPD)

1. G. Smoking cessation.
2. D. Long-term oxygen therapy.
3. F. Non-invasive ventilation.
4. A. Pulmonary rehabilitation.
5. B. Inhaled bronchodilators.

18. Disorders of the interstitium

1. G. Extrinsic allergic alveolitis.
2. C. Asbestosis.
3. F. Caplan's syndrome.
4. E. Progressive massive fibrosis.
5. H. Bronchiolitis obliterans.

19. Malignant lung disease

Bronchial carcinoma

1. B. Adenocarcinoma.
2. D. Palliative care.
3. F. Pancoast's syndrome.
4. E. Paraneoplastic syndrome.
5. C. Small-cell carcinoma.

Malignancy on chest X-ray

1. A. Primary renal tumour.
2. F. Squamous cell carcinoma.
3. D. Mesothelioma.
4. B. Likely soft-tissue sarcoma.
5. C. Small-cell carcinoma.

20. Infectious lung disease

Organisms in pneumonia

1. H. *Legionella pneumophila.*
2. F. *Mycoplasma pneumoniae.*
3. D. *Pseudomonas aeruginosa.*
4. A. *Staphylococcus aureus.*
5. C. *Streptococcus pneumoniae.*

Treatment of respiratory infections

1. A. Isoniazid (tuberculosis).
2. E. Metronidazole (aspiration pneumonia).
3. G. Meropenem (*Pseudomonas*: meropenem is the only antibiotic in the list with Gram-negative cover).
4. D. Co-trimoxazole (*Pneumocystis jiroveci*).
5. C. Clarithromycin (*Mycoplasma pneumoniae*: amoxicillin is ineffective as bacteria lack a peptidoglycan cell wall).

21. Suppurative lung disease

Cystic fibrosis

1. C. Immunoreactive trypsin test.
2. F. ΔF508.
3. G. Liposome.
4. A. Guthrie test.
5. D. DNase.

22. Pleural effusions

Management of pleural effusion

1. A. Diagnostic tap.
2. F. Empyema.

3. D. Therapeutic tap.
4. E. Light's criteria.
5. B. Transudative effusion.

Diagnosis of effusion fluid

1. D. Conservative management.
2. B. Exudate.
3. B. Exudate.
4. A. Transudate.
5. E. Therapeutic tap.

23. Respiratory manifestations of systemic disease

Vasculitis

1. D. Ankylosing spondylitis.
2. F. Sarcoid.
3. B. Wegener's granulomatosis.
4. E. Systemic lupus erythematosus.
5. C. Rheumatoid arthritis.

Glossary

Acinus Airways involved in gaseous exchange, beginning with respiratory bronchioles and ending with the alveoli.

Alveolar dead space Air reaching the alveoli that does not partake in gas exchange, for example because the alveoli are not perfused. This volume is included in physiological dead space.

Anatomical dead space Airways that do not partake in gas exchange, i.e. from the nose and mouth to and including the terminal bronchioles. This volume is usually about 150 mL and included in physiological dead space.

Antitussive An intervention aiming to relieve the symptom of cough.

Asthma An airway disease with symptoms caused by reversible and intermittent airway obstruction. There is underlying inflammation characterized by eosinophilic infiltration. Often associated with other allergic diseases.

Atelectasis Collapse of part of the lung.

Bronchiectasis Permanent dilatation of the bronchi secondary to chronic infection. It is the end stage of many pulmonary diseases, including cystic fibrosis.

Bronchitis See 'Chronic bronchitis'.

Bronchoalveolar lavage A diagnostic test performed during bronchoscopy. Saline is squirted down the bronchoscope into the lungs, then sucked back up and the cells collected sent for cytology. The cellular profiles indicate different pathologies.

Bronchoscopy A diagnostic technique where a (usually fibreoptic) camera is inserted into the lungs to visualize pathology and take biopsy samples.

Chronic bronchitis A disease that is defined clinically by a persistent cough for at least 3 months of the year, for 2 consecutive years. Part of the spectrum of chronic obstructive pulmonary disease.

Chronic obstructive pulmonary disease (COPD) A collective term for inflammatory airway diseases (emphysema, chronic bronchitis and others) occurring almost exclusively in smokers, characterized by irreversible and progressive airway obstruction. Inflammation is characterized by neutrophilic infiltration.

Conducting airways Airways not involved in gas exchange, i.e. airways proximal to respiratory bronchiole.

Continuous airways positive pressure (CPAP) A method of non-invasive ventilation whereby air is blown into the airways (positive pressure) for the whole of the respiratory cycle. CPAP is delivered by mask and is a common treatment for obstructive sleep apnoea.

Corticosteroid (glucocorticosteroid) A commonly used immunosuppressive drug that acts at a nuclear level to inhibit inflammation.

Cystic fibrosis An autosomal recessive condition causing a defect in the cystic fibrosis transmembrane receptor (CFTR), resulting in abnormally viscous lung secretions. In the lung the mutation predisposes to chronic lung infection and bronchiectasis; it also affects the pancreas and can cause male infertility.

Diffuse parenchymal lung disease See 'Interstitial lung disease'.

Emphysema Defined anatomically as destruction of the alveolar septa resulting in permanent enlargement of the air spaces distal to the terminal bronchiole. Part of the spectrum of chronic obstructive pulmonary disease.

Haemoptysis A term to describe the symptom of coughing up blood.

Hypoxic vasoconstriction Constriction of pulmonary blood vessels in response to low alveolar oxygen tension. This mechanism acts to prevent a ventilation: perfusion mismatch.

Interstitial lung disease (ILD) A diverse group of more than 200 different lung diseases affecting the interstitium (the tissue extending from and including the alveolar epithelium to capillary endothelium). May be used interchangeably with 'diffuse parenchymal lung disease'.

Mediastinum The collective name to describe structures situated in the midline and separating the two lungs. It contains the heart, great vessels, trachea, oesophagus, lymph nodes and phrenic and vagus nerves.

Mesothelioma Cancer of the lung pleura, almost always caused by asbestos inhalation.

Obstructive lung disease Diseases which narrow the airways and increase resistance to air flow.

Physiological dead space The total amount of air in the lung that does not partake in gas exchange. Includes anatomical dead space and alveolar dead space.

Pleura An epithelial lining which covers the external surface of the lungs (visceral pleura) and then is reflected back to line the chest wall (parietal pleura).

Pleural effusion Fluid in the pleural space.

Pneumocytes The cells lining the alveoli. They are either type I, which are thin and primarily structural, or type II, which are rounded and secrete surfactant.

Pneumonia Infection of peripheral lung tissue.

Pneumothorax Air in the pleural space; the tension type is a medical emergency.

Pulmonary embolism Thrombi lodging in pulmonary vasculature causing ventilation:perfusion mismatches of varying severity. A serious complication of venous thrombosis.

Pulmonary fibrosis A restrictive lung disease where lung parenchyma is stiffened by deposition of collagen; the end-point of many different lung diseases.

Respiratory tree Another name for the airways, particularly referring to their branching pattern. Does not include alveoli.

Restrictive lung diseases Diseases which stiffen the lungs so that expansion of the lungs is compromised.

Sarcoidosis A multisystem granulomatous disorder of unknown origin that can cause a granulomatous interstitial lung disease.

Surfactant A liquid rich in phospholipids and apoproteins that lines the alveoli to reduce surface tension and defend the host against inhaled pathogens. It is secreted by type II pneumocytes.

Spirometry A diagnostic technique used to measure speed of air flow and the volume of air exhaled from the lungs.

Wheeze The musical sound heard on expiration, caused by airway narrowing.

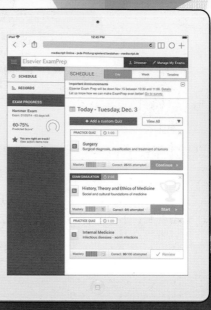

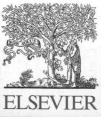